# The care of MINOR HAND INJURIES

# The care of
# MINOR HAND INJURIES

**ADRIAN E. FLATT, M.A., M.D., M.Chir., F.R.C.S., F.A.C.S.**

Professor of Anatomy and of Orthopaedic Surgery and
Director, Division of Hand Surgery, University of Iowa,
Iowa City, Iowa; Hunterian Professor, Royal College of
Surgeons of England; Civilian Consultant to U.S. Air Force
in Hand Surgery; Past President, American Society for
Surgery of the Hand; Past President, Midwestern
Association of Plastic Surgeons

*with forewords by*
**Robert E. Rakel** and **Sir Reginald Watson-Jones**

**FOURTH EDITION**

*with 418 illustrations*

# The C. V. Mosby Company

ST. LOUIS • TORONTO • LONDON    1979

**FOURTH EDITION**

The C. V. Mosby Company
11830 Westline Industrial Drive, St. Louis, Missouri 63141


**Library of Congress Cataloging in Publication Data**

Flatt, Adrian E
    The care of minor hand injuries.

    Bibliography:  p.
    Includes index.
    1.  Hand—Wounds and injuries.  2.  Hand—Surgery.
I.  Title.  [DNLM:  1.  Hand injuries—Surgery.
WE830 F586c]
RD559.F55  1979      617'.1      79-12082
ISBN 0-8016-1581-X


GW/CB/B  9  8  7  6  5  4  3  2  1      01/A/020

# FOREWORD TO FOURTH EDITION

The hand is central to productivity in our society and symbolizes human accomplishment. It also reflects the humanness of the body, equaled only by the face. We use the hand to greet one another, and aside from the eyes and the mouth it is the part on which we focus most of our attention when interacting with other people.

The hand is the most frequently injured part of the body, and all primary care physicians need to be familiar with the principles of appropriate initial management. The term "minor" in the title of this book should not be interpreted as trivial, since problems not managed well at the initial stage may lead to permanent deformity or chronically incapacitating pain. A heavy responsibility is placed on the primary care physician for proper management of the injured hand at its early and most critical stage. For example, if the serious nature of the small penetrating wound of a pressure gun injury is not recognized and treated appropriately, greater damage will result and more extensive surgical débridement will be necessary.

In primary care it is easy for one to be overwhelmed by the sheer volume of material available in the literature. The busy physician must be selective and identify those resources which provide up-to-date practical information of greatest value. Dr. Flatt has done an admirable job of focusing on those problems of the hand most commonly encountered by the family physician and other primary care physicians. Lacerations, contusions, and abrasions are the third most common problem seen by practicing family physicians. The National Ambulatory Medical Care Survey conducted by the Department of Health, Education, and Welfare reveals that problems of the upper extremity rank seventh in frequency among outpatient visits to all physicians.

This is a practical how-to-do-it book written by an experienced hand surgeon whose excellence as a teacher contributes to the organization and clarity of its presentation. Common problems are described in a detail not found in other surgical texts, and the book avoids being cluttered by complicated surgical procedures outside the province of the primary care physician.

This book is an excellent resource for all primary care physicians encountering hand injuries in the office or emergency room, for residents in these disciplines, and all medical students interested in primary care.

**Robert E. Rakel**

*Professor and Head, Department of Family Practice,*
*University of Iowa*

# FOREWORD TO SECOND EDITION

Some surgeons, although ready to use intramedullary nailing for difficult fractures of the neck or shaft of the femur, are reluctant to use the same technique in difficult fractures of the metacarpals or phalanges; although sure of the need to suture a severed radial or median nerve, would not think of suturing a severed digital nerve; and although familiar with cross-leg flaps to replace extensive areas of skin destruction over the shin, have hardly heard of cross-finger flaps to replace small areas of destroyed skin over the palmar surface of the digit. There is still a tendency to regard the first as "major" and important and the second as "minor" and trivial.

Yet surgeons would surely be the first to accept deformity of the thigh with stiffness of the knee in preference to deformity of the hand with stiffness of the fingers. Moreover, the gravity of permanent disability of the hand applies not only to wage earners but equally to housewives and indeed to everyone engaging in recreation as well as some type of work.

The fate of a wounded and fractured hand is usually determined within the first twenty-four hours. Skilled emergency treatment is needed to gain immediate and complete skin cover by wound excision with suture or skin grafting, to reduce and immobilize fractured bones, and to institute immediate measures to prevent joint stiffness.

Whose responsibility is this? Is it the perquisite of an orthopaedic surgeon, a plastic surgeon, or a "general" surgeon? There can be only one answer. It is the responsibility of a surgeon, available by day or by night, who, after experience in general medicine and surgery, has been trained in all the disciplines of orthopaedic surgery and then in the techniques of plastic surgery.

It is for all these reasons that Dr. Adrian Flatt's monograph is so excellent. Written with lucidity and illustrated with clarity, it emphasizes the urgency of treatment of hand injuries, reiterates the basic principles of functional recovery, gives every detail of operative technique, and indicates the essential aftertreatment. Surgeons whose duty it is to treat hand injuries should read it from cover to cover and then have the monograph always ready for reference.

**Reginald Watson-Jones**

*F.R.C.S., F.A.C.S.(Hon.), F.R.C.S.E.(Hon.), F.R.A.C.S.(Hon.)*

# PREFACE

When first published in 1959, this book was offered as a guide for the physician inexperienced in the care of so-called minor hand injuries. There is still no such thing as a "minor" injury to the hand, but for want of a better description I have retained the title, hoping that it will be understood to imply a relatively small amount of tissue damage, outpatient treatment, and freedom from postoperative complications.

I am grateful that this book has been found acceptable; it allows me to publicly thank many who have guided me in my chosen field of surgery. Particularly would I thank my former chiefs. The late Sir Reginald Watson-Jones and Sir Henry Osmond-Clarke of the London Hospital and the late Professor T. Pomfret Kilner of Oxford taught me the principles of orthopedic and plastic surgery. Dr. J. William Littler of New York and Dr. Daniel C. Riordan of New Orleans showed me how to integrate and apply this training in the surgical care of the hand. I shall always be grateful to these five men for their encouragement and forebearance both during and after the years in which I worked under them.

It is hard enough to write a book, but particularly difficult to produce one that is intended to guide the inexperienced. I have tried to follow the precepts of Sir Reginald, who once told me, "In all my writings on orthopaedic, fracture and traumatic surgery I have tried to emphasize the operative procedures that are safe in the hands of surgeons with average experience rather than to describe more adventurous procedures which may be safe in the hands of highly specialized surgeons though with others may be fraught with danger."

No apology is offered for the dogmatic approach. Remembering the quandry that I was in when lack of experience did not allow me to choose between alternatives presented with equal emphasis, I have deliberately concentrated on one method of treatment for each condition. It is not claimed that this is the only, or even the best, specific treatment, but at least it can be said that experience has shown that the method is safe and practical.

In this fourth edition, the original format of two sections has been retained. The first section stresses the important general principles, a knowledge of which is fundamental in good care of the injured hand. The second section contains a detailed discussion of the treatment of the various types of injuries. It has been designed to be delved into as the situation demands. In times of stress, the index and chapter headings are usually searched for appropriate help, and it is hoped that the repetition of some material will obviate the infuriating necessity for repeated back reference to earlier pages.

In the past this book has found acceptance by surgical residents, and I hope I have improved its usefulness for these budding surgeons. However, I have tried to direct many of the new comments to the first line of defense—the family practitioner and the emergency room physician. Dr. Robert Rakel, Head of the Department of Family Practice at the University of Iowa, has made many helpful suggestions and has honored me by writing the foreword.

I have removed inappropriate and outdated material, as well as adding sixty-five new illustrations that I feel stress important points. I have rearranged some of the discussions and entirely rewritten others. Past reviewers had described the chapter on fractures as inadequate. It was. The new chapter is greatly expanded, but in no sense is it a substitute for the larger texts on these injuries. In several areas I have deliberately gone into greater detail than some may consider appropriate. I have done this so that the reader may appreciate the difficulties; it should not be considered an encouragement to "have a try" but rather as an explanation why the problem should be referred to a more experienced colleague.

The final manuscript has been prepared by my secretary, Mrs. Margaret Washburn, with her admirable speed, accuracy, and concern for the English language.

**Adrian E. Flatt**

# CONTENTS

# PART ONE

# General principles of care

To illustrate a principle you must
exaggerate much and you must omit much.

**Walter Bagehot**

# 1 · FUNCTIONAL ANATOMY

**Bones of the hand**

**Joints of the digits**

**The skin of the hand**

**The fascia of the hand**

**Muscles of the hand**
  Extrinsic muscles
  Intrinsic muscles

**Blood supply of the hand**

**Nerve supply of the hand**

**Posture and function of the hand**

This chapter correlates the various anatomical and clinical facts that have a relation to the care of hand injuries. Features that are of practical surgical importance are emphasized, and no attempt is made to repeat the detailed descriptions of anatomical minutiae already published in many textbooks of anatomy.

The hand is a highly sensitive prehensile organ in which both stability and great strength are provided within a very small volume. Function is achieved by coordinating actions of various structures that are usually described separately in anatomical texts. Grasp is dependent on the mobility of the skeleton, the integrity of the joints, and a carefully orchestrated combination of contraction and relaxation of many muscles.

## BONES OF THE HAND

Skeletal mobility of the hand is made possible by slinging its radial and ulnar borders from a central fixed pillar that is firmly anchored to the carpal bones. This pillar is made up of the second and third metacarpals, which are firmly joined through their irregularly shaped carpometacarpal articulations to the relatively immobile carpus (Fig. 1-1). The great mobility of the radial border is supplied by the thumb, which, by virtue of its saddle-shaped joint and strong surrounding intrinsic support, has a wide range of powerful movement. On the ulnar border the carpometacarpal joint of the small finger allows 25 to 30 degrees of motion, and that of the ring finger allows about 15 degrees of flexion and extension. Distal support is supplied at the level of the metacarpal necks by the intermetacarpal ligaments (Fig. 1-2).

Destruction of the central stable pillar inevitably affects the function of the two mobile borders; the thumb may lose its mobility and strength because of interference with the adjacent intrinsic muscles, and, if the ring and small fingers are no longer anchored to the fixed pillar, they tend to drift in an ulnar direction.

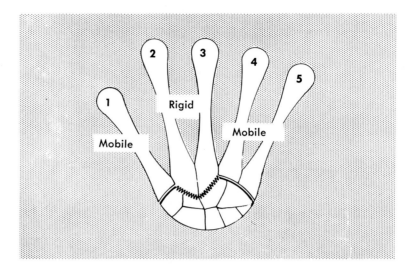

**Fig. 1-1.** *The central rigid pillar of the hand.* The shafts of the second and third metacarpals are firmly joined to the carpus and constitute the central rigid pillar of the hand. The two borders of the hand articulate freely with the carpus, and they are mobile.

To provide a stable base from which grasp and all prehensile activities can develop, the bones of the hand are arranged in three arches: one longitudinal and two transverse. The arch at the base of the hand is rigid and constitutes a sturdy area from which the rest of the architectural pattern can take support. This proximal fixed transverse arch passes through the distal part of the carpus, its two pillars being formed by the ridge of the trapezium and the pisiform. The keystone of this arch passes through the capitate and its articulation with the trapezoid. It is from this point that the central fixed pillar, made up of the second and third metacarpals, takes its firm support (Fig. 1-3). The integrity of this arch is maintained by the intercarpal joint capsules and the strong transverse carpal ligament strung between the two pillars of the arch. The distal transverse arch is at the level of the metacarpal heads and has a considerable degree of mobility. Its integrity is maintained passively by the intermetacarpal ligaments and actively by the interplay between the flattening forces of the extrinsic long extensor muscles and the intrinsic opponens muscles of the thumb and small finger. The longitudinal arch consists of a group of arches, each finger contributing an arch. The keystone of this arch is the metacarpophalangeal joint. The distal limb of the arch is formed by the mobile phalanges and is therefore variable in shape, but the proximal limb is relatively fixed, since it consists of the metacarpal and carpal bones. Like the distal transverse arch, the mobile segments of these longitudinal arches are maintained by the interplay between the extrinsic and intrinsic muscles acting over the metacarpophalangeal joints. Thus, intrinsic muscle paralysis allows a break in both the distal transverse and the longitudinal arches at their keystones and therefore cripples the hand by allowing it to become flattened.

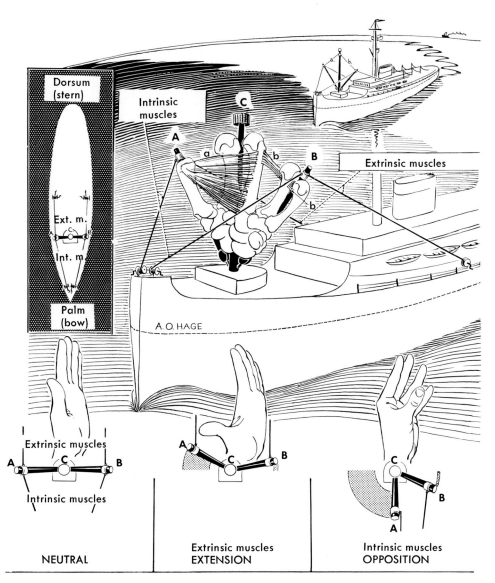

**Fig. 1-2.** *The mobility of the borders of the hand.* A cargo ship has a central mast from which are slung two mobile booms. The hand has as a central mast the second and third metacarpals, represented by **C,** from which are slung the two mobile borders. **A** represents the thumb, and **a** represents the muscle sling that suspends this mobile border. The fourth and fifth metacarpals are represented by **B,** and **b** represents the sling made by the intermetacarpal ligaments. Both borders of the hand are more mobile toward the palmar aspect than toward the dorsum. When the muscles on both aspects of the hand are balanced, the borders lie in the neutral position. When the extrinsic extensors are in action, the range of movement is less than when the intrinsic muscles pull both borders of the hand into opposition.

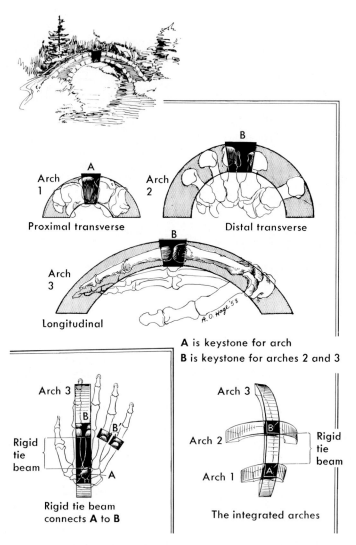

**Fig. 1-3.** *The arches of the hand.* To provide a secure functional base, the bones of the hand are arranged in three arches: one longitudinal and two transverse. The rigid proximal transverse arch passes through the distal part of the carpus. The keystone of this arch lies in the capitate. The mobile distal transverse arch passes through the metacarpal heads. The two transverse arches are held together by the rigid central pillar of the hand acting as a tie beam. The four fingers make up the complex of the longitudinal arch. The longitudinal and distal transverse arches have a common keystone, the metacarpophalangeal joint.

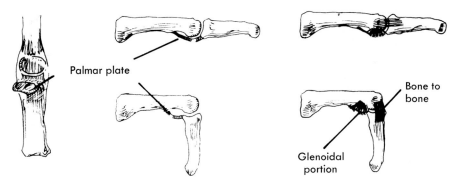

**Fig. 1-4.** *A digital joint.* The palmar plates lie on the flexor aspect of the joint between the flexor tendons and the bones. Each plate has a distal fibrous portion and a proximal membranous portion that is wrinkled and contracted in flexion. Each collateral ligament has two portions: a bone-to-bone and a glenoidal portion that supports the sides of the palmar plate.

## JOINTS OF THE DIGITS

The digital joints connecting the elements of the longitudinal arches all have the same basic anatomical form, which favors palmar flexion. Each joint consists of a capsule and of a pair of strong collateral ligaments that pass around onto the palmar aspect to fuse with the sides of the palmar plate. This plate consists of a tough fibrous portion in relation to the joint surfaces and a proximal membranous portion related to the metacarpal neck (Fig. 1-4). In prolonged flexion of a finger the proximal membranous part "takes up" or shortens by fibrosis, thus fixing the joint in flexion. In some cases this fibrosis may prove an almost insuperable bar to extension. The collateral ligaments each consist of two distinct portions: a strong interbone ligament, which joins the two bones, and the glenoidal portion, which passes from the neck of the proximal bone of the joint to join and support the palmar plate.

### Finger joints

The type of movement in the digital joints differs in the interphalangeal and the metacarpophalangeal joints. The interphalangeal joints are single hinge joints with congruous joint surfaces that travel on the same arc throughout their whole range of movement. The collateral ligaments, therefore, provide constant stability for the joints, since there is the same degree of tension on them in any position of the joint. The stability is greatly increased by the dynamic support of the flexor/extensor apparatus running over the joint. If the flexor and extensor muscles are completely relaxed, a little lateral movement of the joint can be passively produced.

The metacarpophalangeal joint has to provide mobility in two planes, and its mechanism is therefore correspondingly more complicated (Fig. 1-5). The collateral ligaments are slack when the joint is in extension, thereby allowing lateral movement to take place. Strength and stability of the extended joint is provided by the dynamic tone of the extrinsic muscles passing over the dorsal and flexor aspects of the joints.

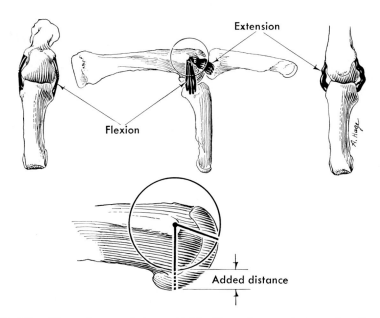

**Fig. 1-5.** *Stability of the metacarpophalangeal joints.* The metacarpophalangeal portion of the ligaments of the metacarpophalangeal joints are attached to the sides of the metacarpal heads. These ligaments are slack when the joint is in extension so that abduction and adduction can occur. During flexion the joint becomes stable because these ligaments are tightened in two planes. In the transverse direction the bulging sides of the head of the metacarpal tighten the ligaments. In the longitudinal direction the tightening is caused by the camlike action produced by the shape of the metacarpal head.

During flexion the metacarpophalangeal ligaments are tightened in a longitudinal direction by the camlike action produced by the shape of the metacarpal head and in a transverse direction by the bulging sides of the condyles. This tightening of the ligaments provides the stability of the joint in flexion. As the metacarpophalangeal joint moves into extension, the ligaments progressively relax, and the joint becomes increasingly unstable (Fig. 1-5). Lateral movement and the lateral stability of this joint in extension are supplied by the intrinsic muscles acting through their insertions into the bases of the phalanges and into the extensor apparatus over the proximal phalanx.

Loss of movement of any one finger joint leaves an acceptable range of function for the digit. Loss of movement of two finger joints will impair but not destroy function, provided that the joints involved are not the proximal and middle joints. If, however, these two joints are stiff, then even full movement in the distal joint is of virtually no functional value.

## Thumb joints

The three joints of the thumb are similar to the three joints of a finger in that the most proximal joint is the most mobile. Anatomically this joint is a carpometacarpal

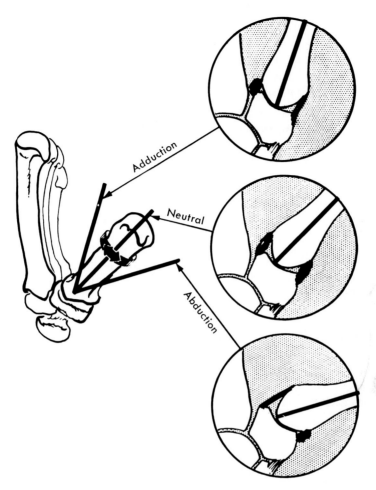

**Fig. 1-6.** *Carpometacarpal joint of the thumb.* This joint has two "positions of function": abduction and adduction. In these positions the joint surfaces are congruous, and they are held together by tense capsular and ligamentous structures. In the midposition the pericapsular structures are slack and rotation of the metacarpal shaft is possible. Rotation of the first metacarpal at this saddle-shaped joint is possible only in the neutral position. (From Flatt, A. E.: Kinesiology of the hand, American Academy of Orthopaedic Surgeons Instructional Course Lectures, vol. 18, St. Louis, 1961, The C. V. Mosby Co.)

joint, which in the fingers would have very poor mobility. In the thumb, however, the range of movement is great, and the joint is almost universal in type. The joint surfaces are saddle shaped, and movement takes place through two main axes: (1) a radioulnar axis for flexion and extension and (2) a dorsopalmar axis for abduction and adduction.

When the proximal joint is in midposition, the capsular structures are slack and the articular surfaces are incongruous. In this state the important additional movement of longitudinal rotation can occur. When the thumb is fully abducted or adducted, the joint's surfaces are congruous and are held close together by tense capsular and ligamentous structures. These two positions are regarded as the "positions of function" of the joint (Fig. 1-6).

Both the metacarpophalangeal and the interphalangeal joints resemble an interphalangeal joint of a finger and have strong lateral stability. However, the metacarpophalangeal joint does permit a few degrees of abduction and rotation that are of great functional importance in the finer movements of prehension.

Loss of movement of any one thumb joint leaves an acceptable range of function. As in the finger, fusion of the proximal and middle joints will severely limit the vital positioning functions of the thumb.

## THE SKIN OF THE HAND

Just as a work glove has a thick tough palmar surface and a relatively thin stretchable dorsal surface, so also does the skin glove of the hand. There is one fundamental difference, however; the work glove surface is insensitive, while the skin of the hand has an extensive sensory supply. Despite the fact that the palmar skin has a thick keratin layer and is upholstered by a tough bolster of fat so that it can withstand the insults of hard manual labor, this skin also has the greatest sensory supply of the body. One fourth of the total pacinian (touch) corpuscles in the body are in the pulp and skin of the hand, by far the greatest part being in the digits, of which the most discriminating portion is the central loop or whorl of the tips of the fingers. The degree of this sensitivity is well shown by the fact that the threshold of touch in the finger tips is 2 g/mm² while in the forearm and abdomen it is 33 and 26 g, respectively.

The subcutaneous fat in the palm is distributed in four strategic sites to aid grasp: thenar, hypothenar, metacarpophalangeal, and digital pulps. These vital pads are retained in place by fascial connections which pass from the skin to the underlying skeleton. Security in grasp is thus provided, since the skin is anchored to the skeleton. The distal palmar crease folds when the ulnar half of the hand is used in grasping, while the proximal palmar crease is used for movements of the index and long fingers. Wounds crossing the palmar creases may produce bowstring scars, and incisions in the palm must be made parallel to the flexion creases but should not actually go through them, since such incisions would ignore the mobility provided by the subcutaneous fat and would tend to broaden the creases unnecessarily.

The skin of the digits is also especially adapted to flexion movements. On the palmar aspect it is fastened almost directly to the tendon sheath over the three sites of flexion, while on the dorsum there is a corresponding redundant fold of skin to allow full flexion.

On the dorsum of the hand the thin loose skin is attached only near the nails and along the sides of the fingers and palm. It covers a surface that becomes increasingly convex as a fist is made. To accommodate for this problem, it is extensile and, instead of creases like those in the palm, there are many minute wrinkles, lying at

90-degree angles to the line of pull, which can be seen when the hand is in extension. When a fist is made, the whole dorsal skin moves distally to accommodate the increased tension and thereby obliterates the minute wrinkles.

Rotation flaps to replace skin loss on the dorsum of the hand must be planned with great care, because the apparent looseness of the dorsal skin in extension is obliterated by a 40% increase in skin tension when a fist is made.

## THE FASCIA OF THE HAND

If the skin glove of the hand could be peeled from its contents, a considerable amount of "packing" would be found to surround the structures running longitudinally. This packing, or fascia, is an important system of connective, fatty, and serous tissues that has several functions. It protects the most delicate structures of the hand from injury, shields its moving parts, and retains both structures and moving parts in definite positions. Apart from these dynamic actions the fascia divides the hand into various functional components. The central part of the palm contains the dense triangle-shaped palmar aponeurosis, the sides of which blend with the fascial covering of the thenar and hypothenar muscles. This triangle is made up of four longitudinally running bands which spread outward from the proximal part of the palm and are held together by many interlacing transverse fibers.

Beneath the skin of the finger webs lies a series of transverse fibers that are in the same plane as the transverse interlacing fibers of the palm. These fibers give distinct support to the web skin, but in addition they contribute fibers which pass distally into the skin cylinders of the fingers with the digital bundle, enclosing the nerve and vessels in a separate fibrous tunnel and protecting them throughout their course within the digit.

These specialized arrangements of the deep fascia help to protect the delicate functioning parts of the hand, yet allow the necessary mobility. To prevent the tendons' bowstringing away from the phalanges the fascia is condensed into tubes or tendon sheaths. Such tubes, when lined with a synovial sheath, allow transmission of the power of flexion around the sharp curves within the narrow diameter of a finger. These tubes, which run from the level of the distal palmar crease to the distal interphalangeal joint, are made up of transversely arranged fibers, except over the joint surfaces where the fibers tend to condense into an X or crisscross formation to allow the finger to flex freely.

## MUSCLES OF THE HAND

The muscles controlling the movements of the hand are conventionally divided into two groups: (1) *extrinsic*—those whose actions on the hand are produced by muscles originating within the arm and forearm and (2) *intrinsic*—those whose origins and insertions are entirely within the hand. This grouping of the hand muscles is convenient for descriptive purposes but has no relation to the functions of the muscles, since any movement is the result of complicated integration of the actions of both groups.

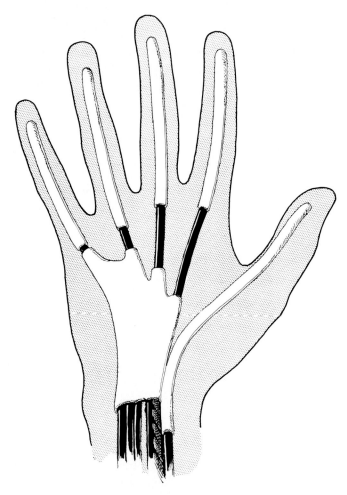

**Fig. 1-7.** *The synovial sheaths of the flexor tendons.* The detailed anatomy of the synovial sheaths of the flexor tendons varies considerably in different people, but the general plan is to provide a greater amount of sheath for the more mobile portions of the hand. The thumb, therefore, has a complete and separate sheath. The small finger and the ring finger have more synovial sheath than is needed by the more rigid second and third metacarpals.

## Extrinsic muscles
### Flexor muscles

Flexion of the interphalangeal joints of the fingers is accomplished by the long flexor tendons, entering the hand within the "ulnar bursa" that begins just proximal to the wrist (Fig. 1-7). This synovial sheath is subject to many variations in detailed plan, but in outline it is of a slanting shape with its maximum size directed to the little finger, the size diminishing for each more radial finger. This shape is directly correlated with the greater mobility of the ulnar border of the hand; thus there is more synovial sheath in the area of greater mobility. The thumb, being the most

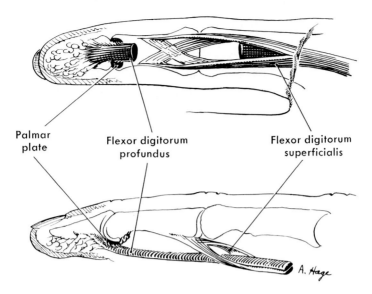

Palmar
plate

Flexor digitorum
profundus

Flexor digitorum
superficialis

A. Hage

**Fig. 1-8.** *The insertions of the flexor tendons.* The superficialis tendon splits into halves, each of which splits again, allowing the two inner quarters of the total tendon to cross each other dorsal to the profundus tendon. These slips are joined by the remaining quarters which have continued on their same side. The conjoined slips insert into the lateral crests of the middle phalanx. The profundus tendon inserts into the base of the distal phalanx, but it also sends fibers of attachment to the adjacent fibrous septa of the finger pulp.

mobile digit, has a separate and very extensive synovial sheath that frequently communicates with the main ulnar bursa.

Of the two long flexor tendons, the flexor digitorum superficialis has its main action on the middle finger joint, whereas the flexor digitorum profundus acts on the distal finger joint. The old name of "flexor perforatus" is a good description of the mode of insertion of the superficialis tendon. At the level of the middle of the proximal phalanx this tendon splits into two portions, each of which splits again, allowing one fourth of the fibers to cross posterior to the flexor digitorum profundus to join its opposite member. The remaining three quarters of the fibers continue on the same side and insert into the lateral crest of the palmar surface of the middle phalanx. The profundus tendon passes through the superficialis tendon perforation to insert into the base of the distal phalanx, and it also sends some fibers into the adjacent fibrous septa of the surrounding finger pulp (Fig. 1-8).

The perforation in the superficialis tendon forms a most efficient pulley that allows considerable independent motion between the superficialis and the profundus tendons. However, the range of the two tendons is different, and to produce full flexion the profundus needs an excursion 1 cm greater than that needed by the superficialis, which needs only 3 to 5 cm for its full action. Should the tendons be stuck together by adhesions, then the action of the profundus must inevitably be hindered, and flexion will be impaired. To test for superficialis action, the profundus tendon to the finger in question must be put completely out of action by passively flexing the metacarpophalangeal joint and hyperextending the adjacent fingers. Hyperextension of these fingers will pull the profundus tendons distally as far as is possible. This apparent lengthening of the profundus tendons will effectively prevent any power from being transmitted to the profundus tendon in the finger that is being examined. Any voluntary flexion of the middle finger joint will then be produced by the action of the superficialis muscle (Fig. 2-7). In tests for profundus action, the finger must be held passively extended at both the proximal and middle finger joints. Voluntary flexion of the distal finger joint will show the presence of profundus power (Fig. 2-8).

### Long extensor tendons

Since there is no intrinsic musculature on the dorsum of the hand, the long extensor tendons lie in a loose connective tissue between the skin and the bones. The synovial sheaths investing the extensor tendons are limited to the carpal region, and the blood supply of the tendons can therefore enter over a large part of their surface instead of being limited to the narrow mesotendons or vincula provided for the flexor tendons.

The most important action of the long extensor tendons is to provide dorsal stability for the metacarpophalangeal joint against the flexor power of both intrinsic and extrinsic muscles. The central portion of the tendon continues distally over the proximal phalanx to insert into the base of the middle phalanx. The central portion contributes to a certain degree to the extension of the middle finger joint, although the major part of this is done by the intrinsic muscles.

## Intrinsic muscles

The intrinsic muscles of the hand consist of a central group containing the interossei and lumbricals and the two lateral groups of the hypothenar and thenar eminences. They are of fundamental importance to the hand, since they are responsible for the delicate joint balance and refinement of movement of the fingers. The intrinsic muscles achieve this control by counterbalancing the activity of the long extrinsic muscles by their primary action in flexing and stabilizing the metacarpophalangeal joints.

### Thenar group

The thenar group is composed of the opponens, flexor pollicis brevis, and abductor pollicis brevis. These muscles are grouped around the shaft of the thumb metacarpal and are responsible for its stability and for the control of all its fine movements.

An additional muscle is the adductor, which arises by transverse and oblique heads. The transverse head arises from the shaft of the third metacarpal and is the active sling by which the radial border of the hand is suspended from the central fixed pillar of the hand. Of the other muscles, by far the most important is the abductor, which alone of all these muscles has the capacity for providing all the functional requirements of good opposition. The other muscles act as their names imply, but Duchenne has shown how the opponens produces less opposition than the short abductor and the superficial head of the short flexor.

### Hypothenar group

The muscles of the hypothenar eminence are concerned with the activity of the small finger. The abductor and flexor aid in abduction and flexion of the finger. The deep-lying opponens aids in rotating and adducting the fifth metacarpal when the thumb and little finger are opposed, thereby helping in cupping of the hand.

### Interosseous muscles

The detailed anatomy of the interossei is infinitely more complicated than standard texts may lead one to believe. In man, the normal primate pattern of seven palmar interossei has been split into four dorsal and three palmar. This is more a division for convenience of description than an established anatomical fact, and therefore these muscles are subject to considerable variations in their origins and insertions. There is, however, no constancy in relationship between anatomical perfection and functional efficiency, and the variations encountered all produce a standard functional pattern.

The muscles arise from the sides of the metacarpal shafts but have differences in their mode of insertion. The palmar group insert almost exclusively into the dorsal extensor apparatus. The insertion of the first dorsal interosseus is virtually 100% into bone. The second and fourth insert mainly into the extensor apparatus, while the third has a varying insertion, though it is largely into the extensor apparatus.

### Lumbrical muscles

The four lumbrical muscles are unique in that they have their origin on a flexor tendon and their insertion into an extensor tendon. They are subject to great variations and may even be absent in large part. For all practical purposes their tendons have 100% insertion into the extensor apparatus, although occasionally fibers do insert into the base of the proximal phalanx.

Many actions have been attributed to the lumbricals, but they have no powerful individual action of their own and can only cooperate with the stronger interossei. When the lumbricals are absent, the interossei take over their actions with no demonstrable loss of efficiency in the hand. Electromyographic studies have shown that the prime action of these muscles is extension of the interphalangeal joints (Fig. 1-9). Since they constitute a direct link between the extrinsic flexor and extensor mechanism, they are used as a moderator or "fine adjustment" between flexion and extension of the interphalangeal joints.

### Intrinsic muscles and finger extension

The interosseous and lumbrical muscles are of fundamental importance in extension of the fingers. These muscles approach the metacarpophalangeal joint from

Lumbrical

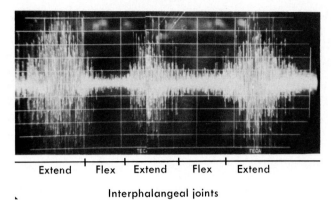

| Extend | Flex | Extend | Flex | Extend |

Interphalangeal joints

**Fig. 1-9.** *Lumbrical action.* This tracing was made after an electrode had been inserted into my second lumbrical. Activity is recorded only during extension of the interphalangeal joints.

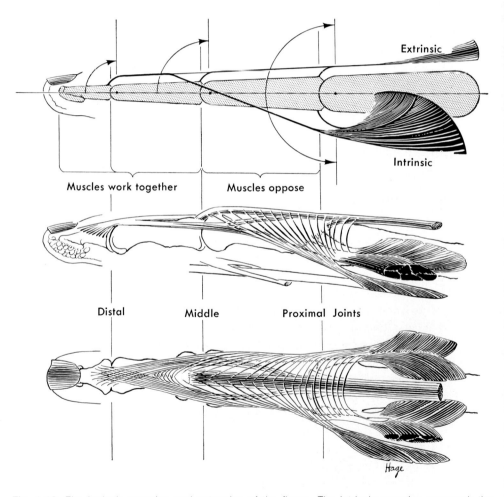

**Fig. 1-10.** *The intrinsic muscles and extension of the finger.* The intrinsic muscles approach the metacarpophalangeal joint from the depths of the hand and lie on the palmar aspect of the axis of this joint. As the tendons enter the finger, they pass dorsally and lie above the axis of the two interphalangeal joints. Therefore, when the intrinsic muscles are in action, they oppose the action of the extrinsic extensor on the metacarpophalangeal joint but reinforce the action of this tendon in extending the interphalangeal joints.

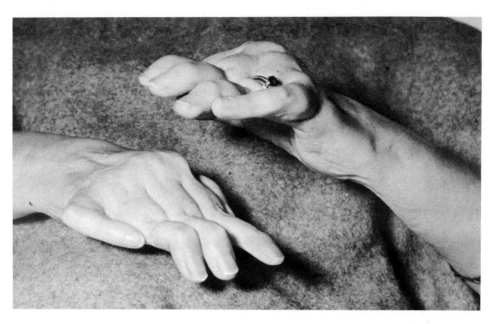

**Fig. 1-11.** *"Swan-neck" deformity.* This fully developed deformity occurred in the hands of a patient with rheumatoid disease, but it can be produced by anything causing permanent contracture in the intrinsic muscles. (From Flatt, A. E.: Geriatrics **15**:733, 1960.)

the depths of the hand and lie on the palmar aspect of the axis of this joint. Therefore, when in action, they flex this joint against the pull of the long extrinsic extensor tendons. The intrinsic tendons pass dorsal to the axes of the proximal and distal interphalangeal joints. They, therefore, extend these joints against the action of the long extrinsic flexors (Fig. 1-10).

Scarring of the interosseous muscle bellies caused by disease or injury will exaggerate their action and produce an imbalance between flexor and extensor mechanisms. The fingers will adopt the "swan-neck" position of hyperextension at the proximal interphalangeal joints (Fig. 1-11).

If similar damage is isolated to a lumbrical muscle belly, it also will lead to scarring and a shortening of the distance between origin and insertion. Clinically this can produce the odd situation called "paradoxical lumbrical action," in which extension of the interphalangeal joints will occur when the flexor profundus is attempting to flex the finger. Immediate relief is obtained when the tendon of the damaged lumbrical is sectioned and full excursion of the profundus is allowed to occur.

## BLOOD SUPPLY OF THE HAND

The blood supply of the hand is largely anterior or palmar in position. All of the arterial supply enters on the front of the wrist, and at least half of the venous drainage leaves by the same route. Both arterial and venous systems are subject to many variations, and the usual textbook pattern is really a description of the most common variations. Age has some influence on the state of the system. Arteriovenous anastomoses are poorly developed in children, whereas in elderly persons both the arteries and the veins become elongated, large, and tortuous. The veins in aged persons can, on occasion, be a particularly trying surgical problem.

### Arterial supply

The superficial and deep palmar arterial arches are so named because of their relationship to the flexor tendons. They are connected to the dorsal carpal arterial arch (which lies deep to the extensor tendons) by a proximal and distal row of perforating arteries that pass between the metacarpal shafts.

The extensive anastomoses between the various vessels allow ligation of an arch anywhere within its length without serious risk to the distal blood supply (Fig. 1-12). Even when both the radial and ulnar arteries are ligated at the wrist, the blood supply can usually be maintained through the collateral circulation, which, in such cases, will pass mainly through the perforating arteries. The digital arteries of a finger are of sufficient caliber to allow survival of the finger tip after complete destruction of one of the pair.

### Venous drainage

The veins draining the hand are grouped into superficial and deep systems. The superficial veins start on the dorsum of the fingers and collect their blood from the plexuses on the palmar and lateral sides of the fingers. They run in several trunks parallel with the long axis of the fingers to drain into the cephalic and basilic veins via the dorsal venous network. There is no constant pattern for this dorsal network, but in general the cross communications are scanty, a fact of some importance when flaps raised by trauma are based distally. Such flaps, even if raised by a surgeon, may die of venous congestion rather than from lack of oxygenated blood.

The deep veins of the hand and forearm are relatively small and do not drain as much blood as the superficial system. They tend to run as venae comitantes with the arteries, but there is no consistency in their pattern.

### NERVE SUPPLY OF THE HAND

The standard textbook description of the nerves of the hand usually is merely a compromise between the more common variations and does not account for the apparently abnormal sensory and motor findings encountered in patients with injuries of nerve trunks. These apparent abnormalities are explained by the fact that the three anterior nerves, the musculocutaneous, the median, and the ulnar, quite commonly anastomose and interchange their distribution. The fourth nerve of supply, the radial, is embryologically distinct from the anterior nerves and does not enter into abundant anastomoses. It does, however, show great variation in its innervation of the thumb, and the line of its junctional borders with the median nerve is often different on the two sides of the thumb. This overlap on the sides of the thumb may lead the unwary to believe that median nerve sensibility is intact, despite a wound over the site of the digital nerves.

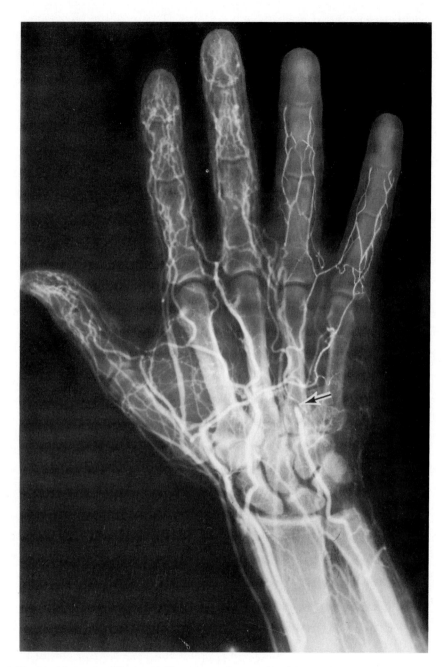

**Fig. 1-12.** *Arterial supply of the hand*. The arrow points to a block in the ulnar artery, but anastomoses with the radial artery branches have maintained the supply to the ring and small fingers.

An important feature of the nerve supply of the hand that gets scant reference in anatomy textbooks is the abundant nerve supply to the finger joints. This is important because the complexity and dexterity of many of the finger movements rely to a large extent on the sense of stereognosis. The principal nerve supply of the joint enters at the point of flexion from the main palmar digital nerves, with additional twigs being derived from the dorsal digital nerves. However, when the nerves of a finger are cut, stereognosis is not completely lost, because there is a very definite additional nerve supply passing through the long tendons.

## Musculocutaneous nerve

The musculocutaneous nerve is a sensory nerve throughout its course in the forearm and hardly supplies any area of skin in the hand. It has extensive anastomoses with the surrounding nerves, and its loss is functionally of little importance.

## Median nerve

Loss of the median nerve leaves a "blind hand" with anesthesia over the primary working area: the thumb and the index and long fingers. The recurrent branch to the thenar eminence supplies the intrinsic muscles, and its loss abolishes the power of opposition and cripples the fine movements of the thumb. Should the nerve be damaged high in the forearm, there will be additional significant loss of extrinsic flexor muscle function.

## Ulnar nerve

Damage to the ulnar nerve causes both a loss of sensibility on the ulnar border of the hand and a loss of the intrinsic muscle power. There is, however, the possibility of an interchange of innervation between the median and ulnar nerves to the intrinsic muscles. This shift can be so great that one nerve takes over supply to the complete exclusion of the other, but such an extreme degree of interchange is very rare. However, it must be remembered that it is unwise to judge the nerve supply of all the interossei on the performance of the most easily palpated first dorsal muscle. Apart from the fact that the long extensors have an element of abduction in their action, 3% of the first dorsal interosseous muscles are supplied by the median nerve. Adduction of the thumb can be produced by the action of the short opponens muscle, and adduction is therefore not necessarily abolished by ulnar nerve injury.

## Radial nerve

The radial nerve is predominantly a motor nerve supplying only extrinsic muscles, and its loss can be readily compensated for by tendon transfers. The motor branch arises above the elbow and supplies the extensor muscles of the wrist and digits. Loss of sensation from interruption of the superficial sensory branches is rarely important to hand function, but damage to these branches over the dorsal radial aspect of the hand frequently gives rise to troublesome neuroma.

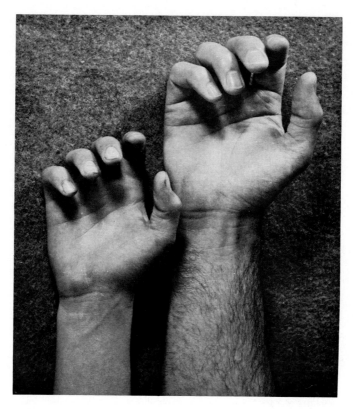

**Fig. 1-13.** *The position of rest.* When the hand lies palm upward on a flat surface, the balance of the tone of the muscles produces a characteristic position. In this position, which is the same in children and adults, the hand shows an orderly gradation in flexion of the fingers. The small finger is the most flexed, whereas the least flexed is the index finger.

## POSTURE AND FUNCTION OF THE HAND

The hand in repose takes a standard position dependent upon the position of the wrist. This position is dictated by the result of balancing the forces in the muscle tone on both sides of the arm. The classical position of rest is one in which the hand lies palm up on a flat surface. In this position the hand shows a gradation of flexion of the fingers, the most flexed being the small finger and the least flexed the index finger (Fig. 1-13). A disturbance of this orderly gradation of the fingers will often be the clue to damage to the flexor tendons (Figs. 2-6 and 11-2).

The hand is used in two fundamentally different ways. The less common and completely unspecialized use is as a fixed end on a mobile arm. The hand acts as the passive transmitter of force, produced by the arm muscles, in such positions as the flattened hand or the clenched fist. The more common skilled use of the hand is as a mobile organ at the end of a mobile limb. Three types of movement are used.

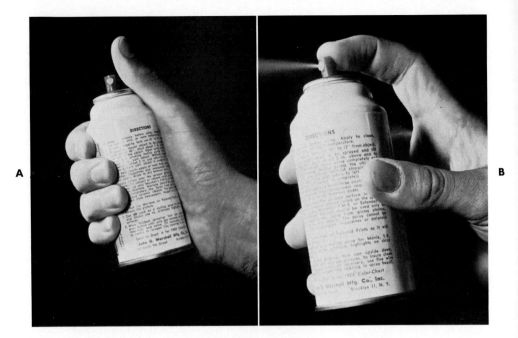

**Fig. 1-14.** *The two patterns of prehension.* In **A** the cylinder is being held in a power grip between the flexed fingers and the palm. In **B** precision handling pinches the cylinder between the flexor aspects of the fingers and the thumb.

1. Slow to rapid movements, with control of direction, intensity, and rate
2. Ballistic or rapid repetitive motions
3. Fixations, including co-contractions yielding prehension

The slow-rapid movements consist of such actions as writing, sewing, and tying knots. Ballistic movements are usually repetitive rapid motions such as are used in typing or piano playing. Muscle power begins the movement and supplies momentum to the limb while the digits remain fixed in the required position. Prehension can be accomplished in a variety of ways, but Napier has shown that there are only two distinct patterns of such movements and has stressed that the fundamental requisite of prehension is that the objects should be held securely. Stability can be combined with prehension in two distinct ways (Fig. 1-14). In precision handling the basic position of the finger is one of flexion and abduction at the metacarpophalangeal joints; the object is pinched between the flexor aspects of the fingers and that of the opposing thumb. The hand is usually positioned on the forearm with the wrist in a dorsal and radial inclination. In a power grip the wrist is often in ulnar and palmar deviation, and the object is held as in a clamp between the flexed fingers and the palm, counterpressure being applied by the thumb lying more or less in the plane of the palm. The two common types of prehension, picking up and holding objects for use, both use precision handling modified into a long pinch-type position.

In this type of prehension the thumb passes through a compound movement

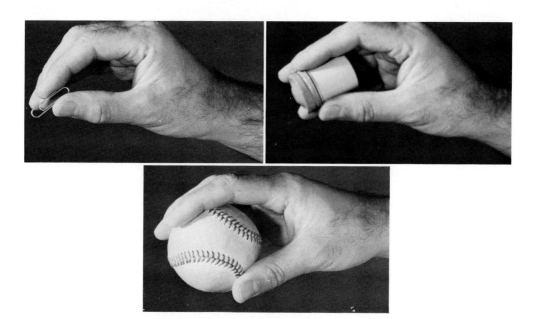

**Fig. 1-15.** *Thumb in prehension.* The fundamental position of abduction and rotation of the thumb relative to the palm is constant in all grasping actions. The basic position remains unchanged despite the variations in size of objects held. (From Flatt, A. E.: Kinesiology of the hand, American Academy of Orthopaedic Surgeons Instructional Course Lectures, vol. 18, St. Louis, 1961, The C. V. Mosby Co.)

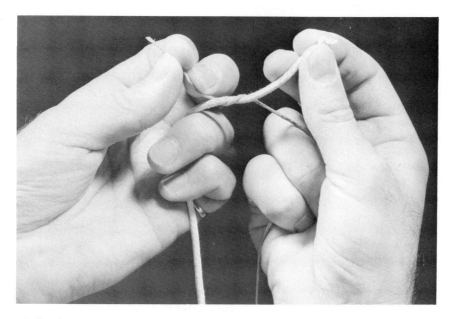

**Fig. 1-16.** *Combined grip.* When a knot is being tied, it is often necessary to grasp the loose ends of the string in a power grip with the ulnar border of the hands while the radial digits perform the precise work of forming the knot. (Modified from Napier, J. R.: The prehensile movements of the human hand, J. Bone Joint Surg. **38-B:**902, 1956.)

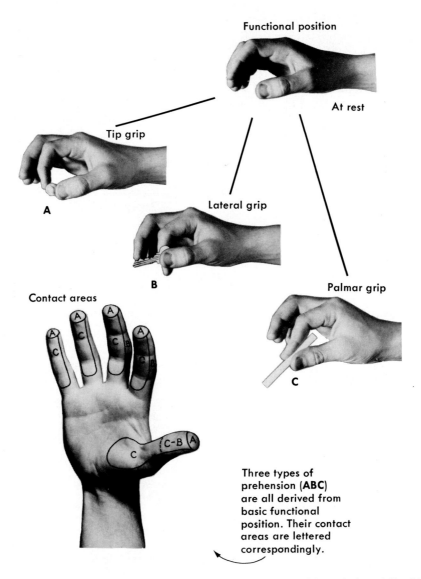

Functional position

Tip grip

At rest

**A**

Lateral grip

**B**

Palmar grip

Contact areas

**C**

Three types of
prehension (**ABC**)
are all derived from
basic functional
position. Their contact
areas are lettered
correspondingly.

**Fig. 1-17.** *The functioning hand.* In the functional position of the hand the wrist is stabilized in moderate extension and the thumb lies in line with the radius, with the metacarpal at right angles to the plane of the palm. The digital joints are held loosely in a semiflexed position. From this basic functional position are developed the fundamental prehensile grips **A, B,** and **C.** Their contact areas are lettered correspondingly. (Copyright by Butterworth, Inc., (1960) and reproduced with permission from Matthew Bender & Company, Incorporated, assignee, from "Hand Deformities" by Adrian E. Flatt, Vol. 2 Traumatic Medicine and Surgery for the Attorney, ¶ 230, p. 157.)

occurring at all three joints. The principal movements of abduction and rotation take place at both the carpometacarpal and metacarpophalangeal joints. This fundamental thumb position of abduction and rotation is constant in all grasping actions. This basic position will remain unchanged despite the size of the object held in the hand (Fig. 1-15). A fundamentally different type of prehension is the hook grip. In this grip the thumb plays a passive role. When objects with handles, such as suitcases, are carried, the demand is for power over long periods of time, and precision requirements are at a minimum. In patients with intrinsic paralysis this coarse grip is virtually the only possible form of prehension.

This division of action of the digits and definition of two prehensile patterns is not absolute. The long finger can take part in either grip, and only rarely does prehensile movement consist of pure precision or pure power elements. Many actions contain portions of both, and it is the predominance of one or the other that will define the type of prehension (Fig. 1-16).

## Functional position of the hand

The functional movements of the hand are dependent upon the integrity of both the longitudinal and transverse arches of the hand.

In the optimum functional position, there is dorsiflexion of the wrist, and the finger tips are at equidistant radii from the tip of the thumb, as if the hand were enclosing a baseball. When the hand is in this position, then both intrinsic and extrinsic muscles are in a position of adequate tone, and no one group is either stretched to its limit or out of action. It is from this position that prehensile movements develop in the normal hand.

Three patterns of prehensile movement can be recognized as most frequently occurring. These types of grip are derived from the basic functional position of the hand (Fig. 1-17) and are classified as tip, lateral, and palmar grips. Collapse of the arches from fractures of either phalanges or metacarpals will totally destroy these prehensile postures. Function can only be returned by restoring the normal arches by appropriate splinting, thereby restoring the balance between flexor and extensor muscles. Bandaging a finger or hand to a flat board is iniquitous and inexcusable and will surely destroy its future function.

# 2 · EXAMINATION OF THE INJURED HAND

Clinical examination

Bone damage

Joint damage

Nerve injuries

Tendon injuries

**A**ccurate diagnosis of the extent of an injury is an essential preliminary to planning treatment. Treatment cannot be properly given if the clinical records are inadequate, but full medical records protect the interests of all concerned.

Despite a natural abhorrence for paper work, any physician who treats more than a few of these injuries would be well advised to use some type of record sheet such as is illustrated in Fig. 2-1. Such a sheet reduces the chances of omitting important details, and the line diagrams will give a good idea of the original injuries long after healing has occurred. Frequently these records have to be produced in court months or years after the injury and if they are inadequate, both patient and physician may suffer.

By far the best form of visual record is the clinical photograph. By using photography, illustrations can be made of the various stages of treatment that are permanently available for future consultation.

## CLINICAL EXAMINATION

To avoid wound contamination, a mask must be worn by the physician and all other personnel at all times while the hand is examined, operated on, or dressed. The problem of staphylococcal infection of wounds is becoming steadily greater, and stringent precautions must be taken to prevent the introduction of infection after the patient reaches the hospital. Virtually half of all hospital personnel are carriers of antibiotic-resistant organisms; therefore, all staff members who will come in contact with the patient during examination and treatment must be masked. Any patient who has any form of respiratory tract infection should also be masked.

There are two parts to the examination of a hand wound. The first must demonstrate any interference with function and is carried out preoperatively; the second is a detailed examination of the wound and the surrounding tissues that can only be done in the operating room under the protection of full sterile precautions. A detailed examination may include probing the depths of a wound; such exploration should never be done during the initial functional examination.

UNIVERSITY OF IOWA     IOWA CITY

*University Hospitals—Department of Orthopedic Surgery*

| RECORD No. |
| --- |

## HAND CLINIC

| CARD PUNCHED |
| --- |

**Name of Patient**................................................................................RIGHT/LEFT HANDED
(Surname first in block letters)

Address ...........................................................................................................Age....................Male/Female

................................................................................................Occupation ...................................................

Date and Time of First Attendance...........................................................Injured at Work.    Yes.  /  No.

Employer.................................................................................................Previous Similar Accident.    Yes.  /  No.

X-Rayed.    Yes.    No.                                    If so, when........................................................

**HISTORY**...........................................................................................................

...........................................................................................................

...........................................................................................................

...........................................................................................................

**CLASSIFICATION OF INJURIES**

| Right: Palm | Dorsum | Thumb | Index | Middle | Ring | Little |
| --- | --- | --- | --- | --- | --- | --- |
| Left: Palm | Dorsum | Thumb | Index | Middle | Ring | Little |

**TYPE OF WOUND.**

| | | |
| --- | --- | --- |
| 1. Crush | 7. Skin Loss | 13. Flexor Tendon Cut |
| 2. " Tidy " Incised | 8. Amputation, Partial | 14. Extensor Tendon Cut |
| 3. " Tidy " Sliced | 9. Amputation, Complete | 15. Digital Bundle Cut |
| 4. " Untidy " | 10. Nail Bed Injuries | 16. Joints Involved |
| 5. Thumb | 11. Foreign Bodies | 17. Discharging Pus |
| 6. Pulp Loss | 12. Bony Damage | 18. Tendon Sheath Involved |

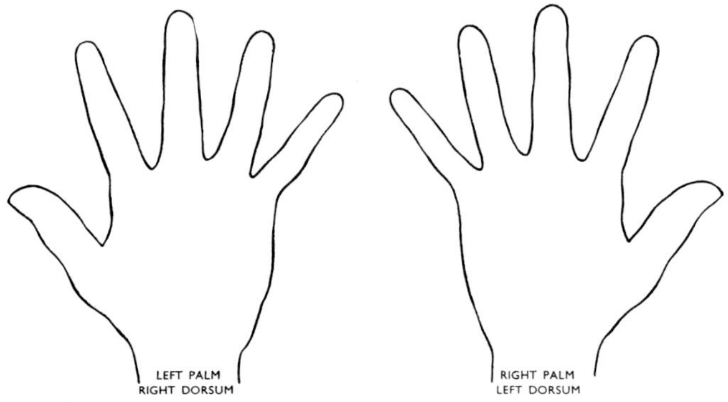

LEFT PALM
RIGHT DORSUM

RIGHT PALM
LEFT DORSUM

*Continued.*

**Fig. 2-1.** *Records of injury and treatment.* Inadequate records may cause unpleasant difficulties for both patient and doctor. A record sheet such as this will help to eliminate omission of important facts and will be permanently available for future reference.

**PRIMARY TREATMENT**

Photographed.    Yes/No                                                    Letter to Doctor.    Yes/No
If Not, Why Not ?...................................................................

                                                                            Signature...................

**FOLLOW-UP ATTENDANCES**

| DATE | CONDITION AND TREATMENT | CHEMOTHERAPY |
|------|-------------------------|--------------|
|      |                         |              |
|      |                         |              |
|      |                         |              |
|      |                         |              |
|      |                         |              |
|      |                         |              |
|      |                         |              |
|      |                         |              |
|      |                         |              |
|      |                         |              |
|      |                         |              |
|      |                         |              |
|      |                         |              |
|      |                         |              |
|      |                         |              |
|      |                         |              |
|      |                         |              |
|      |                         |              |

**DAYS OFF WORK**............              **FINAL CERTIFICATE GIVEN**....../....../.....

**Fig. 2-1, cont'd.** For legend see p. 27.

Since the first, general, examination is really an exercise in applied anatomy, it is best thought of in terms of the question, "What deeper structures could possibly have been damaged through this wound?" The first essential, therefore, is a good history of how the wound was incurred. A small puncture wound at right angles to the skin may cut many essential structures in the line of thrust but is unlikely to cause any destruction in the lateral plane. The more slanting the angle of approach to the skin, the greater the area subject to danger.

Examination of hand function can be rapidly carried out if a methodical plan is followed. Haphazard jabbings with a pin by the physician and uninvited movements of the digits by the patient give little useful information and merely make the hand more painful and less likely to yield accurate information to a properly conducted examination. Errors in diagnosis can occur only because of errors of omission or commission in the examination. One such error is to ignore any possible bone damage until the end of the clinical examination. Even relatively minor bone damage can so distort normal function of the hand that the results of an examination are useless unless they are assessed against an accurate knowledge of the site and extent of bony lesions. Therefore, if there is the slightest indication that the bones or joints may have been damaged, it is mandatory to take x-ray films of the hand before carrying out the full clinical examination. Posteroanterior and lateral views are normally sufficient to show fractures or damaged joints. The x-ray films can be taken without disturbing the first-aid dressings.

The best plan for the examination of a wounded hand is first to assess the extent of the skin wounds. The skeleton and its joints have next priority. After the bone and joint damage has been accurately defined, the integrity of the nerve supply should be determined. Finally, the functions of the muscles should be tested.

## BONE DAMAGE

It is both ethical and professional negligence to fail to do an x-ray examination of a hand that may have bone damage. It is taught that x-ray films should be taken only after a clinical examination has been carried out. Such advice does not apply to hand injuries. There is no justification for forcing fingers through painful arcs of movement when a glance at an x-ray film would show adequate reason for the patient's refusal to cooperate.

Two x-ray films should be taken in planes at right angles to each other. These posteroanterior and lateral views are usually sufficient to reveal bony damage, and only on certain occasions are special views necessary. Fractures of the carpal bones frequently need further views, but routine oblique films usually help little in forming the primary diagnosis. Lateral views of digits are often hard to get, especially if several have been injured, and the use of a small dental film between digits is often helpful.

## JOINT DAMAGE

When movements of the hand are examined, a great deal of time and temper will be saved if the surgeon demonstrates the desired movement with his own hand while encouraging the patient to reproduce the movement with both hands. This helps to eliminate misunderstandings, and an idea of the normal range for the particular patient can be obtained. This is particularly important in finger movements, since the normal range of movement of the finger joints varies widely in different individuals. Stability of any damaged joints must always be gently assessed by applying lateral strains with the joint in a few degrees of flexion.

## NERVE INJURIES

Sensory nerve division results in loss of superficial and deep sensibility and in dryness of the skin due to lack of autonomic function. When examined for this loss, the patient is considerably less apprehensive, and the results of the tests are often

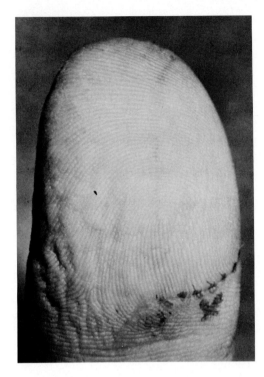

**Fig. 2-2.** *The wrinkle test.* Normally innervated digits or hand will show skin wrinkling after immersion in a pan of warm water for fifteen minutes. This thumb was lacerated at the dotted line X, and the skin distal to it is denervated and did not wrinkle after immersion.

more reliable if testing is done with a wisp of cotton rather than with a large safety pin. In children it is often difficult to do a thorough neurological examination because of apprehension, fear, or even distaste of the hospital scene. The sensory examination therefore has to be swift and accurately confined to the absolute territorial area of each potentially damaged nerve.

Skin sensibility should be tested by comparing touch appreciation of the questionable area with the opposite normal area. It is not necessary to go into the fine detail of two-point discrimination in the first examination, but it should be noted that young children have a 2 mm two-point discrimination but adults have about 3 to 4 mm discrimination in the pulp of the median supplied digits and 5 to 6 mm in the ring and small fingers. These figures are often significantly greater in diabetics.

When a peripheral nerve is severed, sweating or sudomotor activity instantly ceases distal to the lesion. The dryness or lack of sweating in a fingertip can be felt by the examiner, and the absence of sweat droplets can be observed through a magnifying glass or ophthalmoscope.

A particularly useful test is the finger wrinkling test of O'Rianin.* If nerve injury

---

*Observed serendipitously and subsequently reported by Dr. Seamus O'Rianin, a Dublin plastic surgeon.

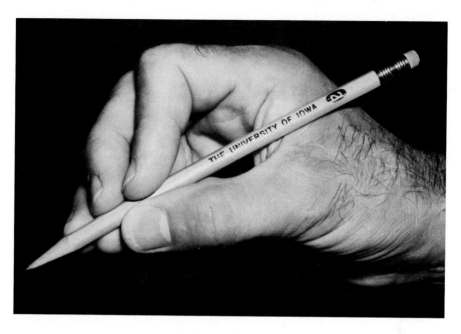

**Fig. 2-3.** *Motor nerve function test.* If the hand can totally surround the shaft of a pen or pencil with all the fingertips, then the three motor nerves are intact.

to a finger or any part of the hand is suspected, the part should be immersed in a pan of warm water for fifteen to twenty minutes. The normally innervated fingers will wrinkle on their palmar surface, but the part supplied by the injured nerve will remain smooth and unwrinkled (Fig. 2-2). Only the palmar aspect of the hand wrinkles in water because it has no sebaceous glands—elsewhere the sebum supplies a waterproofing effect. Children are partial to playing in water, and I have found this test particularly useful in diagnosis and also often use it in adult injuries.

When a complete nerve injury is proximal to or at the wrist, the three nerves have clearly defined absolute individual sensory territories. The median nerve should be tested for on the palmar aspect of the terminal phalanx of the index finger. The same anatomical area of the small finger will give an absolute test for the ulnar nerve, while the radial nerve has exclusive rights to the dorsal thumb web area. More distal injury will not yield such distinct territorial definition, and a more extensive neurological examination will be needed.

Motor activity of the hand is largely controlled by median and ulnar nerves, with the radial nerve supplying postural control of the extensors. A quick and useful test of motor function for all three nerves is to see if the patient can surround the shaft of a pen or pencil with all the fingertips (Fig. 2-3). If he can, then all three nerves and the intrinsic muscles are in good working order. If the tests fails, then each individual nerve must be tested for its motor activity in relation to the site of the wound.

Distribution of the motor branches of the ulnar nerve is not invariable. It is said to supply all the intrinsic muscles of the fingers, but its integrity cannot be tested

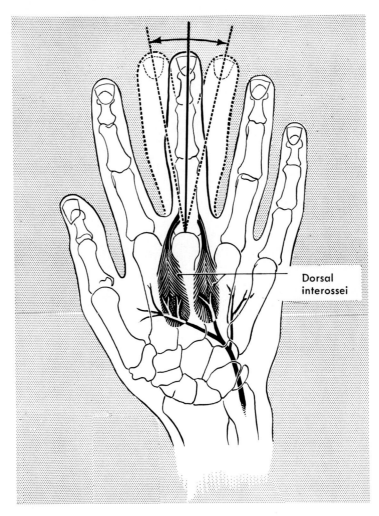

**Fig. 2-4.** *Test for ulnar nerve function.* The most reliable test for function of the ulnar nerve is the demonstration of abduction and adduction of the long finger from the midline when the palm is held down on a flat surface.

by feeling for action in the first dorsal interosseus muscle; at least 3% of these muscles are innervated by the median nerve. Moreover, the flexor digiti minimi muscle in the hypothenar mass is always supplied by the ulnar nerve. To test for its action, put the hand palm up, flat on a table, and invite your patient to flex the metacarpophalangeal joint while maintaining the small finger straight in extension at the interphalangeal joints. This position can only be obtained in a hand with an intact ulnar nerve. Another reliable test is to try voluntary abduction and adduction of the long finger from the midline with the hand palm down on a flat surface (Fig. 2-4). This test will eliminate the possibility of abduction or adduction by the long extrinsic extensors of the fingers.

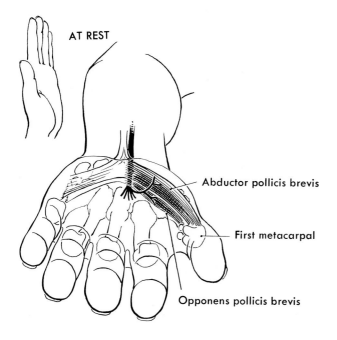

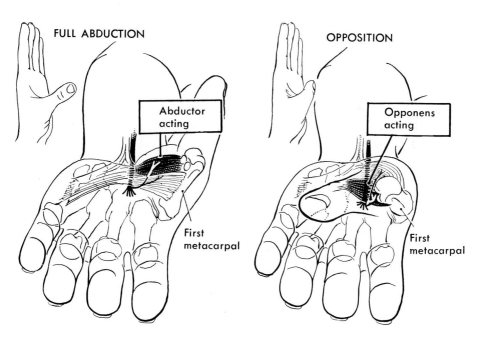

**Fig. 2-5.** *Test for median nerve function.* The abductor pollicis brevis and the opponens muscles are innervated by the median nerve. The nerve is cut if the thumb cannot be raised from the plane of the hand and then moved across until the palmar surface of the thumb and ulnar two fingers are parallel.

The median nerve is tested by observing the actions of the abductor pollicis brevis and the opponens muscles in the thenar eminence (Fig. 2-5). With the hand flat on a table, palm up, the abductor first raises the thumb from the plane of the hand while the nail remains at right angles to the palm; the opponens then moves the thumb across the palm to face the fingers so that the thumbnail becomes parallel to the plane of the hand. If these actions are missing, the median nerve is damaged.

## TENDON INJURIES

No injuries are more commonly missed than tendon injuries, not only because the tests are mostly subjective and the patients are frequently unreliable, but also because the clinical examination is often woefully inadequate. Observation of the position of the finger will give valuable information. The patient's hands should be inspected while at rest, and a disturbance of the normal resting posture, such as an extended finger, may well indicate tendon damage (Fig. 2-6). It is extremely easy to miss an injury of the extrinsic tendons unless each long tendon is tested separately.

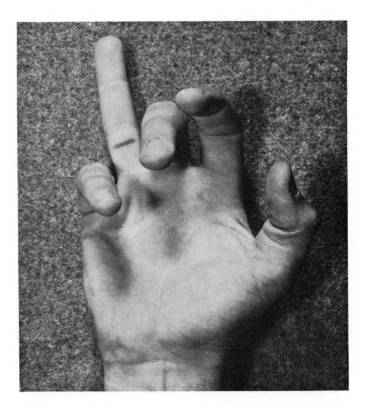

**Fig. 2-6.** *Loss of the position of rest.* Damage to the flexor tendons of a finger unbalances the tone of the muscles controlling that finger and is revealed by the resultant disturbance of the position of rest. The line indicates the site of the original wound.

Tension in a tendon must be tested. It is hard to do without pain, but weakness without significant pain frequently means that a partial division of a tendon has occurred. When testing finger flexor tendons and observing their excursion at the wrist and lower forearm, remember that both the superficialis and profundus tendons lie in the ulnar half of the wrist and to the ulnar side of the palmaris longus when it is present.

The range of tendon excursion varies as much as the range of joint movement, and the capacity for independent flexion and extension of the fingers varies widely in different individuals and at different ages. The only way by which the normal can be defined is to have the patient exercise both hands at your command. When this is done, variations in range will be immediately obvious.

Pain at the site of injury may inhibit or diminish movements, even though the nerves, muscles, or tendons responsible for the movement are intact. Conversely, normal results may seem to be obtained although structures are cut. For instance, if the flexor digitorum profundus tendon to a finger is cut within the tendon sheath, then all flexion of the distal finger joint is lost. If the same tendon is cut in the palm at a point proximal to the final subdivision of the profundus tendon mass, then the cross ties with neighboring tendons allow relatively strong flexion of the distal joint.

The superficialis tendons flex the middle finger joint and are best tested for by putting the profundus tendons out of action by holding all of the other fingers in extension (Fig. 2-7). It must be remembered that many people normally do not have independent superficialis action in the small finger.

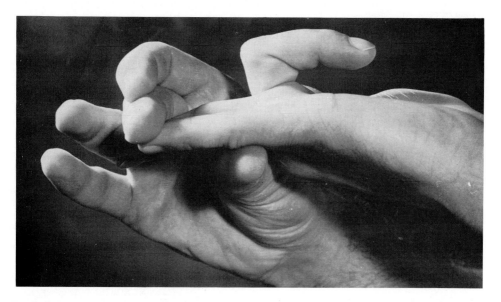

**Fig. 2-7.** *Test for flexor superficialis action.* The flexor profundus tendon to the finger in question must be put out of action by holding the remaining fingers in hyperextension. In this position the profundus tendons are apparently lengthened, and any movements of the flexed finger in the proximal interphalangeal joint must be due to superficialis action.

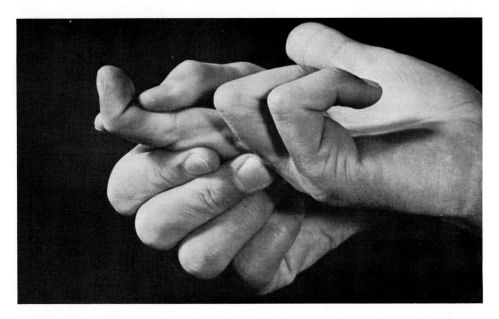

**Fig. 2-8.** *Test for flexor profundus action.* The finger should be held passively extended at the metacarpophalangeal and proximal interphalangeal joints. Flexion of the distal interphalangeal joint will demonstrate action of the profundus muscle.

The profundus tendons flex the distal finger joint, and their actions should be tested for by holding the fingers straight at both the proximal and middle finger joints, and then testing for strong and active flexion of the distal finger joint (Fig. 2-8).

A frequently missed injury is the isolated division of a flexor digitorum profundus tendon. Small lacerations over the proximal or middle phalanges of the fingers may well cut the profundus but leave the split superficialis tendon intact. Thus, superficialis action will be intact, and, unless a specific test is made for active flexion of the distal finger joint, relaxation in this joint following full extension may well be mistaken for active flexion.

The main function of the long extensor tendons is to supply stability to the proximal finger joint. Examination of their function should, therefore, be directed to testing their ability to extend fully and strongly the metacarpophalangeal joint. These tendons are easily damaged and must be assumed to be severed if wounds are in the appropriate places. The presence of many cross connections on the dorsum of the hand enables a finger to extend quite reasonably despite complete severance of its own tendon, but this extension is very weak when tested against resistance. Functional tests to demonstrate a cut of the central slip of the extensor expansion in a fresh injury are frequently not satisfactory, and, if there is a wound in the region of the dorsum of the middle joint of a finger, it must be assumed that the central slip has been severed until exploration reveals the actual extent of the injury. Several apparent "trick" movements of various digital joints may confuse the unwary and unless specifically checked for may lead to incorrect diagnosis.

Extension of the terminal joint of the thumb can be achieved in the face of complete severance of the extensor pollicis longus. This is because the abductor pollicis brevis, an intrinsic thenar muscle, inserts into the extensor tendon distal to the metacarpophalangeal joint and will therefore extend the interphalangeal joint. The extension becomes much stronger if the metacarpophalangeal joint is passively held in full extension.

Two of the four fingers have independent extrinsic extensor tendons. Both the index and small finger have proprius or proper extensor tendons not connected to the communis or common extensor tendon mass, which goes to all four fingers. Extension of either or both of these two border fingers therefore does not show that the communis mass is intact. Integrity of these two proprius tendons is tested for by putting the metacarpophalangeal joints of the long and ring fingers into 90 degrees of flexion. This pulls the communis tendons distally and inhibits their action in the index and small fingers.

# 3 · PRINCIPLES OF CARE

The hand is the most frequently injured part of the human body. Even a trivial wound is an economic disaster to its owner if it prevents an immediate return to work. The length of time lost from work is almost directly related to the skill and care provided during the primary treatment.

The paramount responsibilities of the physician are to prevent infection of the wound and to provide complete skin cover for the wounded area. Gross infection of a wound may lead to sloughing of important structures and subsequent fibrosis. But it is vital to realize that lesser and even so-called subclinical infections can lead to delayed primary healing. This delay in healing will produce fibrous tissue formation and thickening of the wound scar, which may be just as crippling as the aftermath of the more dramatic gross infections.

## THE SKIN OF THE HAND

At the completion of primary care of a wounded hand there must be complete epithelial cover for the whole hand. Replacement of lost skin takes absolute priority over all other treatment. No matter how trivial a wound may appear, if there has been loss of skin, it must be replaced. If the area is left to heal by granulation tissue, scarring will inevitably result, and the function of the hand will be impaired.

Skin loss can be replaced by four types of treatment: (1) free skin grafts, (2) local skin flaps, (3) skin flaps from within the hand, and (4) skin flaps from a distance. Of these four methods, only the use of free skin grafts is applicable to the care of minor hand injuries being treated on an outpatient basis. All other methods of skin supply merit the services of a skilled surgeon working under properly controlled conditions.

### Free skin grafts

In emergency surgery of the hand, free skin grafts are frequently used. This type of graft is the most easily applied method of skin replacement and does not require great experience in its use. Free skin grafts are classified as full-thickness grafts, split-skin grafts, and pinch grafts.

### Full-thickness grafts

Full-thickness grafts are cut to include all of the dermis beneath the epithelium. The technical difficulties in applying these grafts make them quite unsuitable for routine use in acute traumatic wounds.

### Split-skin grafts

Split-skin grafts are cut through the dermis at varying levels. In general they are used either as thick or thin grafts. The average thickness of the skin is 1.3 mm. The thick grafts are cut at about a 0.08-mm level, whereas the thin grafts are between 0.04 and 0.05 mm in thickness.

The rate of successful take of skin grafts depends very largely upon the state of their recipient beds, but it is also influenced by the thickness of the graft. Thin grafts are vascularized more readily and will often survive in areas where a thicker graft would fail. Despite the high rate of success of thin grafts, they tend to scar down in the later stages of healing because the support of the dermis is missing. Because of this risk of contracture, thick split-skin grafts should be used for most defects, and the thin grafts should be reserved for use on areas of doubtful viability.

### Pinch grafts

Pinch grafts are small circular areas of skin of tapering thickness that are obtained by slicing off a piece of skin which has been tented up by a needle point. The graft is thin at its edge and at least full thickness at its center. These grafts cannot be used to cover large skin defects because of their irregular thickness and because the donor site is covered by permanent circular scars. The recipient site is equally bumpy because of the irregular thickness of the grafts. There is no indication for the use of pinch grafts within the hand (Fig. 3-1).

In general there is so little spare skin in the hand that there can only be very limited use of local skin flaps. Two types of flaps that are generally used to treat small losses of skin of the hand are the rotation flap and the transposition flap. Both of these flaps can be used to replace small, generally triangular, defects of skin. Various small triangular flaps can be mobilized on soft tissue pedicles to close the raw end of an amputated finger.

The rotation flap is used on the dorsum of the hand, since some elasticity of the skin is needed to allow the rotation. When the flap is correctly planned, the defect created by the rotation can be closed primarily, and there is no need for a secondary grafting of the surgically created defect. The transposition flap is more commonly used on the palmar skin, which is totally inelastic. The principle of use is to close the primary defect by transposing a flap into the area of skin loss. An equivalent area of skin loss is produced at the site from which the flap was raised. The secondary defect must be covered with a split-skin graft. The transposition flap is used in

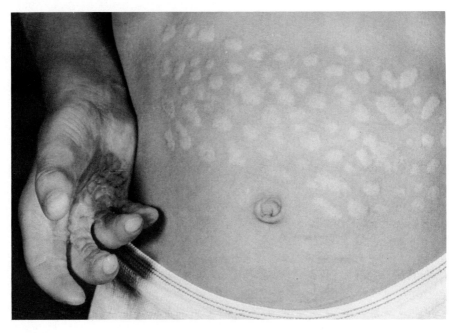

**Fig. 3-1.** *Pinch graft.* The pinch graft is a pyramidal lump of skin that heals in a bumpy fashion and leaves a pockmarked donor site. It should not be inflicted on a wounded hand or an innocent abdomen.

areas where vital structures have been exposed and is designed so that the secondary defect occurs in an area of less importance.

Small triangular flaps raised on a soft-tissue neurovascular pedicle are used to provide full-thickness skin cover on the end of important digits. Great care and judgment are needed in mobilizing these flaps, which, if successful, do provide better two-point sensibility discrimination than free skin grafts (Figs. 9-19 and 9-20, pp. 175 and 176).

The planning and moving of any of these local flaps requires considerable skill and experience, and patients needing such treatment deserve the services of an experienced surgeon.

### Skin flaps from within the hand

Despite the fact that there is virtually no spare skin in the hand, it is sometimes good policy to deliberately raise a flap and to graft the donor site. The skin flap that has been raised can then be used to cover an area which is unsuitable for split-skin grafting with full-thickness skin and subcutaneous tissues. The flexor aspect of fingers is the site where two types of these flaps are most commonly used. The thenar flap is used to provide thick skin and subcutaneous tissues for the pulp of the distal phalanx (Fig. 8-3, p. 136). The cross finger flap is used to cover exposed tendons and bone on the proximal and middle phalanges. The skin from the dorsum

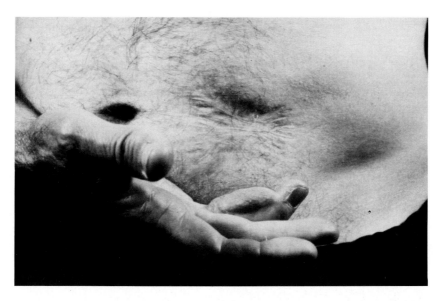

**Fig. 3-2.** *Abdominal flap to finger.* Loss of skin on this man's ring finger was replaced with a "thin" abdominal flap. Some years and beers later the abdomen has enlarged—and so has the flap.

of one finger is crossed over to cover the palmar defect on the adjacent finger. Although the skin is relatively thin, since it comes from the dorsum of a finger, it provides much better protection than a split-skin graft (Fig. 8-9, p. 144).

### Skin flaps from a distance

There is no indication for the use of skin from a distance in the emergency room treatment of minor hand injuries. Many sites are available, but none is really suitable.

Flaps from the opposite arm can provide acceptable skin, but their use greatly handicaps the patient, since, with both limbs immobilized, he can hardly attend to his own toilet requirements. Chest flaps also provide acceptable skin, but the donor site is so obvious that the scarring is unacceptable to women and to a surprisingly high proportion of men. Abdominal skin is a poor substitute and should not be used. The flaps are bulky, and the fat always remains metabolic storage fat. Whenever the patient's abdomen gets fatter, so will the flap (Fig. 3-2).

## OPERATING ROOM ARRANGEMENTS AND EQUIPMENT

The operating room does not need to be large, but the surgeon must be able to shut himself away and get on with the delicate work of repair uninterrupted by the constant traffic of an emergency room. An assistant is a necessity rather than a luxury, but in many instances such help is alleged to be not available. Forceful explanation of the need to staff or nearby relatives is often productive.

An adequate operating room lamp is vital. It does not need to have great power, but it does need great mobility. It is usually necessary to change the position of the lamp several times during the operation, and for this a lamp with a central handle that can be sterilized is excellent and allows the surgeon to locate the light exactly as he requires it. Many surgeons prefer to use a forehead lamp. Both the field of illumination and the power of the light from such a lamp are small, but the light is always under the direct control of the surgeon.

## Instruments

Few instruments are needed, but those used must be appropriate to the small size of the hand structures. Cast-off general surgical instruments, large hemostats, and huge needle holders are useless. No one can undertake repair of the delicate structures of the hand unless they have available small instruments of the size commonly used by plastic surgeons. The instruments most commonly used are straight and curved small scissors, toothed and plain forceps, scalpels with blades of smaller sizes such as 15 or 11, mosquito hemostats, and skin hooks (Fig. 3-3).

Skin hooks are the best form of skin retractors to use, but, for the lone operator, retraction is best supplied by the small ophthalmic type of self-retaining retractors.

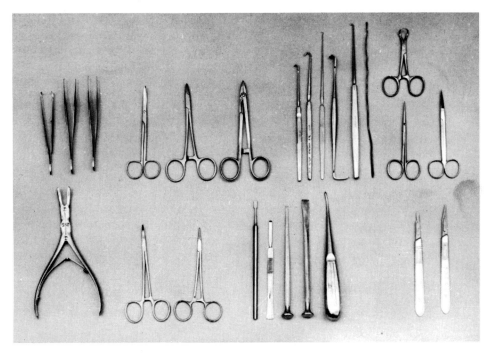

**Fig. 3-3.** *Instruments for hand surgery.* Instruments used to operate on the hand must be appropriate to the small size of the hand structures. The size of these instruments can be judged from the No. 15 and No. 11 blades in the scalpels. Plastic surgery instruments are good. Cast-off general surgical instruments are useless.

When self-retaining retractors are not available, long monofilament sutures should be passed through the wound edge at intervals, and their ends should be clamped by hemostats that are allowed to hang down. The weight of even mosquito hemostats is quite sufficient to supply adequate retraction. Heavy-handed retraction with large instruments can do immense damage and will negate the most careful atraumatic handling of tissues by the surgeon.

Sterilized rubber finger cots or discarded rubber gloves should always be available for all cases of traumatic injury. It is impossible to clean completely under the fingernails of the uninjured digits, and it is better to seal off this possible source of contamination.

## Skin sutures

Suture materials for the skin should be of monofilament construction and should be swaged into an atraumatic needle. The size of the suture is important, and there is no excuse for using sutures larger than No. 4-0 or No. 5-0. Thicker material is harder to work with and more difficult to take out. It is commonly used because it is strong enough to drag together tissues that normally would not meet.

Silk, wire, or synthetic suture can be used. Silk is easy to work with but can sometimes act as a wick to lead infection into the subcutaneous tissues and is therefore not so good as monofilament suture material. Wire is more difficult for the occasional operator to use and is not so suitable for interrupted sutures as is the synthetic suture. In recent years the introduction of fine-braided wire sutures has overcome many of the technical problems inherent in the use of monofilament wire, but for the repair of skin wounds it holds no particular advantages over nylon.

## Catgut

Catgut very rarely, if ever, need be buried in the hand. It acts as a foreign body and is absorbed in an irregular manner. It inevitably leads to irritation and subsequent scarring. For the control of hemorrhage, mosquito hemostats are quite large enough for any vessel in the hand. If they are left in place for some minutes and then twisted off, the vessel will not bleed. Those who have no faith in this advice should throw away all their present stock of large-size catgut and invest in a very small supply of No. 5-0 plain catgut. This fine catgut will control any vessel that can be caught in a mosquito hemostat and is also suitable in size for any subcutaneous sutures that may be needed. No. 6-0 ophthalmic catgut can be used to close skin wounds in young children. It will disintegrate after wound healing with virtually no adverse reaction.

## Drains and packs

Drains and packs are not indicated in the care of minor hand injuries, since they always cause the formation of adhesions and the development of scar. They may be of use in the treatment of hand infections, but their prophylactic use is bad. Drains can act in two directions, and in the hand they act as a pathway for the introduction of skin bacteria just as readily as they assist in drainage from the depth of the wound.

### Tourniquets

A pneumatic type of tourniquet is essential during many operations on the hand. Any surgeon who tries to define and repair the delicate structures of the hand in a pool of blood is truly a traumatic surgeon. Sponging the exposed area is of little use, since wounds of the hand are usually too small and too deep for sponging to be adequate. In any case, every application of the sponge obscures the operative field and tends to remove the surface clotting, thereby encouraging further bleeding.

Routine use of the tourniquet is not recommended. When there is any question as to the viability of skin or deeper tissues, it is wiser to have the tourniquet in place but to delay inflation until all tissue of questionable viability has been inspected and excised as necessary. However, once the viability of tissues has been established, inflation of the tourniquet allows the rest of the operation to be completed quickly and easily. To save time in this way is important, since it reduces to a minimum the time that the wounded tissues are exposed to drying and contamination.

For emergency surgery of the hand, the tourniquet can sometimes be inflated around the wrist. Wherever the tourniquet is placed, the anesthetic used must be appropriate. It is impossible to anesthetize the forearm only and use a tourniquet around the arm without causing the patient a considerable amount of suffering.

The use of a tourniquet is condemned by many because of the potential dangers. There is virtually no risk of "tourniquet paralysis" in a patient with a normal vascular system if the pressure is evenly applied by means of a pneumatic cuff for not more than one hour. The tourniquet must be carefully applied, and care must be taken not to crease the underlying skin. An ordinary blood pressure cuff is perfectly suitable and should be inflated to about 250 mm Hg for adults and to about 200 mm for children. Because the pneumatic cuff distributes the pressure over a large surface area, it does minimal damage, but the same pressure applied over a very narrow band would cause serious damage. For this reason the wrapping of a rubber band or even a catheter tightly around the base of a digit must be condemned. A tourniquet for a single digit can be safely applied for about twenty to thirty minutes if a small Penrose rubber drain is used. The finger should be emptied of blood by squeezing it from distal to proximal. The rubber drain is then wrapped around the base of the finger for two or three turns, keeping the drain flat against the sides of the digit. It can be held tight by clamping the ends with a hemostat (Fig. 3-4).

The greatest problem posed by the use of a tourniquet is when to remove it. Should it be removed immediately after all the deep surgery has been done, or should the skin be sutured and the dressings be applied before the pressure is released? The tourniquet should not be released until the final compression bandages are in place.

A hand that is damaged and then subjected to surgical exploration must inevitably swell. This swelling will be accelerated and increased by the anoxia of the

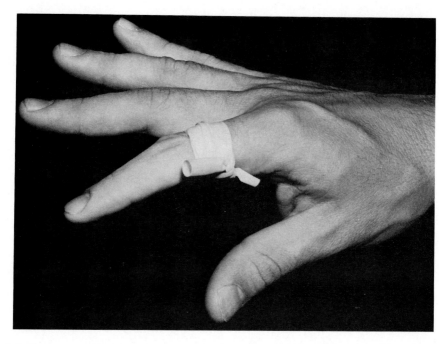

**Fig. 3-4.** *Finger tourniquet.* A small, soft rubber Penrose drain can safely be used as a tourniquet for short time periods if it is carefully wrapped flat, without creases, against the side of the finger. It can be held tight by clamping the ends with a hemostat or tying a half knot. Compare with the bad technique shown in Figs. 9-17 (p. 174) and 15-5 (p. 280).

tissues produced by the use of a tourniquet. But the swelling can only develop after the circulation has been allowed to return. If, therefore, the tourniquet is released so that all bleeding vessels can be clamped and tied, hemostasis is obtained at the expense of a steadily swelling hand. By the time skin suturing is attempted, the hand will be edematous, it will be difficult to close the wound properly, and the bandages will have to be applied to an already swollen hand. If the tourniquet is left in place throughout the operation, there is little risk of serious subsequent hemorrhage. All obvious vessels must be clamped and tied, dead spaces eliminated, the skin wound neatly sutured, and the hand protected by an evenly applied compression dressing.

Whether the tourniquet is removed early or late in the operation, spasm of the digital vessels must be anticipated. A slow return of circulation to the operated fingers is usual, and the blood supply returns without serious difficulty. It is very unusual for it to be necessary either to reapply or even to loosen properly applied bandages.

## ANESTHESIA

The majority of the operative procedures described in this book can be safely carried out under local anesthesia.

Wounds should not be anesthetized by multiple injections directly into the skin edges. Injection of the anesthetic solution at an appropriate site some distance from the wound allows the whole area to be anesthetized after one or two needle pricks.

Local nerve block is satisfactory for most procedures, but its use demands a knowledge of anatomy sufficient to localize the nerves with considerable accuracy before starting the injection. It is cruel to probe around with the point of a needle until paresthesias force the patient to announce localization of the nerve. It is equally bad technique to inject a large volume of solution on a hit-or-miss basis. If the injection site is well chosen, only a few milliliters are needed to affect the nerve. The anesthetic solution acts when it surrounds the nerve. It does not need to be injected directly into the nerve.

For operations that can be completed in about one hour, a 2% solution of either lidocaine (Xylocaine) or procaine is a suitable agent. For procedures that will take more than one hour, it is better to use 0.15% tetracaine (Pontocaine), which will give up to three hours of satisfactory anesthesia. If anesthesia does wear off, there should be no hesitation in reinforcing it by an additional injection.

Whichever solution is used, precautions must be taken to make the injections under full sterile conditions. The injection can be given with absolute safety even before the wound is cleaned if the actual injection site is cleaned. Establishment of anesthesia before the wound is prepared will save the patient a great deal of discomfort. The solution should be injected through a No. 22 needle, which, because of the danger of breaking, must never be plunged in nearly to the hilt. If a needle 6 cm long is used, this danger can be avoided. Anesthetic agents need time to diffuse and develop their full effect. No matter how accurate the injection is, surgery cannot be started for at least ten minutes after the completion of the injection.

For digital injuries, metacarpal block is preferable to injections directed into the finger. The skin and deep fascial cylinder of the finger have very little room for expansion, and raised pressure within this sheath can cause serious interference with finger circulation. For this same reason, vasoconstrictors such as epinephrine should never be added to the local anesthetic solution. Several proprietary preparations have a vasoconstrictor included with the anesthetic solution. Such preparations should not be used in the hand. For more extensive wounds intravenous Xylocaine into the veins on the dorsum of the hand or brachial block anesthesia can be used. When blocking the plexus, the axillary approach is much easier and safer than the supraclavicular route, which can be dangerous in the hands of the inexperienced.

**Intravenous block**

When using the intravenous Xylocaine block, the tourniquet time begins just before the anesthetic is injected, and usually about 1 to 1½ hours of operating time can be obtained. Two parallel tandem tourniquets are placed on the arm. The proximal tourniquet is inflated after a small intravenous catheter has been passed into a suitable vein and the arm exsanguinated by wrapping from distal to proximal with a rubber bandage.

After inflation of the proximal tourniquet the rubber bandage is removed and 30 to 40 ml of Xylocaine injected. Usually about twenty to thirty minutes after tourniquet inflation the patient feels increasing discomfort under the proximal tourniquet. The distal tourniquet should then be inflated over an area that is now anesthetized. Subsequent release of the proximal tourniquet removes the discomfort. Anesthesia is lost almost instantly after deflation of both tourniquets and if the method is used for short surgical procedures, the drug must be admitted to the circulation in small increments by repeated deflation and inflation.

## Metacarpal block

To anesthetize the finger, both palmar digital nerves and the proximal dorsal cutaneous branches have to be blocked (Fig. 3-5). This blocking necessitates a needle puncture on either side of the finger at its base. However, the patient need only feel one needle insertion. Not more than 3 to 5 ml of 2% solution of the short-duration agents is needed.

A wheal is raised on one side of the finger by puncturing the soft skin of the web space just distal to the level of the metacarpophalangeal joint. The needle is directed horizontally and subcutaneously across the dorsum of the finger to its other side to block the cutaneous branches running into the finger from the dorsum of the hand. The needle is then withdrawn until it can be passed vertically toward the palm and

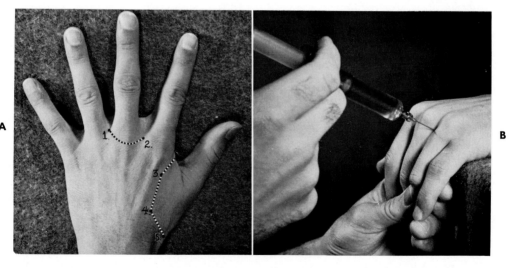

**Fig. 3-5.** *Metacarpal block of a digit.* **A,** Raise a skin wheal at point **1.** While passing the needle horizontally and subcutaneously across the dorsum of the finger, inject solution as far as point **2.** At point **2,** raise a definite wheal. **B,** Then withdraw the needle to point **1** and pass it toward the palm downward and slightly inward toward the head of the metacarpal. When anesthetizing the thumb, the first skin wheal should be raised at **4.** Additional wheals should be deposited at **3** and **5** after the tracks leading to these points from **4** have been anesthetized. (**A** modified from Cullen, Stuart C.: Anesthesia in general practice, ed. 5, Chicago, 1957, Year Book Publishers, Inc.)

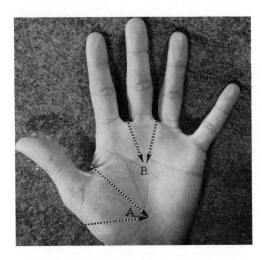

**Fig. 3-6.** *Metacarpal block of a digit.* The area of the palm toward which the needle should be directed is **B** when anesthetizing the finger and **A** when anesthetizing the thumb. The injections for the thumb should be made through wheals **3** and **5** shown in Fig. 3-5. Do not penetrate the palmar skin; the point of the needle should reach no farther than the base of the phalanx. (Modified from Cullen, Stuart C.: Anesthesia in general practice, ed. 5, Chicago, 1957, Year Book Publishers, Inc.)

then slightly inward toward the base of the phalanx (Fig. 3-6). Only 2 to 3 ml need be injected to block the nerve at this site. The injection should be given throughout the time the needle is withdrawn. After withdrawal, the needle is then passed through the already anesthetized skin of the web on the other side of the finger, and a similar amount is injected deeply near the base of the phalanx. A comparable procedure can be carried out to anesthetize the thumb. In cases where several fingers have been injured, it is advisable to block each finger as it is repaired rather than to try to complete the surgery before a total block wears off.

**Radial nerve block**

The radial nerve is the most difficult to block completely because of its tendency to break up into its final branches at varying levels in the forearm. Because of this direct local infiltration anesthesia is often used for small wounds in the distribution of the radial nerve. The branches are best sought in the region of the lower end of the radius on its lateral edge and over the first inch of its dorsal surface. The radial artery and several veins are in the area to be anesthetized, and special care must be taken to avoid injecting anesthetic solution into these vessels. The radial artery should be palpated, and the needle should be inserted into the skin to the radial side of the vessel. It is then passed dorsally and in an ulnar direction through the subcutaneous tissues being kept almost parallel with the skin. The needle should be passed nearly to its hilt and the plunger withdrawn. If the needle is not in a vessel, a total of about 3 to 5 ml of solution should be injected as the needle is slowly withdrawn.

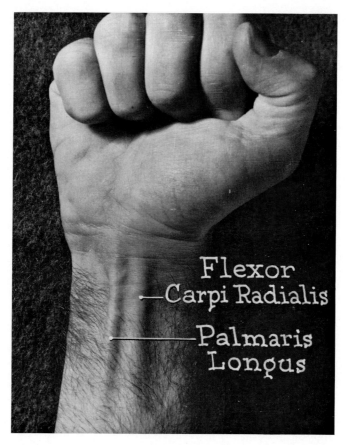

**Fig. 3-7.** *The median nerve at the wrist.* With the arm in supination, the median nerve will be found to lie between the tendons of the flexor carpi radialis and the palmaris longus. These tendons can be made prominent by slightly flexing the clenched fist against resistance. (Modified from Cullen, Stuart C.: Anesthesia in general practice, ed. 4, Chicago, 1954, Year Book Publishers, Inc.)

## Median nerve block

With the arm in supination, the median nerve is usually found to lie between the tendons of palmaris longus and flexor carpi radialis (Fig. 3-7). These tendons can be easily located by asking the patient to touch the small finger and thumb together and then slightly flex the wrist. Two tendons will then be seen to stand out, and the median nerve lies in the hollow between them. In patients in whom the palmaris longus is absent, the median nerve lies about 8 mm medial to the tendon of flexor carpi radialis. A skin wheal is raised 2.5 cm above the wrist at the site where the nerve is expected, and the needle is then passed gently downward until it meets the resistance of the deep fascia. One milliliter of solution is injected here; after a brief pause the needle can be pushed through the fascia and an additional 2 ml injected. If the needle is thrust boldly through the fascia, it will impale the nerve and produce marked paresthesias. These will probably cause the patient to jerk the arm, which may well fracture the needle in the tissues.

## Ulnar nerve block

The ulnar nerve is more readily blocked at the elbow than at the wrist. At the elbow it is easily palpated, and at this level all the sensory supply to the hand will be anesthetized. Injection at the wrist is practical, but more complicated because of the close proximity of the ulnar artery. The needle is placed just dorsal to the ulnar edge of the flexor carpi ulnaris tendon. This tendon can be identified by gentle wrist flexion, and it will be felt to further tense if the small finger is then actively abducted. About 4 to 5 ml of solution are slowly injected with repeated aspirations of the syringe to make sure the ulnar artery has not been penetrated.

At the elbow the nerve is readily felt in the groove at the back of the medial epicondyle, and, after a small skin wheal has been raised, the needle is slowly inserted until the nerve can be felt to roll under the needle point. There is no need to stab the nerve to produce paresthesias. If 3 ml of the 2% solution are injected, good anesthesia will be produced.

## Anesthesia in children

Children eat all the time. The child with an empty stomach is virtually nonexistent, and the parents' knowledge of their child's intake is frequently grossly inaccurate. The use of stomach tubes is barbaric, and it is far better to operate with the child under local anesthesia than to give a general anesthetic and run the risk that the child might inhale some vomit.

Children tolerate the use of local anesthesia remarkably well, particularly if they have been well premedicated with a drug such as pentobarbital. The procedures for blocking the nerves are identical with those used in adults, but allowance must be made for the smaller size of the tissues.

## DRESSING AND RESTING THE HAND

Proper bandaging and splinting of the injured hand is as vital a part of the treatment as the surgical care of the wound. During the early healing of soft tissue wounds immobilization is just as important as it is in the care of fractures. Improper positioning of the hand and inadequate immobilization will let it slip into nonfunctional positions that will rapidly stiffen into irreparable deformity. Only two or three weeks of bad positioning can be sufficient to cause such damage.

The purpose of dressing and bandaging the hand is to provide rest, compression, support, and positioning. Dressings are frequently considered a form of blotting paper wrapped around the operation site to absorb all types of exudate that may occur. Blotting paper is not required in the surgical care of the hand; postoperative dressings should supply an even compression throughout the area and prevent the introduction of infection from outside.

**Primary layer**

Whatever dressing is applied directly to the wound, it must be readily removable and must not stick to the blood oozing from the wound edges. Two types of such dressings are available: mesh gauze impregnated with petrolatum and absorbent cotton covered with a nonwettable plastic.

Wounds covered with an excess of greasy gauze tend to macerate and thereby lead to a moist suture line with the consequent risk of secondary infection. The absorbent plastic-coated dressing known as Telfa functions extremely well. Its perforated plastic sheet does not stick to the skin, yet it allows blood to seep through into the absorbent layer. The whole dressing can be readily peeled off without any risk of its sticking to the wound edges or sutures. These dressings (Telfa) can be bought in conveniently trimmed small pieces and are ideal for use in hand surgery.

In single isolated wounds of a digit, a portion of the palm, or dorsum of the hand, the amount of dressings used can be kept to a minimum. Frequently, a whole hand has to be bandaged even though only a finger or small portion has actually been damaged. In treating multiple wounds, it is better to bandage the whole hand than to try to apply several independent dressings. When a whole-hand dressing is applied, single pieces of Telfa, with the plastic facing outward, should be placed between each digital cleft. By this means, the maceration that occurs in some cases can be avoided. Petrolatum gauze should not be used routinely because maceration frequently occurs beneath it. It is important to ensure that the interdigital dressing does not press proximally on the finger web. Most of the venous and lymphatic drainage of the fingers passes dorsally and proximally in this area, and pressure here can rapidly lead to edematous fingers.

**Hand posture**

Once the primary protective layer has been applied, the position of the hand must be established for subsequent bandaging. The key to hand posture is the position of the wrist. If the wrist is in neutral or a little extension, the digits tend to assume a natural curved arc of flexion. When the wrist is flexed, there is a natural tendency for the metacarpophalangeal joints of the fingers to extend and the proximal interphalangeal joints to flex—a definitely nonfunctional or clawed position. However, the so-called functional position (Fig. 1-17, p. 24) is the position from which function develops in the normal hand. The wounded and bandaged hand is not normal and it should not be placed in the "functional position."

If the whole hand has to be dressed, the most satisfactory position for immobilization is with the wrist in neutral position, the thumb widely abducted, the finger metacarpophalangeal joints in nearly 90 degrees of flexion, and the interphalangeal joints in 5 to 10 degrees of flexion (Fig. 3-8). Some injuries, particularly of the extensor tendons, may demand modification of this position, but experience shows that this position does not lead to irreparable contractures of the digital joints so often seen after prolonged immobilization in other positions.

The explanation for using this position lies in the tendency for the finger joints

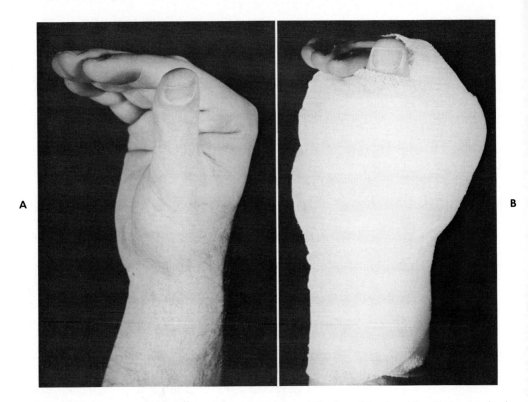

**Fig. 3-8.** *The bandaged hand.* The safe position for immobilization of the hand is with the proximal joints nearly fully flexed and the middle joints nearly fully extended. **A,** The correct position. **B,** The same position after a compression bandage has been applied. (Modified from James, J. I. P.: The assessment and management of the injured hand, The Hand **2:**102, 1970.)

to stiffen in one position but to retain mobility in another. The metacarpophalangeal joints will stiffen if held extended, but when flexed, the bone-to-bone collateral ligament is stretched to its maximum length. By contrast, the proximal interphalangeal joint maintains flexibility when immobilized in extension. This is because although the bone-to-bone ligament is taut in all positions, the glenoidal fibers (Fig. 1-4, p. 7) contract and stick together when the joint is held flexed.

The thumb must be positioned in wide abduction because of the risk of an adduction contracture developing. This is particularly likely to happen if the first web space is blown up with edema, which will subsequently organize into collagen and fibrosis affecting both skin and muscles.

## Compression dressing

With the primary layer placed over the wound and with the hand in the correct posture, a bulky soft resilient fluffed-up dressing is applied to both sides of the hand. It can be made up of fluffed sponges, mechanic's waste, Dacron batting such as is used to stuff pillows, or even ABD pads, but whatever the substance used, it must

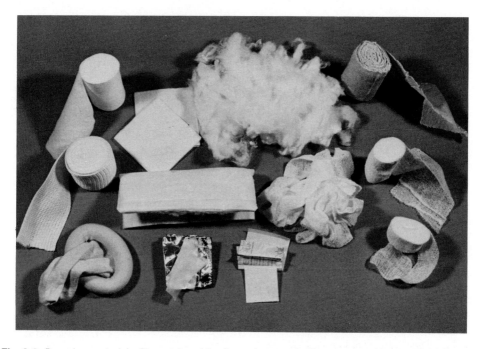

**Fig. 3-9.** *Dressing materials.* The center of the figure is occupied by compression materials, sponges flat or fluffed up, ABD pads, and Dacron batting. At bottom center are petrolatum gauze and Telfa dressings. Along the left side are padding materials to put beneath casts and a rolled-up stockinet for suspension of the hand. The right side top shows bias-cut stockinet and then 4-inch and 2-inch Kling bandages.

contain enough trapped air to yield and conform to the shape of the hand as the external bandage is applied (Fig. 3-9). The bulk of the dressing is usually spread over the palm with the remainder being placed on the dorsum and around the wrist and lower forearm. It is important that the volume of these dressings be evenly distributed over the various areas so that when bandages are applied the ultimate shape will reproduce that of the underlying hand (Fig. 3-10, *A*). Irregular lumpy dressings cannot be tolerated because they will cause irregular distribution of the compression needed to control any tendency to edema of the hand. The fluffed-up material must be applied piecemeal and in general in a longitudinal direction. It must not be circumferential and must pack down firmly yet not occlusively.

Dressing a wounded hand is an art acquired only by extensive practice; the final result depends on the skill with which the external bandage is applied. In selecting the bandage there is no place for ordinary cotton bandages—they are too rigid and unyielding. Strongly elastic bandages or elasticized gauze tubes should be avoided because of the risk of obliterating the venous return and producing circulatory congestion. The best type of bandage is an elastic cotton gauze bandage that

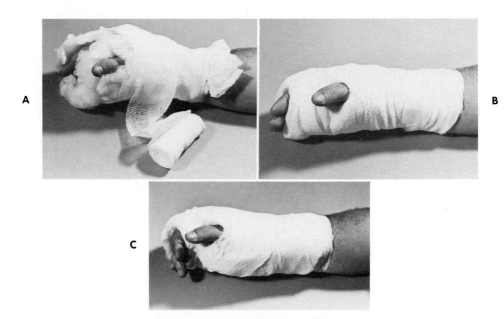

**Fig. 3-10.** *Bandaging a hand.* **A,** Soft resilient Dacron batting is placed in the palm, in the thumb web space, and on the dorsum of the hand. **B,** The Kling bandage supplies an even compression and is held in place with a few strips of tape. The bulk of compression material and the tension on the bandage tapers off toward the wrist. **C,** The completed dressing is supported by a palmar plaster slab held in place with another Kling bandage to prevent subsequent shift in position.

is self-adhering and adapts to the contours of the part around which it is wrapped (Kling). It is available in 2- or 4-inch widths and when properly applied supplies the appropriate compression. The written word cannot explain the tension necessary; it can only be learned by apprenticeship, and in many instances experienced nurses can demonstrate this far better than the average physician. The compression in a well-applied dressing has a decreasing gradation from distal to proximal because a venous tourniquet effect is produced if the bandage is more tightly wrapped around the wrist than the fingers (Fig. 3-10, *B*). Although there should be no worries concerning the circulation of the digits, it is a wise precaution to leave the tips of the digits exposed for inspection. It is very difficult to maintain a limb in the correct position while trying to bandage it, but any position other than the ideal is unacceptable, and the bandages must be reapplied until it is attained.

Even a properly applied bulky compression dressing will continue to pack down over several days so that the support that was originally given to the wrist and hand dissipates and the hand tends to assume the clawed position. Because of this risk most hand surgeons support the wrist and hand position with a carefully moulded lightweight plaster-of-paris splint (Fig. 3-10, *C*). The more modern thermolabile splint materials can be used but in general they weigh somewhat more than their plaster-of-paris equivalent. The plaster splint is usually made of ten to twelve layers placed on the palmar aspect of the forearm and hand. Proximally it should start about 5 cm below the elbow joint and end at about the distal palmar crease. If the fingers are wounded and need immobilization, then the splint should extend to but not over the fingertips.

## A sling

Slings are useful in treating severe injuries, but rarely are they indicated for minor hand injuries. They encourage both stiffness and a martyr complex. Their one advantage, however, is that they do protect the limb from dangling and thereby prevent venous congestion from developing. Luckily, venous congestion is usually not a problem in patients with minor hand injuries, but it can rapidly become one if the hand is allowed to dangle limply over the edge of the sling. Elevation either with or without a sling decreases the blood volume in the hand by approximately 20%. Thus the bandaged hand must always be elevated. The risk of the potential for swelling overcoming the compression supplied by the resilient dressing will be removed if the hand is elevated and the shoulder joint exercised several times a day.

## Bandaging a single digit

A wounded finger or thumb requires a minimum amount of bandaging for the shortest possible time. Immediately following the reparative surgery some form of absorbent dressing must be kept in place for twenty-four to forty-eight hours. At the end of this time the dressings should be removed, and in many cases there will be no further need for any form of covering. Many workers, however, need to protect the wound from contamination in their working environment and therefore have to wear some form of disposable dressings.

The perennial problem of how to keep a bandage on a finger has been solved by the introduction of a stockinet tubular bandage (Tubegauz). This bandage is available in different diameters and, when properly applied, holds dressings securely in place without any risk of strangling the fingers. Various sizes of applicators are available, and very little practice is needed to become proficient in the use of these bandages. They are excellent for the fingers, but they can also be applied easily to the whole palm or dorsum of the hand (Figs. 3-11 and 3-12). A particularly useful feature of these dressings is that the patient can be given several feet of the bandage to take away with him. He can then put on an additional clean outer surface dressing whenever he wishes, and he can change these covers as long as his supply lasts.

## Dressings for children

Dressings for children are a major problem. Practically no form of dressing can withstand their persistent curiosity. It is best to apply the appropriate dressing as if the wound had occurred in an adult and then to apply a separate outer protective layer. In children there is no risk of stiffness following short periods of splinting, and more extensive use can be made of splints than in the adult. There should be no hesitation in completely immobilizing the hand by a large bulky dressing of the

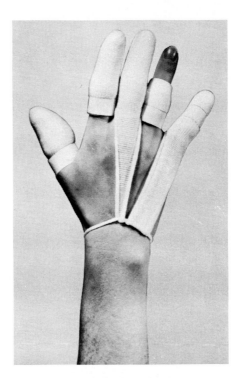

**Fig. 3-11.** *Finger bandages.* Tubegauz bandages can be applied in a variety of ways to the digits. They do not become loose but can be easily changed. (From New techniques of bandaging with Tubegauz, Chicago, The Scholl Manufacturing Co., Inc.)

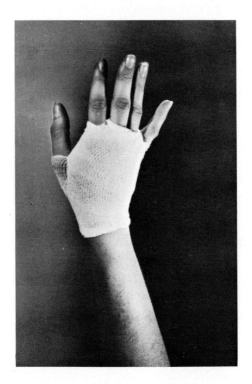

**Fig. 3-12.** *Bandaging the palm or dorsum.* The palm or dorsum of the hand can be effectively covered by Tubegauz bandage, which will remain in place even if the hand is used for work. (From New techniques of bandaging with Tubegauz, Chicago, The Scholl Manufacturing Co., Inc.)

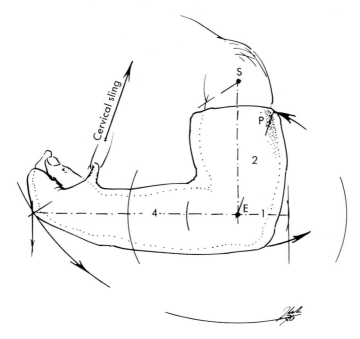

**Fig. 3-13.** *Bandaging a child's hand.* Most children benefit from the rigid secure immobilization supplied by an above-elbow right-angle plaster cast. The posterior aspect of the arm **(P)** should be protected by a felt pad, and pressure is relieved by using a cervical sling through the loop at the wrist. If the sling is not used, the 4:1 lever arm will cause severe pressure at **P.** (From Converse, J. M., editor: Reconstructive plastic surgery, ed. 2, vol. 6, The hand and upper extremity, edited by J. W. Littler, Philadelphia, 1977, W. B. Saunders Co.)

boxing glove type. A light plaster-of-paris bandage can be applied over the outer surface of the bandages to discourage attempts at unwinding.

Most children would benefit from extending this bandage to an above-elbow right-angle plaster support. This should have a plaster loop incorporated at the wrist to accommodate a cervical collar sling (Fig. 3-13). Care is needed in applying these plaster cylinders, and the posterior aspect of the arm must be protected by padding. If the casted arm is not properly supported by the collar sling, the arm will tilt at both the shoulder and elbow, causing severe pressure by the cast on the back of the arm.

If such a cast is not used, a most effective form of protection is a long length of stockinet tubing threaded over the affected limb so that a considerable portion remains distal to the fingertips. This excess stockinet can be pinned to the opposite shoulder, and with the limb in this position elevation is encouraged and exploration discouraged.

## Splinting

Mobility should be encouraged whenever possible, and rigid immobilization should be discarded as soon as possible. Palmar plaster slabs are acceptable as a

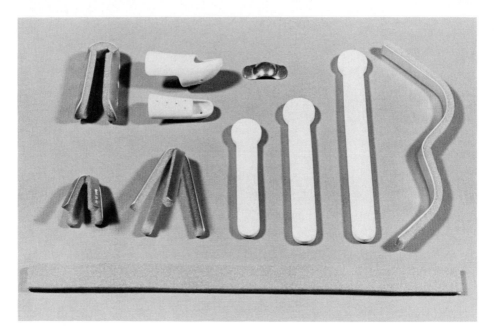

**Fig. 3-14.** *Finger splints*. A variety of commercially made splints are available. Left, end protectors; top, center mallet finger splints, and right and bottom, padded malleable aluminum splints of varying sizes.

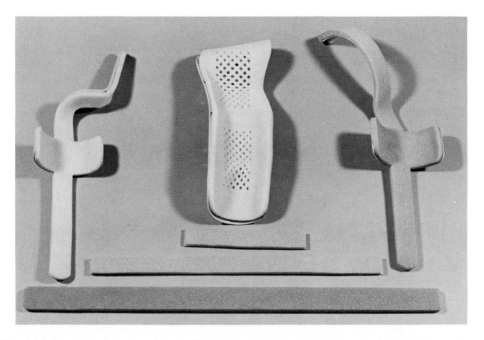

**Fig. 3-15.** *Finger and hand splints*. Left, Burnham thumb splint; right, adjustable Burnham finger splint; center, well-designed padded wrist and hand splint; bottom, varying lengths of malleable aluminum splints.

rigid support hidden in bandages, but full plaster casts should never be used in the care of minor soft-tissue hand injuries in adults. There are virtually no indications for their use, and experience shows that while employers will accept back at work patients whose fingers are bandaged, they often refuse to accept the patient who returns with a plaster-of-paris protection over the dressings because of the risk of liability involved.

Unfortunately, when rigid splinting is considered necessary, it is often left to the ingenuity of the junior intern; equally unfortunately for the hands, there is usually a plentiful supply of tongue blades readily available. The wooden tongue depressor is designed to enable one to look at throats; it is not for splinting sore fingers. To strap the finger to one of these pieces of wood must force it into a non-functional position, with the risk of producing a permanently stiff finger.

Several types of splints can be used to protect wounded digits and in the care of fractures and joint and tendon injuries. Many commercially available splints are designed for use on hands or digits of adults of either sex (Fig. 3-14).

For a single finger or thumb the Burnham digital splint is ideal. These splints are designed so the digit can be rested in the physiological position after restoration of the longitudinal arch (Fig. 3-15). The Burnham finger splint is articulated so that it can be used on any of the four fingers, but separate splints are required for the left or right thumb.

Malleable aluminum splints to which foam rubber padding has been applied can be bought in various widths and lengths. If a simple splint is all that is required, satisfactory substitutes can be made in the home workshop at a fraction of the cost of the commercially available article.

## CONTROL OF INFECTION

Trivial wounds of the hands more often get infected than massive injuries that are treated in the operating room. Good care of wounds of the hands implies meticulous surgical technique and intelligent use of the multitude of anti-infective agents now available. Such care falls into the two main groups of prophylaxis and active treatment.

### Prophylaxis

The only correct prophylactic treatment for clean hand wounds is asepsis. Routine use of antibiotics is absolutely wrong. Present-day antibiotics are powerful agents that can produce many harmful side effects. Their use in patients with clean wounds can do nothing to help wound healing but can produce a resistance to the agent being used in any organisms that may be present. Thorough débridement will do much more than any antibiotic to keep a wound clean. It is particularly important to remove all foreign material from the wound, since its presence may potentiate any pathogens that may be present.

Half or more of all physicians and nurses working in hospitals carry potentially dangerous staphylococci in their noses. To prevent such staphylococci from infecting the wound, masks must be worn when dressings are being applied.

Wet dressings lying on clean wounds may incubate the surface bacteria and any wound contaminants that are present. Nonadherent dressings should be used, they must be kept dry, and they should be changed as infrequently as possible.

## Active treatment

Expectation of severe infection is sufficient justification for the immediate use of a broad-spectrum antibiotic. Choice of antibiotic is discussed on a later page, but in general, it is best to select one which previous experience has shown to be successful in your local environment. Infection can be reasonably suspected when wounds have occurred through already infected areas or when dirty materials have been handled. In this connection it must be appreciated that "dirty" means infected rather than socially unpleasant. A wound that is full of street dirt is relatively clean when compared with one contaminated with hospital dust or dirt. When large surfaces have been exposed for prolonged lengths of time, the use of prophylactic antibiotics is permissible.

## Antibiotics
### Risks of treatment

Several severe complications can arise following treatment with antibiotics. Among these complications are anaphylactic reactions, procaine reactions, serum sickness, and superinfections.

### *Anaphylactic reactions*

Anaphylactic reactions are by far the most dangerous complication of antibiotic treatment. Their important feature is that the previous sensitizing dose has usually been a parenteral injection. However, the reaction itself can occur no matter what route is used to give the antibiotic. Reactions have occurred following the use of ointments, nasal sprays, ophthalmic drops, injections, oral penicillin, or other preparations.

It is therefore very important when treating children with antibiotics that they should be given oral preparations only. By this means the risk of future anaphylaxis will be greatly reduced, possibly even entirely eliminated. Patients experiencing anaphylactic reaction first have itching of the palms, soles, and perineum and then become cyanotic and faint, their respiration rate slows, and there is a fall in blood pressure. Death may follow rapidly. The treatment is administration of 0.3 ml of 1:1000 epinephrine subcutaneously. If this initial dose of epinephrine is not effective, it should be repeated in five to twenty minutes. An adequate airway must be established and maintained. If the injection of penicillin has been into an arm or leg, a tourniquet can be applied proximal to the injection to cut down further absorption of the drug. Cortisone and antihistamines are of no value in treating this reaction. Anaphylactic reaction is rarely caused by the tetracyclines or other broad-spectrum drugs because they are not usually given parenterally.

### Procaine reaction

If a blood vessel is inadvertently entered during the administration of procaine penicillin, a reaction may occur, since each 600,000 units of procaine penicillin contains 240 mg of procaine. Such a reaction can be avoided if the elementary precaution of pulling back on the plunger of the syringe is carried out to ensure that the needle is not in a vessel before the intramuscular injection is given. If this precaution is not carried out and if the injection is given at a speed that will deliver a greater quantity of procaine than 8 mg per minute, then there will be a generalized reaction consisting of flushing, dizziness, and numbness.

### Serum sickness

Serum sickness usually occurs about one week after the beginning of treatment, although it can occur at much shorter periods of time. The patient will complain of urticarial skin rash and may complain of pain and swelling of the joints. There is marked pruritus, possibly lymphadenopathy, and possibly edema of the face. Blood studies may show an eosinophilia. This reaction does respond to treatment with cortisone or prednisone, which should be given in doses such as 100 mg four times a day, the injections being tapered off as soon as a response is seen. Many milder reactions will respond to antihistamines alone.

### Superinfection — staphylococcal enteritis

Staphylococcal enteritis, a serious complication of antibiotic therapy, usually occurs with a staphylococcus resistant to the antibiotic and usually happens when the patient is being given tetracycline or some other broad-spectrum drugs. It is unlikely to occur in the type of patient whose hand injury is being treated on an outpatient basis; however, because of its very real dangers, it is mentioned in this discussion. Superinfection can occur after a very small dose of the drug has been given, but it is more likely to occur after prolonged treatment with 2 g per day of tetracycline. Because of this, tetracycline is usually given in doses of 1 g per day.

Superinfection is more likely to occur in hospitals where antibiotic-resistant staphylococci or gram-negative rods are frequently encountered. The staphylococcal organisms should be identified on gram-stained direct smears of the stool. The stool should be cultured on blood agar as well as the usual media used for stool cultures, since these latter media are inhibitory to staphylococci.

Treatment should consist of immediate cessation of all broad-spectrum antibiotic therapy or a penicillin-streptomycin mixture and replacement with an antibiotic thought to be effective against the currently occurring staphylococcus. The antibiotic may have to be changed again when culture and sensitivity tests are made on the organism isolated from the stools. If the patient is severely ill, parenteral therapy by the intravenous route may be necessary, and for postoperative patients with large amounts of secretions in the upper gastrointestinal tract, parenteral therapy is recommended.

The gram-negative rods (*Escherichia coli*, *Pseudomonas*, *Proteus*, or *Klebsiella-*

*Enterobacter*) may cause severe pneumonia in hospitalized patients receiving prolonged or mixed antibiotic treatment. Again antibiotics should be discontinued, and an effective anti–gram-negative rod agent such as gentamicin substituted.

### Rules for use

The following rules should be observed for the use of antibiotics:
1. Antibiotics should be used only when clearly indicated.
2. Parenteral penicillin treatment should be avoided whenever possible and especially in children who have never previously been given penicillin.
3. Pus must be drained before or at the time treatment is started. If the response to treatment proves to be inadequate, it may be because the pus has pocketed, and it must be released.
4. Treatment will have to be started empirically. However, the organism must be identified and then tested by in vitro sensitivity tests. Such tests cost about as much as one day in hospital and are thoroughly justified in good patient care.
5. Accurate treatment with a well-chosen narrow-spectrum drug is better than the use of a wide-spectrum antibiotic.
6. Bactericidal antibiotics are preferable to the bacteriostatic types. The more common bactericidal antibiotics are the penicillins, the cephalosporins, streptomycin, gentamicin, tyrocidine, bacitracin, and neomycin. Erythromycin is bactericidal if given in high dosage.
7. Full doses of the antibiotic must be given for an adequate length of time. Proprietary cocktails containing a half dose or less of two otherwise useful antibiotics should be avoided.
8. Evaluate the effectiveness of the antibiotic every forty-eight hours by monitoring the temperature chart. It will tend to fall like a bouncing ball, and the antibiotic should be continued for an adequate length of time.

### Choice

The following choice of antibiotics is recommended: gentamicin, kanamycin, and carbenicillin.

Antibiotics active against gram-negative bacilli include tetracycline, streptomycin, and chloramphenicol.

In order of preference, antibiotics active against staphylococci are nafcillin (cloxacillin or methicillin), penicillin G, the cephalosporins, erythromycin, and clindamycin. Kanamycin can be given only intramuscularly. Vancomycin can be given only intravenously. Tetracyclines are not recommended. Gentamicin is usually given intramuscularly three times daily in a dose of 1 mg/kg body weight.

### Dosages

The following dosages of antibiotics are recommended for adults:
Penicillin—it is best to use procaine penicillin, 600,000 units twice daily intramuscularly.

Nafcillin—it is best given 1 g orally q4h or methicillin 2 g IV q4h.

Cephalosporins—Cephalothin is given 1 g IM q6h, and cephalexin is given 1 g
by mouth q6h.

Erythromycin is usually given in divided doses by mouth to a total of 1 to 2 g
daily.

Clindamycin is usually prescribed as 150 mg orally four times daily.

## Steroids

Cortisone and other steroids are mentioned only to be condemned. During the
last few years they have been used in every conceivable situation, and extensive
studies have shown that in treatment of infection, with rare exceptions, their use
is of no obvious benefit. At best, steroids will produce a temporary feeling of well-
being, and at worst, in the presence of an organism resistant to the antibiotic being
used, may lead to a fatal septicemia.

## Specific infections
### Tetanus

Tetanus does not necessarily develop only after deep traumatic wounds; it can
occur after relatively minor lesions, and about 20% of cases develop without any
identifiable site of injury or break in the skin. It is relatively frequent in children
under 15 years of age. In the very young and the very old, it is a serious condition.
Prophylactic treatment, when there is a reasonable risk of tetanus infection, is mandatory. A single injection of 500 units of tetanus immune globulin (human) administered intramuscularly is recommended. For children a smaller dose based on body
weight should be given; approximately 8 units per kilogram is recommended.
Recent experience suggests that these doses, which are somewhat higher than some
previously suggested, will maintain a satisfactory amount of circulating antitoxin for
at least a month. The reaction rate to tetanus immune globin (human) is unknown,
but it is probably very low.

Three doses of 0.5 ml tetanus toxoid are given intramuscularly or subcutaneously with an interval of 3 to 4 weeks between injections. A reinforcing dose of 0.5
ml is administered within one year after the third dose of toxoid.

Booster doses of tetanus toxoid (preferably with absorbed tetanus toxoid) should
be administered routinely at fairly regular intervals, and a ten-year interval is currently thought satisfactory. A routine booster (0.5 ml) at any time up to ten years
may restore immunity, and a booster dose of tetanus toxoid may be relied upon in
an emergency in any fully immunized person up to ten years after the last previous
toxoid injection. However, the simultaneous administration of antitoxin along with
the toxoid is justified in the patient with multiple, contaminated injuries (especially with associated head or neck wounds), when there is uncertainty regarding
previous tetanus immunization, or if there is delay in administering the emergency
booster injection. Emergency boosters should be given no more than one year apart.

Antibody response is suppressed in adults receiving long-term prednisone
therapy of 200 or more mg but not in those receiving 5 to 30 mg daily. In children

the suppressive dose is 40 mg, and it is recommended that it be reduced to 10 mg at the time of immunization. Concentrated use of immune serum globulin and vaccine is suggested in patients receiving corticosteroid therapy. This combination is also recommended for persons with wounds which indicate an overwhelming possibility that tetanus will develop or for immunized persons with wounds other than clean minor wounds. The tetanus immune globulin and tetanus toxoid must be administered from separate syringes and given at different anatomical sites.

Patients who suffer from tetanus do not become immune to the infection, and active immunization with toxoid must be carried out. A past history of tetanus without active immunization does not allow one to forego prophylactic treatment for possible infection.

### Gas gangrene

Gas gangrene infection is rare; it occasionally occurs after small puncture wounds or larger areas of damage in the hand. In actual numbers it is probably more common in elderly debilitated patients, in diabetics, and in patients receiving chemotherapy. This devastating infection must be treated with adequate surgery. The operations must relieve all tissue tension, excise all dead infected tissues, and provide adequate drainage. Hyperbaric oxygen treatment, when available, may be a valuable adjunct to treatment.

Antibiotics are not effective against the spores of these organisms, and they cannot substitute for adequate surgical care. Bacitracin, penicillin, tetracycline, and chloramphenicol are all effective in vitro against the clostridia. Prophylactic antiserum must be given and, as in the case of tetanus, must be preceded by a skin test to rule out sensitivity. The usual prophylactic treatment is 9000 I.U. of *Bacillus welchii* antitoxin, 4500 units of *Vibrio septicus* antitoxin, and 9000 units of *Bacillus oedematis* antitoxin. Prophylactic treatment is given intramuscularly, but, if there is any degree of urgency about the case, it may be given intravenously. The therapeutic treatment is given intravenously in at least three times the strength of the prophylactic dose. If the organism has been identified, a monovalent serum can be used when appropriate. Some believe that modern treatment methods when combined with antibiotics may make the protection supplied by antitoxin superfluous. In diabetics the clinical and radiological signs of gas are more commonly caused by a mixed aerobic and anaerobic infection than by gas gangrene.

### Staphylococcal infections

Staphylococcal infections are the most common infections of the hand. Infection occurs by contamination from another infected source or by droplet or hand transfer from a nasal carrier who may be the physician, nurse, or even the patient. Staphylococci are classified by their ability to clot human or rabbit plasma with an enzyme called coagulase. Coagulase-positive *Staphylococcus aureus* is considered to be a potential human pathogen.

Staphylococcal infections are usually localized and rarely show spreading cellulitis, lymphangitis, or lymphadenitis.

### Streptococcal infections

Streptococcal infections of the hand are less common than staphylococcal infections. The streptococci are usually introduced by droplets originating in the infected throat or tonsils of the patient or a carrier.

The classical picture of erysipelas is an area of bright red inflammation with a sharply defined raised palpable edge between the area of infection and the normal skin. Characteristically, there are red lines of lymphangitis, and regional lymphadenitis is present.

### Infections caused by other organisms

*Escherichia coli* infections respond well to gentamicin, kanamycin, or colistin. In less serious infections ampicillin or tetracycline may be used if sensitivity tests are positive. *Enterobacter* infections also respond to gentamicin, kanamycin, or colistin treatment. *Pseudomonas* infections occur very rarely in the hand and more commonly are seen around the sites of an infusion puncture wound. Occasionally a *Proteus* organism will cause an infection in the hand. Antibiotic sensitivity tests are mandatory before treatment of infection by these organisms, since it is impossible to predict what antibiotic should be used. Gentamicin is a suitable initial therapy in doses of 1 mg/kg intramuscularly every 8 hours, but careful monitoring of levels is mandatory. Streptococci will not be covered by this agent, and penicillin G or cephalothin can be added.

## POSTOPERATIVE THERAPY

Both physical therapy and occupational therapy can be of value in rehabilitation of the injured hand. These forms of treatment are complementary to each other and not mutually exclusive. Both are of great importance in the postoperative care of major injuries to the hand. For the more minor wounds they can also be of very definite, though limited, value in the after-treatment.

The hand therapist provides continuity to the care initiated by the physician. Specifics of treatment will vary, but the fundamental plan must enlist the active cooperation of the patient. Although the therapist plans the program and supervises its execution, it is the patient who will *do* the treatment. Therapy once or twice a day is useless; a program to be done at home between therapy sessions is essential, and each day the patient's progress must be monitored.

### Passive and active exercises

The two types of exercises possible are passive and active. Passive exercise is movement produced by the therapist without resistance or assistance from the patient. Active exercise is carried out entirely by the patient with varying degrees of encouragement from the therapist and is the only treatment that yields lasting benefit.

Passive movement produces very little change in the blood flow of the limb but does tend to prevent adhesions between muscle planes and to maintain the range of movement of the joints. In active movements the blood flow in the limb varies directly with the degree of activity of the muscle. The neuromuscular inhibition that follows injury is more easily overcome by active than by passive exercises.

Exercise must be prescribed for a definite purpose; vague wavings of the limb in midair accomplish nothing and produce a stiff limb that the patient is reluctant to use. Stiffness of itself is not a contraindication to continuing purposeful exercise. If, however, the stiffness is extreme, or if there is actual muscle soreness, then the amount of exercise should be reduced. Such discomforts can be avoided by progressive increase in the degree of exercise demanded and in the later stages by slow but steady increase in the resistive component of the exercises.

All uninjured parts of the hand should be put through their normal range of movement several times a day, with care being taken that the limits of flexion and extension are reached. Swelling can be controlled by these active movements and by elevation of the limbs. The fingers that have not been injured rapidly become stiffened by edema if the fluid is not dispersed by regular exercise. Even persistent swelling responds better to this treatment than to application of various forms of heat, which frequently seems only to prolong the condition.

Violent manipulation of a stiff joint by either therapist or patient can produce disastrous results. Adhesions and scar tissue will yield to gentle persistent force; sudden "cracking" of the joint will tear tissue and produce bleeding and ultimately more scarring than was caused by the original injury.

Gradual application of a persistent force is whimsically illustrated in Fig. 3-16. Most patients can readily recognize the principle from this illustration and can subsequently be taught to apply the appropriate force for short periods of time many

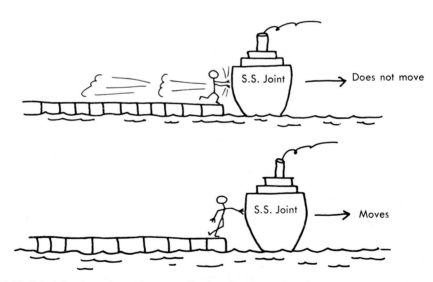

**Fig. 3-16.** *Principle of persistent force application.* Sudden violent force applied to a stiff joint will not increase the range of movement in the joint. If, however, a gentle, persistent force is applied, the scar tissue will yield without excessive reaction. (From Howard, L. D.: Fractures of the small bones of the hand; booklet circulated privately.)

times a day. The key to such self-treatment is the appreciation of the difference between discomfort and pain. The discomfort of properly applied force is virtuous
and should be tolerated, since the tissues will gradually yield to such treatment.
The pain is a warning and must be respected; the amount of force and the duration
of its application must be reduced until the discomfort is tolerable.

Prolonged formal therapeutic programs have little place in the treatment of
minor hand injuries. The best therapy is to return the patient to work at the earliest
possible moment. Since, however, many of the patients with hand injuries are
eligible for workman's compensation, the prospect of litigation often inhibits the
recovery process. In such cases, occupational therapy can be of great help in demon-
strating to the patient (and his lawyer) that the injury does not prevent the normal
performance of his work. Frequently, the necessary muscle and joint movements
can be produced as a demonstration of capability by an ingenious therapist devising
tasks that resemble but do not actually reproduce the actual work conditions.

## Treatment for specific conditions
### Dislocations and sprains

In a dislocation the articular surfaces of the joint are completely displaced from
one another by violence and may or may not remain displaced. In a subluxation
the joint surfaces remain partially displaced, and in a sprain the joint surfaces,
although momentarily separated from each other by the violence, return to their
normal position. In all of these conditions the trauma that caused them produces
stretching and tearing of the structures surrounding the joint. There is a general
extravasation of blood from the vessels in these injured structures. Therapy is directed to dispersing the hematoma and tissue fluid around the area of injury and
later to increasing gradually the range of movement without causing further trauma.

### *The wrist*

Sprains and dislocations of the wrist are treated by the same physiotherapeutic
measures, but in the case of sprains the progress is more rapid and treatment is
started earlier than in dislocations.

A "sprained wrist" is an uncommon injury. Many so-called sprains are later
correctly diagnosed as a fractured scaphoid. If there is the slightest suspicion that
a fracture may have occurred, x-ray films must be taken. Plaster-of-paris immobilization of the wrist in all doubtful cases is the best treatment. If the second set of
x-ray films shows no fracture and all symptoms have disappeared, then the patient
has received good treatment and been spared the risk of months of immobilization
that might be necessary if he had been moving a fractured scaphoid.

In both sprains and dislocations of the wrist, adequate time must be allowed for
soft tissue healing to occur before movements of the actual joint are commenced.
In the case of sprains, these can be started in three to five days, but in the case of a
true dislocation of the wrist it is advisable to allow at least three weeks of immobilization before wrist movements are started. The first stage of treatment is massage

to the area proximal to the site of injury from the wrist to elbow, followed by general massage to the elbow and shoulder regions. After this, the elbow and shoulder joints should be put through a full range of movement. Gentle massage to the fingers and dorsum of the hand and also over the wrist joint itself is helpful and can be done when compresses are being changed. Active movements of the fingers and thumb should be encouraged from the start of treatment of both dislocations and sprains.

The next stage of treatment is to increase the degree and duration of massage for the forearm and upper arm. The amount of movement demanded of the fingers and thumb should be increased, and attempts should be made to reach a full grip. When the inflammatory edema has subsided and when little pain is felt on movement, exercise of the wrist joint can be added to the finger exercises. Stiffness in both the fingers and the wrist should not be an indication for passive movements by the therapist. The patient must be encouraged to increase the range of these joints by active movements.

### The digits

The principles of care of the digits are the same as those used for the wrist. Treatment may have to be modified and delayed because of the slow rate at which the edema subsides from the digits.

Sprains will eventually cure themselves despite any therapy. The symptoms can be prolonged by inadvisable treatment and by too active use, but there is little definitive in the way of therapeutic care that will accelerate their healing. The patient must be warned that minor symptoms may persist for many months.

Dislocation of the finger joints is frequently treated by operative repair of the torn structures. Movements cannot, therefore, be started until the wound is healed. In many cases it is advisable to wait until the edema has begun to subside. There is so little room for inflammatory edema within the cylinder of skin that the additional swelling caused by premature movement could impair the circulation of the finger.

Active movements are the best means of promoting drainage of the edema; however, until they can be started, gentle massage in a proximal direction may be of great help.

### Fractures

Postoperative therapy has a very definite role in the treatment of fractures of the hand and digits. It is not concerned with the care of the fracture, but with the rest of the limb. Prophylactic treatment should be given to all the joints of the extremity that are not immobilized. This must include the shoulder and elbow joint because many times these joints will be found to be stiffened because the limb was being held immobile in a sling for a prolonged period of time.

Massage in an attempt to disperse the inflammatory reaction around the fracture is inadvisable because of the risk of further displacement at the fracture site. After the removal of the immobilization, active movements in whirlpool baths is a very efficient form of aiding recovery, but if such baths are not available, movements in warm water should be encouraged. In either case the hand must not be allowed to be dependent; edema fluid cannot drain uphill.

The emphasis must be on active movements. Passive movements of the immobilized part can do nothing but harm. Even if the fracture site is sufficiently healed to withstand the manipulation, the periarticular tissues will react violently, and the resultant edema may lead to permanent limitation of movement.

## "DISABILITY"

An important and fundamental principle concerning the assessment of disability is emphasized in a publication by the American Medical Association.* Much stress is placed on the scope of medical responsibility in evaluation of permanent disability and in differentiating between "permanent disability" and "permanent impairment."

Evaluation of permanent *disability* is an administrative function and is not part of a physician's responsibility. Disability is affected by many nonmedical factors such as age, sex, education, and economic and social environment. All these factors have to be considered by the administrator after receiving the physician's report on the patient's permanent *impairment*.

Permanent impairment is a purely medical condition, and the physician is solely responsible for the accurate assessment of this part of the patient's disability. Because it is impossible to measure objectively many of the nonmedical factors, the assessment of permanent impairment is frequently used as the basis for awarding the disability. Thus, although the final decision does not actually rest with the physician, his assessment of impairment must be based upon some permanent and unaltering scale of measurements.

Proper evaluation of permanent impairment is based upon a complete physical examination that records accurate, objective measurements of function. These measurements are absolute and are not relative to such factors as geography, the patient's age, sex, social status, or employability.

This assessment of permanent impairment must be based upon demonstrable functional impairment substantiated by evidence of pathology, loss of structural integrity, or pain attributable to clinical findings. When the clinical examination has been completed, its findings must be assessed against the patient's ability to carry out the activities of daily living. These activities are self-care, normal living postures, ambulation, elevation, traveling, and nonspecialized hand activities.

It must be emphasized that this assessment of impairment is based on the patient's ability to perform normal social acitivites. A hand that has lost two fingers has the same degree of impairment whether it belongs to a watchmaker or a lumberjack. The percentage of disability to be awarded to the two people would be greatly different because of the difference in their subsequent ability to carry out their occupations.

---

*Committee on Medical Rating of Physical Impairment of the American Medical Association: AMA guides to the evaluation of permanent impairment, Chicago, 1971, American Medical Association.

The difference between impairment and disability can be illustrated by considering an amputation through the proximal interphalangeal joint of a finger. Even though treatment may have produced a pain-free stump with excellent movement and therefore little impairment, many states arbitrarily classify such an injury as a 100% loss of the finger.

When considering impairment of function in the end result of a hand injury case, many factors have to be considered. Some of these factors, such as range of movement and muscle power, can be measured objectively, but others, such as sensibility, security of grip, and dexterity, defy measurement. Because of these difficulties, any physician who does not see many end results of these cases would be well advised to refer such patients to a more experienced colleague.

# 4 · SURGICAL TECHNIQUES

**Débridement**

**Stopping bleeding**

**Closing the wound**
Subcutaneous tissues
The skin

**Skin grafts**

**Tendon suture**

**Nerve suture**

The craft of surgery is accomplished in many ways, and the methods described in this chapter are not the absolute and only way of carrying out the intent of a procedure. All that can be said of them is that at least one surgeon knows they work.

Textbooks of general surgery usually contain detailed descriptions of the techniques of surgery, and this section stresses only the various points of technique that may be of value in treating minor hand injuries.

## DÉBRIDEMENT

Débridement is a convenient word to describe a variety of cleaning-out and throwing-away processes that should be carried out before a skin wound can be closed. It is a process that demands great judgment on the part of the physician. To err on the side of cleanliness and cut out far too much healthy tissue may make the problem of closing the wound almost insoluble. On the other hand, it is equally dangerous to leave behind tissue that is contaminated or that has lost its blood supply. Such tissue can lead only to subsequent infection and very delayed healing. When the skin edges of the wound are being trimmed, a strip only 1 to 2 mm wide should be removed. Removal of such a small amount of skin does not cause any serious loss of function, but it does ensure good and rapid healing of the skin wound.

If the trauma has raised small flaps of skin, these should be carefully inspected, and, if they are considered viable, they should be retained, because they may be of great use as rotation flaps when the skin wound is being closed. All foreign bodies and dirty crusted tissue must be excised, even if this implies excision of a small amount of tissue to get rid of ingrained dirt.

## STOPPING BLEEDING

In most instances bleeding will cease if enough time is allowed to elapse. Capillary ooze is not of serious consequence and will cease almost immediately after the adjacent raw sides of the wound are stuck together. Pressure applied by a moist

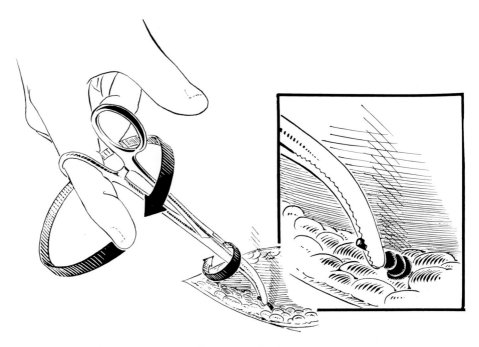

**Fig. 4-1.** *Twisting off bleeding vessels.* Catgut is a foreign body and, if possible, should not be buried in the hand. The majority of vessels can be twisted off rather than ligated. If the tip of one finger is left in the handle of the hemostat and the instrument is wound ten to fifteen times, the intima of the vessel will curl up and form an effective block to bleeding.

sponge held in place for several minutes will control most forms of hemorrhage, and only the most obviously spurting vessel should be caught by hemostats. A moist sponge must always be used in treating wounds of the hand. A dry sponge is too rough and coarse to be dragged across tissues; if it is left in place as a pressure dressing, a clot will form in its interstices and will be torn away from the vessel ends when the sponge is removed. Even if hemostats are used, it should seldom be necessary to tie catgut ligatures around them. Even the finest catgut is a foreign body, and foreign bodies should not be buried in the hand, unless it is absolutely unavoidable.

The caliber of all vessels in the digits, except the main digital artery, is such that the vessels can be held in a hemostat for three to five minutes and then "twisted off." The twisting off consists of putting a finger through one end of the handle of the hemostat and with a twisting motion winding the vessel around the tip of the hemostat for ten or fifteen turns and then removing the hemostat (Fig. 4-1). This apparently traumatic method of dealing with a cut vessel is in fact relatively mild and causes much less reaction in the tissues than catgut knots. The twisting damages the intima of the vessel sufficiently to encourage rapid clotting and provides a good framework in which this clotting can take place. Even the main digital arteries can be treated quite readily by twisting off, but the physician usually sleeps better if he has tied a ligature around an artery of this size.

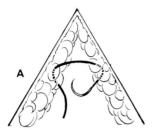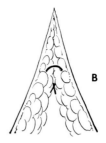

**Fig. 4-2.** *Suturing methods.* Subcutaneous catgut sutures should be inserted reversed so that, when the knot is tied, the ends point into the depths of the tissues, **B.** The needle must be inserted from the depths of the wound toward the superficial tissues, pass across the wound, penetrate the superficial tissues on the opposite side, and finally come out through the deep tissues, **A.**

When a bleeding vessel has to be clamped, its ends should be caught clearly by mosquito hemostats, with no extra fatty tissue included. Occasionally, a vessel will have a longitudinal slit in its length. Do not try to hold this by one ligature. Two hemostats should be put across normal parts of the vessel and the damaged portion between them cut out before ligatures are applied. If a ligature is tied around both fatty tissue and the vessel, there is the risk that the fat may let the ligature slide off the end of the vessel. Even if this does not happen, the fatty tissue is strangled by the ligature and will subsequently necrose, thereby delaying healing in that area.

## CLOSING THE WOUND
### Subcutaneous tissues

If a wound has considerable depth, and particularly if there has been disruption of tissue planes, it may be advisable to put in a few catgut sutures to help retain the subcutaneous tissues in more normal relationships. Plain catgut, No. 4-0 or No. 5-0, is usually quite strong enough. It should be inserted in the reverse way so that, when the knot is tied, the cut ends of the ligature point downward into the depths of the wound rather than push up beneath the subcutaneous tissues (Fig. 4-2). In order to tie the suture in this manner, the needle has to be started in the depths of the wound on one side and then pushed up and withdrawn through the more superficial layers of the subcutaneous tissue on the same side. The suture is then passed across the wound, and the needle is probed into the superficial layers of the subcutaneous tissues. The needle should be slanted so that it comes out of the deeper tissues opposite the original point of entry of the suture. The catgut should then be tied and cut off short. The ends of the suture will slowly tend to twist out of sight and point into the depths of the wound. Only the minimum number of these sutures necessary to close the tissue planes should be used. There should be no wholesale burial of catgut.

### The skin

Choice of skin suture is important but not nearly as vital as proper placement of the suture. Small-sized monofilament synthetic sutures are best; 4-0 or 5-0 pro-

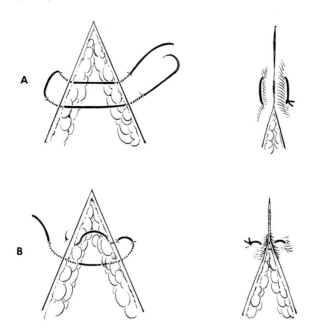

**Fig. 4-3.** *Suturing methods.* Mattress sutures for the skin can be either horizontal **(A)** or vertical **(B).** This type of suture gives good eversion but must not be pulled too tight because of the risk of skin necrosis.

line or nylon suture can be used in adults, but in children 5-0 or 6-0 catgut is more suitable. There are many different ways of suturing the skin, and certain standard types of sutures have advantages in different situations. The most commonly used and probably the best for general use is the ordinary "through-and-through" suture. It is important when tying this not to pull too hard, since too great a pressure will produce a linear necrosis beneath the suture. Subsequent scarring will then ultimately leave the familiar ladder effect seen all too often on many abdomens.

The problem in suturing the skin of hand wounds is to maintain an adequate eversion of the edges of the wound and yet not close the wound so tightly that accumulating hematoma cannot escape. Because of the importance of this eversion, many times a mattress suture is more suitable than the usual through-and-through stitch. In most instances Steristrips are not an adequate substitute for sutures because of the tendency for the skin edges to invert.

Mattress sutures can be used in either the vertical or horizontal plane (Fig. 4-3). The vertical or end-on mattress suture gives good opposition of the deep tissues and is more generally used. The horizontal mattress suture gives good eversion and can be used when a considerable length of wound is to be closed. If mattress sutures are used, the temptation to pull them too tight must be resisted. If they are pulled too tight, there is grave danger of necrosis developing along the line of the skin edge enclosed by the suture.

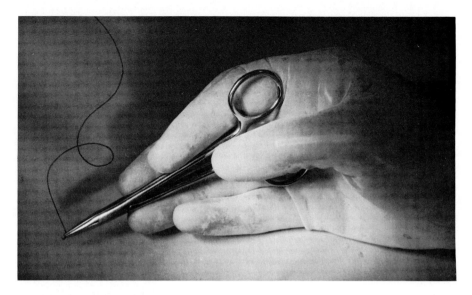

**Fig. 4-4.** *Grasping a needle holder.* The needle should be held in a self-locking needle holder. When this instrument is used, a powerful closing grip is not needed and muscle power can be concentrated on accurate control of the instrument.

## Passing skin sutures

When placing skin sutures, there is often difficulty in passing the needle through the skin. If an ordinary needle with an eye is being used, there may be considerable difficulty in passing the eye with the looped suture. It will be found to be much easier to pass either an atraumatic or an ordinary needle if the following technique is used.

The point of the needle is passed into the very superficial layers of the skin so that it is just caught. The direction in which the needle is to go is then selected by adjusting the position of the needle holder. The needle is then pressed a little more firmly downward and in the desired direction; it will pass easily if a firm but quick movement of supination is made. This movement is made easier and the needle holder is controlled more readily if the instrument is held loosely in the palm rather than if the fingers are placed in the handle holes (Fig. 4-4). By this means the rotation power needed to pass the needle is produced by a combination of forearm and hand movement and is very accurately controlled.

The needle must always be completely withdrawn from one skin edge before it is passed through the other side. If attempts are made to pass the needle through both skin edges at once, it is quite probable that the needle will be broken, and, even if it is successfully passed through both edges of the wound, the edges will not be everted. This failure of eversion may lead to delayed healing, a depressed scar, and tethering to the deeper tissues.

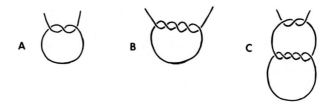

**Fig. 4-5.** *Suturing methods.* The surgeon's knot is necessary when using fine monofilament nylon sutures. **A,** Because of the slippery surface of the nylon, a single half knot will not lock. **B,** A double twist on the first half of the knot is needed to prevent slipping; **C,** a single twist is sufficient to complete the knot.

## Tying knots

Catgut and silk sutures have an inherent roughness on their surfaces that gives adhesion when a knot is tied. It is therefore necessary to do only one half turn to lock the suture in place before completing the knot. Should the first half of the knot slip, it is not the fault of the suture; rather, it is the result of too much tension on the tissues, causing them to pull apart. The suture should be removed and two or more sutures substituted instead of the single stitch. By this means a more even distribution of the tension will be achieved.

Monofilament synthetic sutures have a smooth slippery surface and cannot be made to lock on a single half knot. The surgeon's knot or a double twist on the first half of the knot is essential to stop slipping; only a single twist is needed to complete the knot (Fig. 4-5).

For areas in which there is not much movement, a frequently used stitch is the treble twist. In this stitch the first half of the knot is made by three twists. If the ends of the suture are then tightened, the stitch will not slip. When tightening the stitch, the ends should be pulled parallel with, rather than at right angles to, the skin surface. When the twists are pulled in this direction, they will be laid flat against the skin surface and will remain locked.

## SKIN GRAFTS
## Cutting a skin graft

Skin grafts are either full thickness or split thickness. A full-thickness graft consists of all the epidermal layers together with the dermis. It is not often used in the treatment of acute hand injuries. A split-thickness graft consists of all the superficial epidermal cells and cuts through the dermis, hair follicles, and sweat glands. Different thicknesses of the graft are cut, but the variation lies in the thickness of the dermis. It is impossible to cut a graft that consists of only epidermis either by hand or by machine.

The thickness of a graft influences the rate and the likelihood of its survival. A split-skin graft is kept alive during its early days by tissue fluids soaking into it from the depths. However, granulations rapidly grow in and provide a good blood supply. An adequate blood supply for the epidermal cells is therefore established

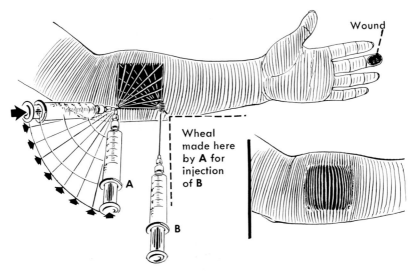

**Fig. 4-6.** *Split-skin grafting.* Anesthetizing the donor site. An area 8 cm square on the proximal forearm can be infiltrated through two skin punctures. Two tracks, at right angles, should be established through one skin puncture and the area between them infiltrated in a fan-shaped manner. A second fan-shaped infiltration should cross the first group, thereby defining the donor area.

more quickly in a thin graft than in a thick one. In selecting the thickness of a graft, the likelihood of survival of a thin graft must be balanced against the fact that thin grafts contract from subcutaneous scarring to a much greater degree than thicker split-skin grafts. Full-thickness grafts do not contract, because they have the support of their whole dermis.

When selecting a donor site for skin to be moved to the hand, it is better to try to take the skin from a hairless area. Patients also appreciate it if the donor site is in an inconspicuous area, since after healing there is usually some discoloration that may show throughout life. Ease of access is an important factor in choosing the donor site. A site that meets most of these requirements is the flexor aspect of the forearm of the injured hand. The donor site is readily available, the skin is relatively hairless, and the discoloration after healing is less noticeable than it would be on the extensor aspect. However, some patients do object to the cosmetic defect at this donor site, and all are entitled to be warned of its possibility. The bikini area is about the only site that meets present-day mores on nonexposure.

Grafts of the size needed for the injuries dealt with in this book can be readily cut with the patient under local anesthesia. An area about 8 cm square on the upper part of the forearm should be outlined with indelible ink marks at the four corners. This precaution helps avoid the embarrassing possibility of cutting the graft from an unanesthetized area (Fig. 4-6). Using 2% procaine a needle puncture is made at one corner, and two tracks at 90-degree angles to each other are infiltrated subcutaneously. The area enclosed by these two tracks is then infiltrated in a fanlike manner by the same needle, which should be left in place if the syringe has to be refilled.

The needle should then be withdrawn, and a second puncture should be made at the extremity of one of the original tracks. By this means, the second needle puncture is not felt by the patient. Another track at a 90-degree angle to the original track is then infiltrated, and further fan-shaped infiltration of the enclosed area is carried out (Fig. 4-6). By this means, a square anesthetized plateau is raised from the surrounding forearm skin. The tension produced by the injected fluid firms the tissues, making it easy to cut the graft from the surface of the plateau.

It is possible to anesthetize the donor site by applying cold for 45 to 60 minutes. Crushed ice in a plastic bag can be strapped in place over the donor site until the skin becomes raised, reddened, and numb. I very rarely use this method because of the long time involved in obtaining anesthesia.

Many intricate machines are available for cutting skin grafts, but they are not necessary for cutting the small area of skin needed in the care of hand injuries. An "old-fashioned" skin-grafting knife is the ideal instrument for cutting such grafts. Two types of grafting knives are available: the naked blade type and the type that has a roller in front of the leading edge of the knife. The latter type of knife is easier to use, and varying thicknesses of graft can be cut by adjusting the height of the roller. A good average thickness for general use is between 0.04 and 0.05 mm. Thicker and thinner grafts can be cut by roller adjustment, but care must be taken when increasing the thickness that the grafting knife does not cut through the dermis into the subcutaneous fat. The knife illustrated in Fig. 4-7, *A*, is lengthy and can cut a graft much wider than is usually needed. The Silver knife has been introduced to overcome this difficulty (Fig. 4-7, *B*). It incorporates all the good features of the larger knife, yet is designed to hold a regular razor blade and is the ideal instrument for this type of work. If neither knife is available, a razor blade held in a hemostat can also be used to cut a split-skin graft (Fig. 4-7, *C*).

Cutting a skin graft with a hand-held knife is remarkably easy and requires very little practice. The greatest difficulty will be encountered in trying to keep the knife at an even depth and, consequently, the graft of an even thickness. When cutting the graft, the forearm must be laid on a stiff surface so that a firm backing is given to the forearm muscles when the knife is in use. The knife should be held so that its flat surface remains parallel to, and in contact with, the skin surface. It must be pressed against the forearm skin so that the skin bulges slightly against the sharp leading edge. If the height of the hand is varied, a seesaw motion will be transmitted to the knife, and a ragged edge of irregular depth will be produced.

Two hands are needed to cut a skin graft, since the hand that is not holding the knife should hold a wooden board with a rounded edge about 8 to 12 mm in front of the knife's roller (Fig. 4-7, *A*). This wooden edge will flatten the skin that approaches the knife's edge and allow an even graft to be cut. Petrolatum gauze should be used to cover the donor site after the graft is cut, and both the edge of the wooden board and the back of the knife should be lubricated with a piece of this gauze or with sterile mineral oil. The cutting edge of the knife must not be lubricated because the grease would contaminate the undersurface of the graft and interfere with its healing.

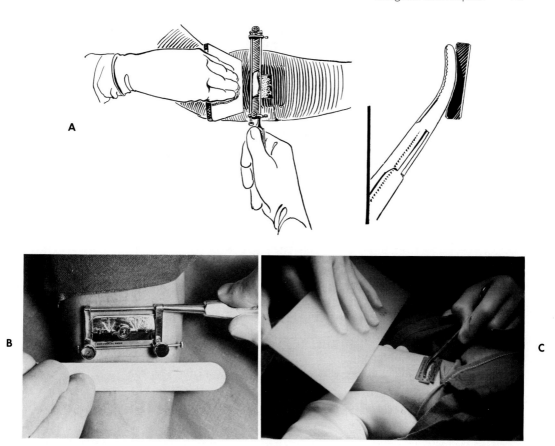

**Fig. 4-7.** *Split-skin grafting.* Two hands are needed to cut a skin graft. The instrument should be held horizontal to the skin in one hand while the other holds a wooden spreader just in advance of the cutting edge. **A,** Full-size grafting knife used for cutting large grafts. **B,** The Silver knife holds a razor blade and can cut suitably sized grafts for minor hand injuries. **C,** If proper instruments are not available, a razor blade held in a hemostat can be used to cut small pieces of graft.

When cutting the graft, short, quick, transverse strokes should be used with very little forward progress of the knife. The forward progress should be slow, and both hands should move in unison, so that the distance between the wooden board and the roller remains constant. Immediately after the graft is cut, the edge of the knife should be washed clean. If blood is left on the knife, it will rapidly corrode and blunt the cutting edge.

**THE DONOR SITE.** Immediately after the graft is cut, the donor site must be covered with petrolatum gauze, several layers of dampened sponges put on, and a sterile cotton elastic bandage wrapped around the forearm to seal off completely the donor site from outside contamination. By this means the clean wound created by cutting the graft is immediately sealed and protected from contamination by the wounded area. The graft should be stored in a saline-dampened sponge until it is needed.

AFTERCARE. If serum soaks through the bandages during the healing period, additional dressings should be put on top as a further protection. It is important to prevent outside infection from reaching the donor site via soaked dressings.

The donor site for a thin graft will heal in about ten days, whereas ten to twenty-one days will be needed for healing of a medium-thickness donor site. The donor site should not be disturbed for ten to twelve days. At this time, all the layers of dressings can usually be gently peeled off the new epithelium that has grown out to cover the area. If the dressings are stuck in certain areas, use scissors to trim away the loose portions and let the adherent portions separate later. Rough removal of adherent dressings is likely to tear off the delicate new epithelium.

Small, unhealed areas should be covered with Telfa and dry sponges. Even if the area is completely epithelized, it is wise to protect and support it with a dry dressing and a stretchable bandage for an additional week.

## Placing a skin graft

All skin grafts should be sewn into the defect they are to cover. Such suturing is essential because survival of a skin graft depends upon the necessary blood vessels being supplied by the granulations that grow into the graft from its deep surface. Movement of the graft during this critical period could jeopardize the chances of success.

Since the elastic tissue within a graft will cause it to contract, the graft should be sutured in place under slight tension, but it should not be placed drum tight over the recipient site.

Usually a split-skin graft is cut larger than the actual size of the recipient site. This is an advantage because it allows a margin through which sutures can be passed. The graft should not be placed on the recipient site until bleeding has been controlled. Minor capillary oozing is acceptable, but anything more vigorous than this must be controlled before the graft is sutured in place. Controlling the hemorrhage can be troublesome, but no ligatures are permissible unless there is a large spurting vessel in the depth of the wound. Even these vessels can usually be controlled by waiting a sufficient length of time after clamping. Direct pressure on the raw surface will stop most of the bleeding, provided that a moist sponge is used and sufficient time is allowed for clotting to take place.

The sutures used to anchor the graft should be placed so that they pass through the graft just inside the circumference of the raw area, through the wound edge from its raw or deep surface, coming out through its skin surface, and finally penetrate the excess skin graft from its deep surface. The knots should be placed so that they lie on the excess graft tissue and not within the perimeter of the area to be grafted. It is wrong to put in so many sutures that a watertight fit is achieved. The sutures are to prevent the graft from slipping on its bed and must not be so numerous that they prevent any hematoma from draining out. One end of the suture should be left long to be used as a tie over the dressings. When sutures are passed this way, they will penetrate the graft cleanly in the area where it is to be used (Fig. 4-8). As the

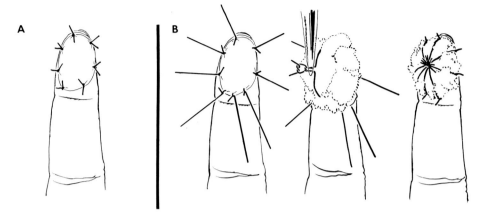

**Fig. 4-8.** *Split-skin grafting.* **A,** A skin graft must be anchored in place by stitches placed at intervals around its circumference. **B,** If one end of each suture is left long, the ends can be used to tie over fluffed-up dressings that will supply even pressure to the graft.

needle passes through the excess graft from its deep surface, the skin may be tented up and torn. Tearing of the overlapping excess skin does not matter. If the needle is passed in the reverse direction, there is a risk that the important part of the graft may be torn.

DRESSINGS. After the graft has been sewn into place, a firm compression dressing must be applied. Such a dressing is essential to maintain a good contact between the raw surfaces of the graft and the recipient site. By this means all dead space is obliterated, and hematoma formation is avoided.

The surface of the graft should be covered with a layer of petrolatum gauze or Telfa. If petrolatum gauze is used, it should be wiped with a dry sponge to remove a large part of the grease, since grafts covered with too much grease tend to macerate. A second layer of similarly treated petrolatum gauze should be placed on the first. On top of this a mass of cotton balls should be built up. The cotton balls should be soaked in saline or mineral oil and then shredded into pieces of about 6 mm in diameter. By pressing these small pieces onto the graft, a mold can be built up that will exactly fit any irregularities in the surface of the area to be grafted. When sufficient bulk has been built up to cover the whole area to a height of about 1.25 cm when compressed, an opened-out dry sponge is laid over the top to hold the pieces of cotton together.

The necessary compression is applied to the graft by using the long suture ends as tie-over sutures. The sutures are laid over the top of the heaped-up dressings and tied to their opposite number around the circumference of the wound. By this means compression is obtained that remains constant and does not depend on the integrity of outer layers of bandaging (Fig. 4-8, *B*). This type of dressing is useful for any graft placed in an area where movement is likely to occur; it should certainly be used on large grafts but is equally suitable for grafts as small as those used on a fingertip.

When attempting to make the first half-knot of the tie-over sutures, it is often found that the resilience in the cotton balls forces the knot apart. This resilience can be overcome by pulling the first half of the knot to the desired tension and then, while maintaining the tension, pulling the two ends vertical to the half-knotted suture. While the suture is held in this position, an assistant holds the outside of the half-knot in a pair of nontoothed forceps. While the knot is being held in this way, the tension on the suture ends can be released and the second half of the knot tied (Fig. 4-8, *B*). As the knot is pulled tight, the assistant releases pressure on the forceps in time with the tightening. In this way, the knot is tied without any slipping, and the jaws of the forceps, which are on the outside of the knot, cannot be trapped as the knot is completed.

AFTERCARE. All skin grafts should be inspected on the fourth day after grafting. If a graft is going to "take," it will do so by this time. If it has died, it should be removed and the area regrafted. After the outer bandages are removed, it will be found that the cotton balls have dried into a hard mass but that this mass can be kept intact by separation between the two layers of petrolatum gauze or between the plastic and cotton layers of the Telfa. If tie-over sutures have been used, the knots on top of the cotton mass should be cut. By cutting here, several of the sutures will still be long enough to retie when the dressing is reapplied. The deepest layer of dressing should be peeled off the surface of the graft and the graft inspected.

## Successful grafts

In successful grafts small pink or red areas will be seen scattered over the surface at the time of the first dressing. These areas show where the granulations are beginning to penetrate into the graft. The excess graft lying on the intact skin around the grafted area will be beginning to mummify and will not need to be disturbed. If, however, portions of the excess graft are moist and look as if they might be a good nidus for infection, they should be excised at this time. The sutures around the graft need not be removed at the first dressing.

After the petrolatum gauze or Telfa has been renewed, the cotton ball dressing should be replaced. If this dressing was tied in, the sutures should be retied wherever possible. In a successful take, there is no need to inspect the graft for another six days. At that time all dressings should be removed and the sutures taken out. A line of demarcation will have developed between the excess graft and the successful graft. Frequently, the ring of excess skin will peel off, since the graft will already have joined the normal skin edge of the wound. In some areas the separation may not be complete, and excess skin must be cut off with scissors. Pulling at this skin might cause the graft to be lifted from its bed. If the graft has successfully taken, only a small protective dressing is needed for the next four to five days, after which time the area should be exposed as much as possible to allow it to consolidate.

Even two weeks after grafting, the new skin is somewhat delicate, and it cannot withstand violent trauma or constant soaking. Occupations involving these hazards should be avoided for an additional two weeks. The sebaceous glands will take a considerable time to regrow, and during this interval the surface of the graft should be protected by daily application of lanolin.

## Graft failures

Little blisters and small areas of failure need not cause concern. The blisters should be punctured and the small areas of failure opened with sharp-pointed scissors. Often a small bead of hematoma exists beneath such areas. This hematoma should be shelled out and the edges of the incision made with a scissors cut into an ellipse. The areas of apparent failure should not be excised, since during the next few days lateral growth of granulations within the thickness of the graft will allow some of this seemingly dead graft to revive. The aftercare of grafts with such minor complications is the same as for successful grafts, except that the dressings will have to be kept on for four to five days longer than a 100% successful take.

There is no place for a wait-and-see policy in cases of total failure. The original indication for grafting still exists, and to allow the area to granulate because the graft has failed is wrong. Common causes of failure are hematoma under the graft or infection. In either case, all sutures should be removed, the area cleansed by soaks and dressings for twenty-four hours, and the grafting procedure repeated, using a thin split-skin graft.

## Full-thickness grafts

Full-thickness grafts are not deliberately chosen for use in emergency surgery of the hand. However, sometimes the patient brings in the amputated finger tip or detached portion of skin. If the skin is in good condition, it can be trimmed and used as a full-thickness graft to cover the skin defect. It is not a wise practice to cover part of a defect with a full-thickness graft and the remainder with a split-skin graft. It is better to cover the whole area with a split-skin graft. The skin that the patient brings in can be used only if it is in good condition. Skin that has been cut off by a clean slicing wound is suitable, but it would be unwise to use skin that has been avulsed by tearing or crushing injuries.

To make a full-thickness graft from the skin, all the subcutaneous fat has to be removed from its deep surface. This is best done by placing the skin upside down on a hard surface and cutting away the excess tissues with a pair of curved scissors (Fig. 6-6). The dead white dermal tissues can be easily distinguished from the more yellow subcutaneous fatty tissues. The graft should be sewed into place with interrupted sutures. One end of each of the sutures should be left long to allow a dressing to be tied over the grafted area.

DRESSINGS. Two layers of petrolatum gauze or a layer of Telfa should be cut to the correct size and placed on the graft. Small pieces of damp cotton balls should then be built up sufficiently high to allow an even pressure to be applied when the long ends of the sutures are tied over the top of the dressing.

AFTERCARE. The first dressing of a full-thickness skin graft need not be done for a week. At the end of this time all the dressings should be removed, and in most cases the sutures also should be removed. Full-thickness skin grafts take longer to establish their blood supply than do the split-skin grafts. Because of this time lag the superficial layers of the skin die and are shed during the second week after grafting. If the graft is from the palmar aspect, there will be a thick keratin layer that will be cast off. This death of the superficial cells can appear most depressing, and it may be thought that the underlying graft has died. Even though full-thickness grafts do not survive as readily as split-skin grafts, this discoloration and wrinkling of the surface layers is normal. When these layers have separated, it will be found that good skin lies underneath. After any surface portions of the graft that have begun to separate have been excised, the two layers of petrolatum gauze and the cotton mass are reapplied. The dressings should be changed again at about the tenth postoperative day. At this time any remaining sutures should be removed, and further surface layers of the graft that are ready to separate should be excised.

During the first few days after separation of the superficial layers, the remaining portion of the graft may appear moist, granular, and raw. The epithelial elements lying in the dermis will rapidly proliferate and supply an epithelial cover for the whole grafted surface.

Full-thickness grafts can usually be exposed without dressings during the third week after injury. Their ultimate function is more satisfactory than the thinner split-skin grafts.

## TENDON SUTURE

End-to-end junction of cut tendons can be accomplished with either silk or wire sutures. Wire sutures can be buried and left in place indefinitely, but silk sutures stimulate a foreign body reaction over a period of time and are not so satisfactory as wire. Braided-wire sutures, No. 5-0, are now available with a straight needle swaged onto each end and are ideal for this work.

TECHNIQUE. The tendon ends should be first trimmed off square, so that reasonable surfaces are available for the junction. The wire is first placed in the distal cut end of the tendon. A needle is passed transversely through the tendon about 2 cm beyond the cut end. It is pulled through until there is an equal length of wire on each side. The end of the tendon is then held between the thumb and index finger of one hand, and each needle in turn is passed back through the tendon, entering a slight distance nearer the cut end and leaving at a point about halfway to the cut end. The second needle is then passed in a similar manner from the opposite side so that the wires cross within the tendon (Fig. 4-9).

It is best to pass both needles through the tendon before withdrawing either of them. This eliminates the possibility of passing a needle through the substance of one of the wires. Should a needle be passed through the wires, the wires will not

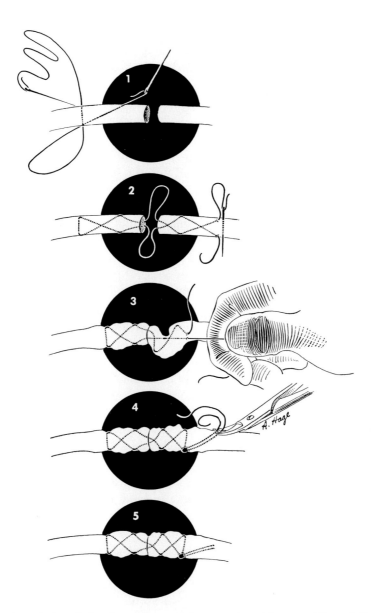

**Fig. 4-9.** *Tendon suturing.* **1,** A suture with a needle on each end is passed through the distal cut end of the tendon; the two ends cross over inside the tendon. **2,** After the sutures have crossed, they are brought to the surface and then passed back into the tendon so as to come out through the cut end of the tendon; they are then passed into the proximal cut end and crossed within the tendon as in the distal tendon. **3,** After the suture has been passed, the tendon ends must be bunched up by pulling on the two ends of the suture. **4,** After the ends have been tied, they should be passed into the substance of the tendon for about 2 cm before they are cut off by scissors pressed firmly onto the surface. **5,** After the ends are cut, they will spring back within the substance of the tendon, leaving a smooth outer surface.

run freely, and it will be impossible to pull them tight before tying the suture. After the wires have been pulled through, the needles are once again passed back into the tendon, this time with the points directed so that they come out through the cut end of the tendon equally spaced across the cross section.

The proximal end of the tendon should then be pulled down and transfixed with a thin Keith needle. This needle should be passed through the tendon some 5 cm proximal to the cut end. Transfixing the tendon in this manner abolishes the pull of the muscle tone and immobilizes the tendon end while the suture is being inserted.

The wire should be passed through the proximal tendon in exactly the reverse order to that in which it was passed into the distal end. The two needles are first passed into the cross section of the cut end of the tendon and are brought out of the same side of the tendon on which they enter. They are then passed back into the tendon, crossing each other in a similar manner to that used in the distal end of the tendon. The wires are now held taut and both the tendon ends milked down the wires so that they are crinkled on the wires. This bunching up of the tendons will look bulky and untidy, but it serves a useful purpose. During the healing period, the wires will cut through the tendons, and the bulky junction site will eventually heal with a nearly normal diameter throughout its length. If the tendons are not bunched up, the wires will cut through and allow a relative lengthening of the tendon during the healing phase.

One needle is then passed horizontally across the tendon so that it emerges about 3 mm from the point of exit of the second wire. After a final tightening of the tendon ends on the wires, the knot is tied at the point where the two wires leave the side of the tendon. Instead of cutting the wires short, it is better technique to pass the needles independently of each other through the tendon obliquely in a proximal direction. They should travel at least 1.5 cm within the tendon substance. Each wire should then be pulled taut and the wire-cutting scissors pressed flush with the tendon surface before cutting off the wire (Fig. 4-9). This technique pulls the knot into the substance of the tendon, and the wire ends spring back within the tendon so that no rough or lumpy foreign body is left on the surface of the tendons.

When the tendon junction is complete, the transfixion needle through the proximal tendon should be removed. When closing the skin wound over the tendons, it is essential that at least the junctional area be covered by subcutaneous tissues as well as skin.

**AFTERCARE.** Sutured tendons must be supported by splinting for three weeks. When extensor tendons have been sutured, it may occasionally be necessary to modify the functional position and retain the finger in some degree of extension to allow the maximum relaxation of the tendon junction.

After three weeks of immobilization active movements should be encouraged, but passive movements are definitely contraindicated. Full range of movement should not be expected immediately after the immobilization is removed. There is frequently a considerable amount of inflammatory reaction around the site of tendon suture, and three weeks is too short a time to allow complete resolution. In addition, the muscle that controls the tendon may need an appreciable length of time to regain its tone and power.

## NERVE SUTURE

Mixed nerves do not respond well to primary suture, but, on the other hand, pure motor or pure sensory nerves frequently show excellent recovery after primary suture. Stereognosis may not be regained, but light touch and pinprick sensations usually return. The conditions of the wound should be ideal before primary suture is attempted. Ragged lacerated wounds that may be contaminated are not suitable sites for primary repair. Clean incised wounds of recent origin with a clean cut across the nerve are suitable for attempted repair.

It should be realized that even a pure nerve such as a digital sensory or the motor branch of the median cannot give a good recovery unless the actual repair is technically well done. To do a good primary repair of a small nerve even with the aid of a microscope is a difficult surgical procedure. To do such an operation in the average emergency room is impossible. Because of these great technical difficulties, it is well to realize that the chances of success in this operation are not high, but that if the operation succeeds, the results are excellent. On the other hand, if the final result is not satisfactory, some good has still been done for the patient. The primary anastomosis will hold the nerve ends together and prevent retraction, thereby making it easier to perform a secondary anastomosis. Immediate suturing of the nerve sheath cuts to a minimum the inflammatory reaction within the nerve, and large tender neuromas are not very often formed.

TECHNIQUE. There is nothing inherently different about suturing a cut nerve. The problem is that the tissues are so thin and small that passing and tying the sutures are extremely difficult.

The nerve ends must be isolated and the nerve mobilized a short distance proximally and distally. The ends must be inspected, and if they are in any way ragged and not clean cut, they must be cut across with a large sharp scalpel or a razor blade. The suture used must be small (Nos. 6-0 to 9-0), with a round-bodied needle swaged on. As it comes from its package, the suture is so long that it is unwieldy to use, and half of its length should be sacrificed. Before use the suture should be passed through the nearby fatty subcutaneous tissues several times in order to lubricate it.

The nerve ends must now be matched up as well as possible and suturing started (Fig. 4-10). In a fresh injury the nerve sheath, though a very definite structure, is thin and tears easily. However, it is through this structure that the suture has to be passed. The needle must be passed through one side, and the suture must be drawn through as far as necessary before the needle is passed into the other side. After the suture has been passed through each end of the nerve, sufficient length should be left for tying purposes before it is cut and held by hemostats. A similar technique should then be used at a point opposite the first suture. Before these sutures are tied, the two ends of the nerve should be held closely together by a combination of

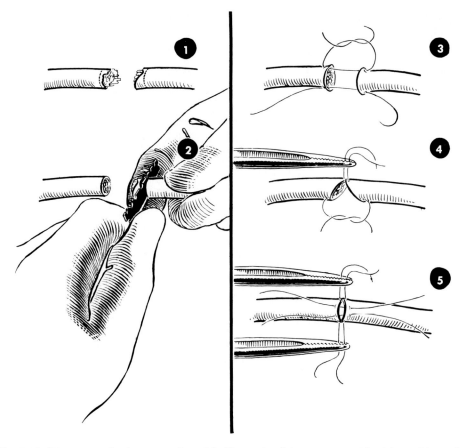

**Fig. 4-10.** *Primary repair of a nerve.* **1** and **2,** The ends of the nerve must be trimmed to a clean cross section by gently cutting across with a new razor blade; it is advisable to place one's fingertip beneath the end being cut since this encourages the necessary delicacy of touch. **3** and **4,** Sutures must be placed on opposite sides of the nerve before either is tied. **5,** The ends should be left long so that they may help in holding the nerve while the remaining sutures are placed.

relaxation of joints and actual holding of the nerve sheath in nontoothed forceps.

When the sutures have been tied, the ends should be left at least 5 cm long and held in fine mosquito hemostats. If the hemostats are held gently apart, the nerve sheath can be stretched and flattened. Additional sutures can then be put more easily into the superficial surface. The deeper surface can be sutured in a similar manner after one of the original two long sutures has been passed beneath the nerve and pulled upon. This twists the nerve, and, if the hemostats are now stretched apart, the undersurface of the nerve will be exposed and additional sutures can be put in. After all the sutures are in place, the long ends should be cut back very short. For a digital nerve and the motor branch of the median nerve, two to four sutures are sufficient.

AFTERCARE. The hand or digit must be immobilized so that all tension is taken off the suture line for at least three weeks. After this period of time the hand or digit can be gently mobilized by active exercises, but all passive movements should be absolutely forbidden.

Although Tinel's sign has fallen into disrepute in some quarters, it has actual clinical value. Tapping along the course of the nerve to determine the stage of actual recovery will usually show progressive improvement.

# 5 · BASIC TREATMENT

**General principles**
First aid
The time factor
Sterile precautions

**Cleaning the hand**

**Classifying the wound**

**Essentials in treatment and planning**


## GENERAL PRINCIPLES
## First aid

First aid is synonymous in most lay minds with hemorrhage and "pressure points." Stress is still laid on the use of tourniquets despite their obvious dangers, and it would be better by far for hand injuries if the emphasis could be on prevention of contamination of the wound.

Gross hand injuries usually receive reasonable attention; a large dressing is "slapped" on the wound, and the patient is hurried to the hospital. It is in the minor and neglected small lesions that most of the complications from infection arise.

There is no hemorrhage from an injured hand that cannot be stopped by the application of direct pressure over the wound with a sterile dressing. If the hand is then splinted into a comfortable position, the dressings are very unlikely to move during transport of the patient to the hospital.

It is better treatment for the patient to protect the hand from contamination by his surroundings and by the breathing and coughing of friends and neighbors than it is to clamp something around his arm and twist it tightly. Hemorrhage from hand wounds is usually slight, and the body can readily tolerate such losses, but crushing injuries from tight tourniquets or infection of the hand may well be considerably more serious.

Infection of a simple hand injury converts it into a major problem with markedly increased morbidity. One half of all hand injuries with permanent physical impairment are infected, and the average compensation expense of a hand injury is doubled if it becomes infected.

### The time factor

Six hours was formerly considered the longest time after wounding in which it was safe to close wounds primarily. Experience shows that this arbitrary time limit can be safely exceeded in many cases. Time alone is not the factor that dictates the type of primary care given to a wound.

Certain wounds are never treated by primary closure, even when they are seen within a few hours of wounding. Among these wounds are animal or human bites and wounds contaminated by animal or human excreta. Wounds that have been open for twenty-four hours or more are almost inevitably infected and should not be closed primarily. In other injuries the time factor is less important than the state of the wound. The amount of tissue damage, the presence and number of foreign bodies, and the likelihood of infection must all be assessed when deciding on the primary treatment. Clean tidy wounds can be closed at least twelve hours after injury, and in many cases suturing has been successful twenty or more hours after wounding.

Although time is not an important factor in deciding on the type of treatment to be given a wound, it is of vital importance *during* treatment. Injuries of the hand cannot be treated in a hurry. Their care demands that sufficient time be allowed for meticulous surgery to be carried out. If adequate time is not available when the patient is first seen, it is better treatment to postpone surgery until it can be undertaken free of interruption.

## Sterile precautions

The inspection or treatment of a wound must not be undertaken unless the physician is wearing a mask.

The patient's hand will have to be thoroughly cleansed, but similar cleansing is not sufficient for the physician. Sterile gloves must be worn. No matter what solutions are used to "scrub up" the hands, it is impossible to sterilize the skin. Scrubbing the hands mechanically removes the surface dirt but leaves untouched the depths of the creases, hair follicles, oil glands, and sweat glands. In these deep recesses are many organisms, and they will rapidly come to the surface as the hand is used. Both ethically and medicolegally, it would be wrong to operate on patients with acute hand injuries without the protection of sterile rubber gloves.

The operative repair of hand injuries must be undertaken in the proper surroundings. It is utterly wrong to attempt to "put in a few sutures" in the patient who is lying on a cart in the emergency room corridor. Hand wounds demand and deserve the best possible care. This care implies that adequate space is available in which the physician can operate under sterile conditions.

## CLEANING THE HAND

Most injuries to the hand occur when it is in a state of surgical dirtiness, and it is usually even socially dirty. For this reason, extensive cleansing is necessary before surgery can be undertaken. It is unnecessarily cruel to attempt such cleansing before the wound has been anesthetized. To inject the anesthetic agent directly into the wound edges may introduce infection into previously uninfected tissues and usually produces inadequate anesthesia. The appropriate nerve block should be performed before the wound and its surroundings are cleansed.

The most satisfactory method of cleansing is for the patient to undertake all the preliminary cleansing himself. Most patients can also be trusted to shave the defined area with a safety razor. It is useful to define the area that has to be cleansed by marking off the limb with some form of dye such as methylene blue. Be generous with the area to be cleansed; a wound of the hand needs a skin preparation to the level of the elbow. More than a quarter of a century ago Koch and Mason showed that excellent results can be obtained by the use of soap and water. Despite the recent introduction of a variety of detergents for skin cleansing, no dramatic advantage has been demonstrated over the use of ordinary soap and water. Detergents may help to dissolve surface grease and shift adherent debris, but they are often extremely difficult to remove from the depths of the wound. For those who prefer detergents, the forearm and hand should be soaked for fifteen to twenty minutes in a warm saline solution of the detergent. However, the use of an ordinary neutral white soap is recommended. The patient should be seated in front of a sink and told to wash the limb for at least fifteen minutes under warm running water. No matter which of the two methods is used, the patient can materially help in the cleansing process if he is given a supply of sterile sponges to be used as washcloths. Some bleeding from the wound is inevitable, but unless it is actual arterial spurting the only treatment necessary is reassurance. It should be stressed to the patient that there is no need for him to attempt to clean the depths of the wound, and in fact he should be told definitely to avoid washing the surrounding dirt into the depths of the wound.

After the preliminary cleansing, the limb should be wrapped in a sterile towel, and the patient should be placed on the operating table. The surgical cleansing must be done in two stages by the surgeon after putting on sterile gloves. The cleansing of the tissues surrounding the wound and those at a distance from the wound is done while sterile dressings are held over the wounded area. The wound itself should not be cleansed by rough scrubbing but rather by irrigation and gentle washing with soft sponges.

Many solutions are available for cleansing, but a good combination is first to clean the arm with ether, thereby removing any remaining grease, and then to give the limb a thorough washing with 3% hexachlorophene, which should be allowed to enter the wound. A suitable final solution for cleaning up to the wound edges is 70% alcohol. Whatever final solution is used, it is important that it be colorless. Tinted solutions may look impressive, but they obscure the normal skin color and make it impossible to judge the viability of skin flaps or the state of return of circulation after release of the tourniquet.

## CLASSIFYING THE WOUND

It is said that wounds are of such an infinite variety that to attempt to classify them is to attempt the impossible. This dictum is probably true if every feature of the wound has to be considered. However, certain major features are sufficiently constant to allow generalizations concerning diagnosis and treatment to be safely made. The classification of wounds of the hand used here is quite arbitrary and certainly is not complete (Fig. 5-1). However, it is of practical value in treatment.

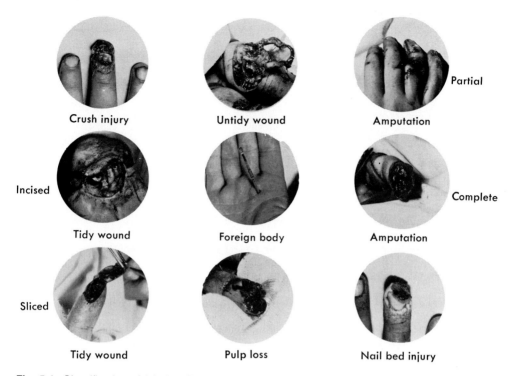

**Fig. 5-1.** *Classification of injuries.* Examples of the more common injuries classified by the major feature of the wound.

### Tidy wounds

Tidy wounds have clean and well-defined edges and are usually made by a sharp instrument. They are of two major types:
1. *Tidy incised wounds*
   Tidy incised wounds are linear and may or may not be straight.
2. *Tidy sliced wounds*
   Tidy sliced wounds cover an appreciable area. The slice of skin that has been raised may or may not be attached by a basal pedicle.

In both tidy incised and tidy sliced wounds the essential feature is that the wound is produced by a sharp edge with minimum death of nearby cells. These wounds can be expected to heal primarily and to leave a minimum of scarring.

### Untidy wounds

Untidy wounds are produced in many ways, but they are frequently inflicted by tools with serrated edges. They have uneven edges with many small flaps that may have a very poor blood supply. Some of these flaps can be expected to die during the first week after injury.

### Crush wounds

Crush wounds are diagnosed from the history of how they were sustained, and their full extent does not become defined until several days after the injury. They are injuries with depth, and the edema that results from the penetration of the force into the depth of the tissues may lead to thrombosis and massive death of tissue.

### Pulp loss

In this injury there is loss of skin and pulp from the palmar side of the terminal phalanx, but the rigid supporting structures, such as the nail and bony phalanx, are intact. This injury must be considered quite different from a partial amputation, because the nail and terminal phalanx are intact.

### Amputations

1. *Partial amputation*

   A wound that appears to sever a finger will, on many occasions, be found to have spared a bridge of skin containing one of the neurovascular bundles. If careful inspection of the distal portion of the finger reveals satisfactory bleeding, then the amputation is partial, and every attempt must be made to save the finger tip.

2. *Complete amputation*

   An amputation is complete when the distal portion of the organ is severed from all blood and nerve connections with its proximal portions. It does not have to be completely disconnected. There may be a small skin bridge connecting the two, but, if this does not contain a neurovascular bundle, the wound must be considered a complete amputation.

### Nail bed injuries

A distinction must be made between nail bed and nail root injuries. In the latter group the actual area from which new nail grows is wounded. Inevitably, after a wound to this area there is death of nail-forming cells, and at best the ultimate result must be a deformed and irregular nail. In nail bed injuries there is a slicing injury of the dorsum of the tip of a finger so that a portion of the nail, its underlying bed, and the distal part of the finger tip are lost.

### Foreign bodies

Diagnosis of an injury caused by a foreign body is not difficult; it will depend upon the history given by the patient, an inspection of the wound, and usually an x-ray film.

### Fractures

Many fractures can be suspected on clinical examination, and they are self-evident if they are compound. It is essential to take x-ray films in two planes so that an accurate diagnosis of the extent of injury can be made.

### Degloving injuries

The term degloving injuries includes all wounds in which there is major loss of skin of the hand by a peeling-back process, such as that used in removing a glove. Frequently the skin is still attached to the part. The majority of these lesions are too extensive to be graded "minor," and the patient should be admitted to a hospital for definitive treatment. However, outpatient care is suitable when only a single finger has been degloved. Almost invariably this injury is produced when a ring worn on the finger is caught on some projection; for instance, when a person jumps down off a truck.

### Thumb injuries

Because of its overwhelming importance, the thumb is entitled to a separate category. It can, of course, suffer any form of injury to which the rest of the hand is subject.

## ESSENTIALS IN TREATMENT AND PLANNING

Even after a wound has been placed in a category in the classification, certain questions must be answered before an intelligent plan of treatment can be outlined. If a standard group of questions such as the following is applied to all patients, there is little risk of important features being missed.

**SEVEN ESSENTIAL QUESTIONS**

1. What is the patient's *occupation?*
2. What is the *cut/crush* ratio?
3. Is the wound *tidy* or *untidy?*
4. Is there any *skin loss?*
5. Is the *neurovascular bundle* injured?
6. Are the *tendons* injured?
7. Are the *bone* and *joints* involved?

### The patient's occupation

It is of paramount importance to establish at the outset the relationship of the wound to the patient's occupation. No matter under what circumstances the wound occurred, it is important to find out exact details of what the occupation involves in order to be able to give a reasonable prognosis of future work ability. If the wound has been sustained at work, a history should be taken concerning any previous similar accidents to help establish whether or not the victim is accident prone.

### Cut/crush ratio

Cutting injuries cause a minimum death of tissue, and only the cells immediately adjacent to the wound will die. Crush injuries are injuries in depth, will produce massive edema, and may lead to massive death of tissue.

The butcher's knife that slips and the carpenter's misguided hammer produce injuries of opposite extremes, but many injuries are a combination of cutting and crushing. Depending on the proportion of each, the treatment and prognosis will be varied. A detailed discussion concerning these features is given in the appropriate treatment discussion.

### Tidy or untidy

The edges of a tidy wound are clean and well defined, since they are generally made by sharp instruments drawn across the area. These wounds will heal rapidly if the edges of the incision are trimmed to a 90-degree angle. Untidy wounds always heal badly in comparison with tidy wounds. This poor healing is a result of the general disturbance of tissues over a much larger area and the death of several of the small flaps, leaving areas of skin loss that may need secondary treatment.

## Skin loss

Skin loss is usually self-evident on inspection of the wound. In an untidy wound there is frequently loss of skin in the width of the wound, but, unless it is specifically looked for, this loss may not be apparent until closure is attempted.

Particular attention must be given to the viability of any skin flaps that have been raised by trauma. In many instances, these flaps of skin, when replaced, will be based distally, and very often their pedicles are narrow in proportion to their length and width. The circulation in a distal-based flap is frequently in jeopardy because the venous drainage in the hand is poor and the flap becomes congested with venous blood. This complication is particularly common in degloving injuries and crush injuries in which there has been avulsion of the skin. In both instances there is a very poor chance that the skin will survive if it is simply replaced and sutured in position.

## Neurovascular bundle

Spurting arteries are obvious, but nerve damage has to be tested for carefully. It must be remembered that there is an intimate association between the nerves and vessels in the fingers; if one is divided, the other is almost certain to have been damaged. The digital nerves lie very close to the sides of the flexor tendon sheaths, and if there has been a wound sufficiently severe to cut the flexor tendons, a special point must be made of testing the digital nerve supply in that finger.

## Tendons

There is no excuse for failing to diagnose tendon injuries, but they will be missed unless a methodical plan of testing each tendon in each digit is always carried out.

## Bones and joints

Injuries involving the bones and joints are usually easily diagnosed, but the extent of the damage cannot be assessed without x-ray examination.

# PART TWO

# The care of specific injuries

Too many man hours are wasted waiting
for conservative treatment to produce
second-rate results.

**John Barron, F.R.C.S. (Ed.)**

# 6 · WOUNDS OF THE SKIN

**Superficial cutaneous wounds**

**Subcutaneous wounds**

**Lacerating wounds**
    Tidy wounds
      Tidy incised wounds
      Tidy sliced wounds
      Puncture wounds
    Untidy wounds

**Degloving injuries**

**Skin flaps**
    Rotation flaps
    Transposition flaps

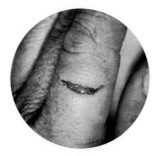
**Tidy incised wound**

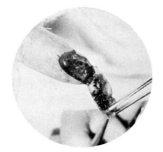
**Tidy sliced wound**

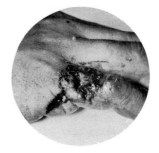
**Untidy wound**

The skin of the hand can be injured in many ways. Portions may be actually missing, the skin may be lacerated, or the lesion may be only superficial in nature.

Blisters are intradermal vesicles distended with serum that appear in skin subjected to irritation and friction. They are common on the hands of the weekend gardener and on several areas of the weekend athlete. The best treatment is prophylactic in the sense that gloves provide an intermediate layer between the soft skin and the handle. If an area of irritation has developed, a protective layer of petrolatum gauze under the glove will often be sufficient protection.

Many methods are recommended to relieve the pain in the taut blister, and most have drawbacks. At all costs the area must be saved from being infected by the treatment. Probably the most effective treatment is to widely open the blister for over one-half its circumference to provide full and continuing drainage. The outer skin must be left in place, since it is the best possible dressing. An antibiotic ointment and a Band-Aid complete the treatment. In three to five days the tender deeper skin will toughen up. The outer layer will dry up and can be completely removed within one week.

If the blister is infected, it must be completely unroofed and the outer skin thrown away. Irrigation cleansing, an antibiotic ointment, and a small protective dressing will usually ensure rapid healing.

Superficial abrasions and lacerations can be readily treated, but areas of skin loss need careful treatment. There is little excuse for not replacing an area of skin loss with a skin graft. If a large wound is left to heal by granulation, the area will eventually be covered by a very thin epithelium. This epithelium has very low resistance because it is based on a layer of scar tissue instead of normal dermis. The whole area will be contracted, tender, and probably disabling. The contraction of the scar tissue may lead to edema of the hand, and in some patients it may even be associated with sympathetic vascular disturbances that produce atrophic changes in the digits.

The rate of healing of lacerations of the hand depends largely upon the type of wound. Cleanly incised wounds heal well, whereas bursting wounds caused by crush injuries take a considerable time to heal. Good healing will result if care is taken in closing the wound. Frequently, the skin creases of the hand will be crossed by a wound. If the cut edges of these creases are matched, the wound will heal rapidly, and no "dog ears" will be left at either end. The subcutaneous tissues do not usually require many stitches, but fine plain catgut should be used to obliterate any potential dead spaces in the depth of the wound.

The dorsal skin is relatively thin and elastic, but the palmar skin is thick, attached to the deep tissues, and nonelastic. Palmar skin is often difficult to suture because of the hardened keratin layer on the surface. This keratin tends to invert the skin edges and frequently becomes macerated under dressings. If the superficial layers are shaved off for about 0.5 cm around the periphery of the wound, it will be easier to evert the edges when the wound is sutured, and the risk of maceration is greatly reduced.

## SUPERFICIAL CUTANEOUS WOUNDS

Superficial cutaneous wounds do not penetrate all layers of the skin. They are usually caused by scraping, scratching, or friction (Fig. 6-1). The brush burns produced by friction are usually more serious than other abrasions. However, even these friction burns usually involve only the superficial layers, penetrating as far as the papillary layer. The area is painful, and the patient will complain of a burning stinging pain in the reddened weeping area from which serum exudes.

TREATMENT. Thorough cleansing of the wound is the best treatment. Anesthesia is rarely needed. Surface dirt should be removed by gently scrubbing with a sponge or a very soft brush. If the surface is deeply tattooed with spicules of dirt, it is better not to attempt to clean the area completely. Some of the particles will remain in the deeper tissues, but many will be shed as healing proceeds.

DRESSINGS. Some form of sterile antiseptic dressing should be used to cover the area until it has crusted over. The dressing should not be sealed in all around the periphery by adhesive tape. If this is done, the area will remain moist and will

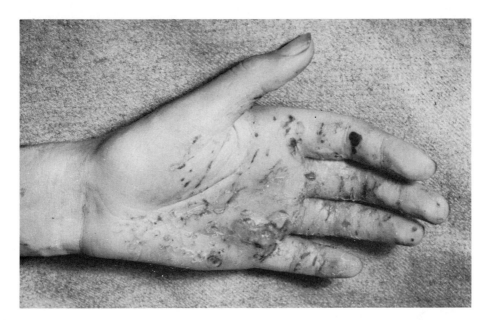

**Fig. 6-1.** *Superficial cutaneous wounds.* Abrasions and scratches do not penetrate the full thickness of the skin. They will heal rapidly if they are kept dry and superficial infection is prevented.

not crust over. Immediately after a dry crust or scab is formed, the dressings should be left off. Salves and ointments should not be used, since they perpetuate the moist state of the wound and thereby increase the risk of surface infection.

## SUBCUTANEOUS WOUNDS

Blows or pressure can damage the skin quite extensively without producing a break in continuity of the skin. Severe crushing forces produce gross examples of this type of injury, but the common examples are bruises from direct blows to the area.

A bruise usually swells rapidly because of hemorrhage from ruptured subcutaneous blood vessels; occasionally there is a more generalized hemorrhagic infiltration throughout the bruised area. The raised tension in the tissues usually causes a dull throbbing pain, but in severe bruises there may be partial anesthesia of the tissues and little pain.

TREATMENT. If there appears to be any likelihood that the skin of the bruised area will break down, the surface should be cleansed with soap and water and a mild antiseptic. Rest, elevation, and a cold compress are useful during the first twenty-four hours. After this time all bleeding will have stopped, and subsequent treatment should be directed toward helping absorption of the extravasated blood. This can best be done by continuing the rest and elevation but substituting hot packs and gentle compression bandages for the cold compresses. From about the third day, massage and active and passive movements should be carried out, since they frequently accelerate resolution of the area.

## LACERATING WOUNDS
### Tidy wounds

DEFINITION. Tidy wounds are produced by sharp edges, are neatly incised, and have no element of crush in their production. Three major types are distinguished: tidy incised, tidy sliced, and puncture wounds. The common feature of these wounds is that they are produced by sharp edges with the minimum of disturbance to nearby tissues. Because of this, they heal rapidly and with the minimum of local reaction.

ANESTHESIA. Wounds of the digits should be anesthetized by a metacarpal block using a 1% or 2% solution of lidocaine without epinephrine. For other areas, circumferential blocking with 2% lidocaine is best. Circumferential blocking implies the use of multiple needle punctures to produce adequate anesthesia. If the wound is seen within a short time after its occurrence, the damaged tissues may still be going through the period of relative insensitiveness that frequently occurs after trauma. During this phase, and even afterward, the number of needle punctures needed for anesthesia should be balanced against the number of sutures that will be needed to close the wound. If there is considerable length to the wound, there is no doubt that preliminary anesthesia is necessary, but, if the wound is relatively small, it may be quicker and, in final analysis, less traumatic to the patient to suture the wound without preliminary anesthesia.

### Tidy incised wounds

Tidy incised wounds are made by such things as knives, razors, or broken glass. If the cutting edge that caused the wound was relatively clean, the bleeding from the wound will probably be sufficient to flush out the depths, and very little additional cleansing will be necessary before closing the wound.

It must be remembered that it is essential to carry out a full clinical examination before treating these wounds. There may be considerable depth to the wound. A thorough examination will demonstrate the damaged parts, and their relationship in the depths of the wound can be determined before surgery is undertaken.

TREATMENT. Suturing without anesthesia is suitable only for the most superficial wounds. If this method is chosen, brand-new needles with really sharp points are essential. Needles that have never been used but have lain around in sterilizing solution for some time are likely to have lost the fine edge of their sharpness and are not suitable for this type of suturing. It is kinder and easier to use atraumatic needles with swaged-on sutures.

Any wounds other than the most superficial must be adequately anesthetized, and a thorough exploration must be made of their depths. Very little if any débridement is needed in this type of wound, but it may be necessary to twist off or even tie off bleeding vessels with No. 5-0 or No. 4-0 plain catgut. The same size catgut can be used if necessary to reconstitute any tissue planes, such as deep fascia or muscle bellies, that have been severed and are separated. Interrupted sutures should be used, and only as many as are needed to close the tissues should be put in.

If the edges of the wound are not at a 90-degree angle to the skin surface, the edges should be trimmed with sharp scissors before the sutures are placed. Ordinary interrupted sutures of No. 5-0 nylon are perfectly suitable for the closure of these wounds. In long straight wounds it is permissible to use a continuous suture, which should be locked at intervals.

TREATMENT FOR CHILDREN. In children, many tidy incised wounds can be closed with "butterfly sutures" made of adhesive tape. There are several commercially available versions of these adhesive dressings which strap the two sides of a wound together very efficiently and obviate the struggles inherent in multiple skin punctures either for local anesthetic or for actual sutures. However, the edges of skin wounds do tend to curl inward, and the edges must be perfectly dry so that the adhesive will hold them up and prevent a depressed scar from forming later. If stitches are needed for proper closure, No. 6-0 plain catgut sutures on an atraumatic needle should be used, since they will fall out spontaneously in about two weeks.

DRESSINGS. Tidy incised wounds require the absolute minimum of dressings. A small dry dressing should be held in place with adhesive tape for twenty-four or forty-eight hours. After this time the wound edges will have crusted, and dressings are no longer necessary. If dressings are continued, they may be a liability, since, if they become damp, they will macerate the wound edges.

## Tidy sliced wounds

Tidy sliced injuries are similar to tidy incised wounds, but the blow that produces them comes in at a slanting angle so that a flap of tissue is raised. If there is a "carry-through" to the blow that produces the flap and if the blow is at a sufficiently acute angle to the skin, the flap will probably be completely detached and a raw area of skin loss produced.

### Tidy sliced wounds with the skin flap attached

TREATMENT. If the injury leaves the flap of skin attached, the appropriate treatment is to suture it back in place. However, if there is a considerable amount of fat in the flap, it is wiser to remove some of this from the deep surface. The blood supply of the subcutaneous fat tends to enter from its deep surface, and, if a considerable amount of fat has been left on a flap, it is likely to have a poor blood supply and may undergo dissolution that will delay healing.

The base of the flap can be situated at any point on the periphery of the wound. If the flap is situated laterally or proximally in relation to the axis of the limb, the wound heals readily. Wounds in which the base of the skin flap is distal sometimes give considerable trouble (Fig. 6-2). The arterial supply of such flaps is good, and they bleed freely from the cut edges. Unfortunately, not all this bleeding comes

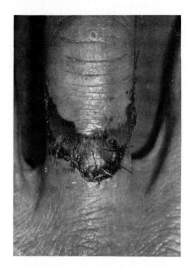

**Fig. 6-2.** *Distally based skin flaps.* The arterial supply of flaps that are based distally is good, but, because the venous drainage is cut off, the resultant congestion may cause skin necrosis.

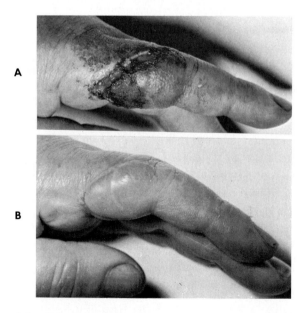

**Fig. 6-3.** *Swelling of distally based skin flaps.* Many flaps with distal bases will survive, but the interference with venous drainage may cause the wound to split open, **A.** The flap may remain swollen long after healing has occurred, **B.** (From Flatt, Adrian E.: J. Bone Joint Surg. **37-B:**117, 1955.)

from the arteries. Much of the blood comes from the veins that have been cut across but are still draining toward the heart. When the wound is closed, these veins will rapidly be sealed off, and the venous blood will pool in the flap. New venous drainage will then have to be established in a retrograde fashion along the sides and around the base of the flap. In small flaps this pooling may not necessarily interfere with healing, but it will probably produce a long-term swelling of the flap (Fig. 6-3). If, however, the flaps are large, the venous congestion can be a very serious problem, and it may cause necrosis of the distal portion of the flap. Such necrosis almost certainly occurs if the angle at the tip of the flap is very acute (Fig. 6-4). In injuries such as this, it is extremely difficult to give an accurate prognosis and therefore correspondingly difficult to prescribe the correct treatment. If it is certain that the tip of the flap is nonviable, it must be removed, and the defect must be treated as an area of skin loss. In doubtful cases only experience can help, but as a generalization it can be said that the more acute the angle of the tip and the longer the sides of the flap, the more certain it is that the distal portion will die from necrosis caused by the tissue congestion.

If the nature of the wound leaves little doubt that part of the flap is doomed, the correct treatment is amputation of that portion which is likely to die and its imme-

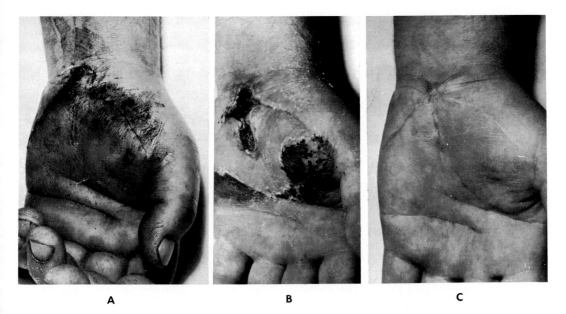

**A**     **B**     **C**

**Fig. 6-4.** *Large distally based flaps.* The venous congestion of these flaps is a serious problem, and necrosis of the tip is almost inevitable. If the angle of the tip is acute, as in this case, **A,** it is certain that necrosis will occur. **B,** Area of skin loss that resulted from necrosis. **C,** Final scarred result that is produced by allowing secondary healing to occur. This was the wrong treatment; skin grafts should have been applied to the raw area seen in **B.** (From Flatt, Adrian E.: J. Bone Joint Surg. **37-B:** 117, 1955.)

diate replacement with a skin graft. In most instances it is impossible to be so wise, and the best treatment is to suture the flap back into place, keep the limb elevated, and await events. If an area at the tip begins to discolor and is obviously going to die, it is wrong to wait for a fully established line of demarcation. If the tip of the flap is left in place, the necrotic tissue will get infected, the surrounding tissues will become inflamed, and the whole area will eventually heal by second intention with gross scarring to all adjacent tissue (Fig. 6-4).

If it is obvious that there is going to be loss of tissue, the patient should be taken back into the operating room. All the discolored tissue together with a thin margin of normal tissue should be excised, and the area of skin loss should be treated with a split-skin graft. Such early replacement of skin will produce a minimum reaction in the deeper tissues and very little scarring, and the patient can return to work much sooner than if he had been treated by a wait-and-see policy.

### Tidy sliced wounds with the skin flap separated

**GENERAL REMARKS.** Areas of skin loss in these wounds cannot and must not be closed by attempting to drag the tissues together with interrupted sutures. It is becoming increasingly fashionable to treat "small" areas of skin loss by "skillful neglect." This deliberate lack of management can succeed, but it can also produce very sensitive scarred areas. Its proponents have never yet successfully defined "small" for all the various sites and ages. I still believe that in most of these wounds the area of actual skin loss is sufficient to justify replacement from a distance. In general it is wiser to use a split-skin graft than to use a full-thickness graft. The thinner the split-skin graft, the more certain it is that it will survive and grow. However, the thinner the graft, the more the likelihood of subsequent contraction and scarring. As a corollary, although full-thickness grafts are incorporated with virtually no scarring, their chance for survival is much more precarious than that of a split-skin graft. As a compromise, therefore, it is best to use a split-skin graft of medium thickness if the original skin cannot be used. Do not be afraid that because these grafts are "split-skin" they will not be able to stand hard work. As the years go by they respond to the demands placed on them and resemble the adjacent skin (Fig. 6-5).

### Tidy sliced wounds with the skin available

**TREATMENT.** A full-thickness skin graft should not be cut deliberately to be used in these wounds. But occasionally the patient will produce the sliced-off piece of skin wrapped in a handkerchief. If the skin is in good condition, it should be thoroughly washed under running water and used as a graft. The fat on its deep surface should be trimmed until the dermis is exposed, and the skin can then be sutured back into place. The easiest way to remove fat from the undersurface of the flap is to place the skin, raw surface upward, on a hard surface and then cut off the fat with curved scissors. Cutting should be continued until the white felty surface of the dermis is exposed over the entire surface (Fig. 6-6).

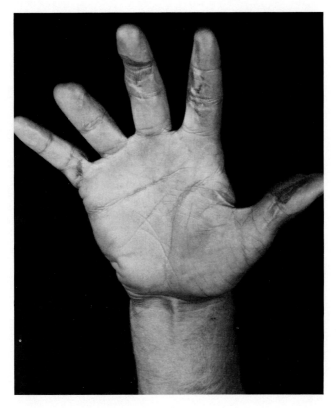

**Fig. 6-5.** *Split-skin grafting.* Three years before this photograph was taken a blasting cap mutilated this boy's fingers. Skin loss was replaced by medium-thickness skin grafts. They have responded to the demands placed upon them, thickened, and developed the appropriate creases.

The area of the wound must be inspected, and any dead or loose tissue must be excised before the skin is replaced. All bleeding must be stopped. Pressure with a damp sponge will rapidly control most hemorrhage, but bleeding vessels should be caught in mosquito hemostats. If these vessels are twisted off (Fig. 4-1), no catgut ligatures are needed. Catgut is a foreign body, and, if the skin is sewed back in place over catgut ligatures, a tissue reaction will occur, causing the graft to fail in that area.

When the wound is dry, the skin should be sutured back in place. Anesthesia may not be needed if the wound is treated shortly after its occurrence. If the area is very sensitive, it may be necessary to use a ring or metacarpal block using 2% lidocaine. The injections should be made well clear of the wound edges and through skin that has been thoroughly cleansed.

The skin can usually be replaced very accurately by using the skin creases or finger whorls as markers. Interrupted No. 5-0 nylon sutures should be used, and it is helpful if several are left long so that the ends can be used to tie over the dressings (Fig. 4-8).

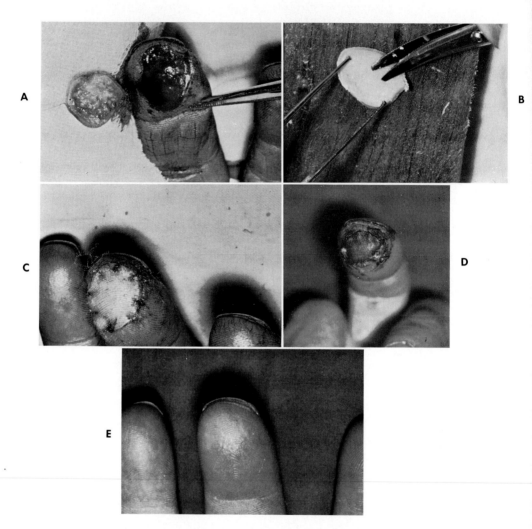

**Fig. 6-6.** *Full-thickness skin graft.* **A,** If the patient retrieves the sliced-off piece of skin, it can be replaced as a full-thickness graft. **B,** Showing how curved scissors should be used to remove all the subcutaneous tissues down to the level of the dermis. **C,** Showing how the skin should be sutured in place using the fingertip whorls to align the skin in the correct position. **D,** After ten days the graft looks terrible because of death of the superficial layers of the skin. **E,** The eventual excellent result obtained after the dead superficial tissues have been shed.

DRESSINGS. Full-thickness grafts need very careful immobilization and after-care, but the ultimate functional result is better than that produced by split-skin grafts.

The graft should be covered with a small piece of petrolatum gauze or Telfa. Small pieces of saline- or mineral oil–dampened cotton ball should be carefully placed on top of the graft so that, when the sutures are tied over them, the pressure will be evenly distributed over the surface of the graft. The finger or hand should be bandaged in the functional position, and the patient should be told to keep the hand elevated in a sling to chest height for twenty-four hours.

AFTERCARE. The sling can be discarded after twenty-four hours, and the hand can be used for light tasks; but direct use of the grafted area should be avoided if possible.

The dressing should be changed one week after the grafting. All the sutures should be taken out and the dressing renewed. At this dressing, the graft often looks black and dead, but, unless it is obviously infected, it should be left in place. The discoloration is due to death of the superficial layers of the epidermis and the keratin. At subsequent dressings, which should be done at three-day intervals, the discolored layer will peel off, leaving the new epithelium beneath it. Dressings will be required for about twelve to sixteen days. They should be left off when the superficial layers have completely separated from the graft. Occasionally when separation occurs, the deeper tissues will look moist and raw. If the area is protected with a Telfa dressing, epithelium will rapidly grow out from the deeper elements in the dermis. The area should be kept covered until the new epithelium appears.

*Tidy sliced wounds with the skin missing*

TREATMENT. When the skin is not available for replacement, a split-skin graft will have to be used to cover the defect. If the raw area of loss is potentially dirty, if it consistently oozes and hemorrhage is hard to stop, it is often wise to postpone immediate skin grafting. Instead, apply a moist compression dressing for about forty-eight hours. This will allow hemorrhage to stop and any latent infection to be controlled and will encourage formation of a fine network of granulation tissue, which is the ideal bed on which to place a skin graft. In addition, the raw area is usually pain free by this time. Many donor sites are available from which to take the graft; the flexor aspect of the forearm, although convenient for both physician and patient, does tend to leave a visible scar. If the forearm is to be used, the graft is usually cut from the flexor aspect of the forearm of the same side as the injured hand (Fig. 4-6) before any treatment is given to the hand injury. The forearm should be cleansed, and if necessary the flexor aspect should be shaved. The correct site for injection of the anesthetic to block the wound must also be cleansed. The size of the skin defect must be measured either by the eye or with a ruler, so that an area of appropriate size can be anesthetized on the forearm. An area 8 cm² is usually sufficiently large (Fig. 4-6). After the anesthetic has been injected into the forearm, the wound should also be anesthetized. The actual wound should not be cleansed at this time, and, after all the anesthetic solution has been injected, the hand and lower forearm should be wrapped in sterile towels. The graft should invariably be cut larger than the size of the defect on the hand. This will allow the graft to overlap the edges of the defect and thus make it easier to sew the skin into place around the periphery of the wound.

After the graft has been cut, the donor site should be dressed with petrolatum gauze, and a considerable number of dampened sponges should be fluffed up and held in place by a gentle compression bandage. The graft should be stored in a saline-dampened sponge until it is needed.

After the donor site on the forearm has been bandaged, the hand can be un-covered and the wound, which is now insensitive, can be adequately cleansed. Débridement of the wound must be thorough, and any obviously dead or loosely attached tissue must be trimmed away. Bleeding will occur from the skin edges, but pressure from a dampened sponge for a few minutes should be sufficient to stop the flow of blood. A dry sponge should not be used, since the blood clot will form in the meshes of the sponge and will be torn away when the sponge is removed, and the bleeding will start once again.

Vessels in the floor of the wound that are actually bleeding should be caught in mosquito forceps, which must be left in place long enough for the blood to clot in the vessel. No catgut sutures should be used, since the graft will fail to take in any area where such a foreign body holds it away from the deep tissues.

Since the graft is larger than the defect, it should be laid completely over the area. The overlapping edges serve as a good layer through which interrupted nylon sutures can be passed. Sufficient stitches should be placed all around the periphery of the wound to hold the graft firmly in place. One end of each suture should be left long, in order that the dressings may be tied in place (Fig. 4-8).

**DRESSINGS.** The surface of the graft should be covered with an appropriately trimmed piece of Telfa or petrolatum gauze. Saline- or mineral oil–dampened pieces of cotton ball or very small sections of gauze sponge should be carefully placed over the whole area. These must be piled up sufficiently high to supply an even pressure to the whole area when the long ends of the sutures are tied over the top.

The dressings on a finger should be protected by a Tubegauz bandage, and those on a hand should be protected by a Tubegauz or a stretchable compression bandage.

**AFTERCARE.** The hand should be kept in a sling for twenty-four hours to allow the graft to become adherent to its bed. After this time the hand can be used for light work.

The graft should be inspected four days after surgery. The sutures should be removed and all the dressings carefully peeled off. The graft should have taken satis-factorily, but if small areas show blisters, these should be punctured.

Telfa and small pieces of dry sponge should be built up on the graft and mild pressure applied to the whole area by bandaging. Dressings should be changed about every three days and can usually be left off between the tenth and fourteenth postoperative day (Fig. 6-7).

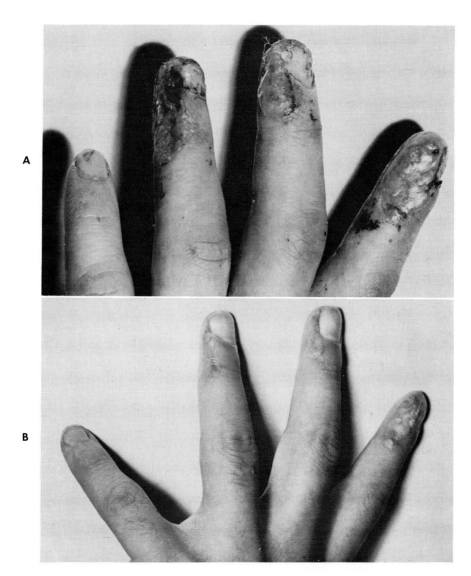

**Fig. 6-7.** *Split-skin grafting.* The skin loss on the ulnar side of the index, long, and ring fingers has been replaced by split-skin grafts. **A,** Condition ten days after grafting. **B,** The fingers one month after injury; the doubtful looking areas on the ring finger were due to thicker areas of the graft, and it can be seen that they consolidated satisfactorily.

Such small grafts recover sensibility in approximately six months. If the graft is a total failure, the whole process will have to be repeated after a few days of dressings have established a clean granulating surface.

## Puncture wounds

Penetrating injuries of the hand or fingers vary in size from those caused by a needle prick to the extensive perforating wounds produced by a knife or bullet. There is a strong possibility that foreign bodies such as metal, wood splinters, or pieces of cloth may be retained in the depths of the wound, and an x-ray examination is frequently an essential part of the clinical examination.

Because these puncture wounds are deep and narrow, they may damage essential neurovascular structures, tendons, or even bone. Palmar wounds often penetrate the thin skin over the flexion creases. At these sites the skin lacks the bolstering of the palmar fat, and the underlying structures are readily injured. A thorough clinical examination is mandatory, but complete assessment may have to be delayed until the wound is explored in the young or uncooperative patient.

Puncture wounds drain poorly because of their shape and depth and frequently become infected. They are potential sites for tetanus infections, and a booster dose must be considered if the patient has not been immunized with tetanus toxoid within ten years. It is a wise precaution to take a bacteriological swab for culture from the depths of all wounds that are explored.

Prophylactic chemotherapy should be given in all but the most minor cases. It is important that a high blood level be present at the time of surgery so that the blood clot in the wound will contain an effective level of broad-spectrum antibiotic. The first dose should therefore be given before the anesthetic is started.

ANESTHESIA. A regional block anesthetic will have to be used for a wound of the palm or dorsum of the hand, and a metacarpal block for a wound of a digit. The anesthetic solution should be injected before any attempt is made to cleanse the wound. The block must be established in healthy tissue at some distance from the wound. It is quite wrong to inject the anesthetic solution directly into the wound edges, because the solution will expand tissue planes and allow any infection that is present to spread in a centrifugal manner.

### Small splinter wounds

TREATMENT. After thorough cleansing of the skin around the entry site, the direction of the wound should be determined by probing. This probing must be done gently with a blunt-tipped probe—if a sharp instrument is used, it is likely that a false track will be made. When the track has been identified, it should be exteriorized by slitting it open to the surface with a sharp scalpel. A No. 11 blade is usually most satisfactory. Judgment must be used when opening these splinter tracks; wholesale cutting of important structures in order to open the track to the surface is not justified. If the wound penetrates into vital anatomical areas, it should be excised in a cone-shaped manner so that adequate drainage is established.

A thorough search must be made for foreign bodies, and particular care must be taken to make sure that nothing is left at the far end of the wound. After the wound has been explored, it should be irrigated with hydrogen peroxide followed by saline solution.

DRESSINGS. The wound should be protected with petrolatum gauze or Telfa and some fluffed-up sponges held in place by adhesive tape. On a finger a Tubegauz bandage is more efficient than adhesive tape.

AFTERCARE. These wounds granulate and heal very rapidly. They need protection for only a few days. During the healing period there is no reason why the patient should not continue to work, provided that the dressings are kept dry.

### Larger penetrating wounds

TREATMENT. After the area of skin around the wound has been cleansed, the skin and subcutaneous tissue edges should be excised. Any obviously devitalized tissue should be removed and a careful search made for foreign bodies in the wound. Hemorrhage must be stopped, but catgut ligatures should not be buried in the wound; the hemostats should be twisted off (Fig. 4-1). After irrigation with hydrogen peroxide followed by saline, the depths of the wound should be lightly packed with petrolatum gauze. No attempt should be made to close the skin wound at primary operation. Secondary suturing of the wound is good treatment, and several fine nylon sutures should be passed through the skin edges but should not be tied.

DRESSINGS. The wound should be lightly packed with petrolatum gauze and then covered with several fluffed-gauze sponges. The dressings should be held in place by a gentle compression bandage, and the hand should be retained in a position of function.

AFTERCARE. If infection is established within the wound, it will become evident within the first few days. Cultures should have been made so that the appropriate antibiotic can be chosen.

Normally, these wounds heal readily, and the secondary suturing can be carried out by tying the sutures three to four days after the primary operation. After the sutures are tied, the hand can be used for light work, but the dressings must be kept dry. The sutures should be retained for about ten days after they are tied. It is often wise to remove the sutures over a period of several days because of the slower rate of healing in secondarily sutured wounds.

## Untidy wounds

DEFINITION. Untidy wounds have ragged irregular edges as a result of lacerating injuries by such things as edges of tin cans, saws, and other irregular sharp edges. These wounds usually have several small, ragged, narrow-based flaps around their periphery that are unlikely to survive. There are usually areas of skin loss. Deciding on the best treatment for these wounds is often difficult. Though wholesale sacrifice of tissue is not justified, it is better to replace obviously devitalized tissue with a good graft than to hope that the tissue will live and then be faced subsequently with a discharging, infected wound.

In certain areas, such as the dorsum of the hand, it may be possible to replace the skin loss with a rotation flap, but such a procedure is usually not possible, and to attempt such a flap on a finger is unwise unless considerable experience justifies such treatment.

Inspection of the wound usually shows whether a split-skin graft is needed to cover any areas of actual or potential skin loss. If there is a probability that such a graft will be needed, the flexor aspect of the forearm of the injured hand should be shaved and the skin prepared.

**ANESTHESIA.** The wound should be anesthetized with 2% lidocaine either by a metacarpal block or by a ring block. If a graft is to be taken from the flexor aspect of the forearm, it should also be anesthetized. A square area with sides 8 cm long will be needed (Fig. 4-6).

**TREATMENT.** If it is certain that a skin graft will be needed, the hand should be draped off with sterile towels and the forearm cleansed. The size of the graft needed can be judged by the eye, and, after a medium-thickness graft is cut, it should be wrapped in a saline-dampened sponge and kept until required. The donor site must immediately be covered with Telfa or petrolatum gauze, a thick layer of dampened sponges, and a gentle compression bandage.

If it is not certain that a skin graft will be required, the forearm should be cleansed and wrapped in a sterile towel, which should be held in place by a bandage. The hand and wound should then be thoroughly cleansed. By this time the anesthetic will have taken effect, and the wound can be cleansed without causing pain.

After the wound has been cleansed, débridement must be done. Only a few millimeters of skin should be excised from the wound edge, but more trimming can be done in the depth of the wound if there are many loose pieces of fibrofatty tissue.

When only viable tissue has been left in the wound, the problem of obtaining primary epithelial cover must be assessed. If it is possible to close the entire wound with local flaps, this should be done, even if a few millimeters have to be resected. The skin flaps must be viable and should be replaced or rotated so that they lie in position without tension (Fig. 6-8). The sutures must be put in without tension on the skin edges. If it is impossible to cover the whole wound with local flaps, no attempt should be made to drag the tissues together. The flaps should be arranged to cover raw bone and as much of the palmar surface as is possible. The remaining raw area should be covered with a split-skin graft, which must be sewed into place with interrupted sutures. One end of each suture should be left long so that a dressing can be tied into place.

**DRESSINGS.** If a graft has not been used, the wound should be covered with Telfa and gauze sponges held in place on a digit by Tubegauz bandage and on a flat surface by an elastic compression bandage.

If a graft has been used, a small piece of Telfa must be cut to cover the grafted

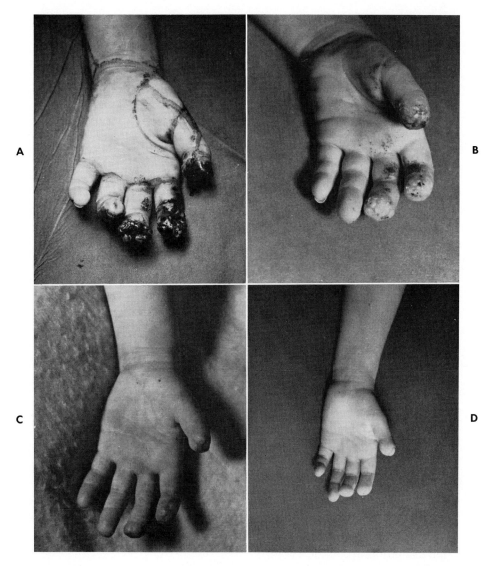

**Fig. 6-8.** *Untidy wounds.* This 7-year-old girl held a dynamite cap in her left hand and hit the cap with a hammer. Local flaps could be mobilized sufficiently to cover all the raw surfaces without tension on the flaps. **A,** The original wounds. **B,** The degree of healing when the sutures were removed fourteen days later. **C,** Follow-up at one year. **D,** Follow-up at three and a fourth years.

area, and small pieces of dampened cotton ball placed over the area in sufficient quantity to press evenly over the grafted area when the long suture ends are tied over the top. The rest of the wound should also be covered with Telfa and dry gauze dressings. The dressings should be held in place either by a Tubegauz bandage or a stretchable compression bandage.

    **AFTERCARE.** These wounds will tend to ooze more than tidy incised wounds, and they should therefore be carefully immobilized. The patient should be cautioned against attempted movements during the first few days. The graft must be inspected not later than the fourth day. If the graft is going to take, it will have commenced to do so by this time. At this first dressing, all layers should be changed, because the blood-soaked dressings might encourage local infection to develop if they are left in place too long. If the graft has failed, there is no alternative to repeating the grafting. The original indication for the use of a graft still exists, and there is no justification for a wait-and-see policy. The longer one waits, the greater will be the reaction in the local tissues and the greater the eventual amount of scar tissue and contracture. Before the skin grafting is repeated, the bed of granulation tissue on which the dead graft lies should be gently scraped to remove any florid or infected granulations and to leave a firm base for the new graft. It is often necessary to wait a few days before repeating the grafting. The aftercare is the same as that for primary grafting.

## DEGLOVING INJURIES

Degloving wounds of the hand are major problems, and the patient must be admitted to a hospital for suitable care. Often several fingers as well as portions of the palm or dorsum will be degloved. The patient should not be given piecemeal outpatient treatment but rather inpatient care in a hospital. On occasion a ring-bearing finger may be degloved when the ring becomes caught on an obstruction.

### Degloved finger

Degloving of a finger usually occurs as a result of a ring being caught on an obstruction when a person jumps off a truck (Fig. 16-12, p. 316). The force is sufficiently great for the ring to strip the skin distally off the finger and possibly to turn it completely inside out. This stripping of the skin and subcutaneous tissues leaves the tendons, joints, and bone undisturbed. The digital vessels are torn away, but occasionally the digital nerve remains in position. Sometimes the entire terminal phalanx, together with the profundus tendon, may be torn off at the level of the distal interphalangeal joint; the tendon will remain attached to the bone and avulse at its point of origin in the muscle of the forearm.

Examination of such a degloved finger shows that there is very little bleeding from the proximal skin stump because the vessels have been sufficiently traumatized to cause contraction and clotting. Sometimes the skin is still attached to the finger tip, and on other occasions the patient will bring the detached skin with him.

TREATMENT. Temptation to replace the skin is great, but the usual results of such treatment are dreadful (Fig. 6-9). Several authors have reported successful replacement of avulsed skin after it has been cleansed. Some recommend the removal of all fat from the skin before it is replaced. Others recommend direct repair of the cut arteries and veins. Such treatment is occasionally successful in the hands of very experienced surgeons, but the chances of infection are so great and the skin is usually so badly traumatized that routine replacement of the skin is bad treatment.

If an isolated finger has been degloved and the rest of the hand is normal, the

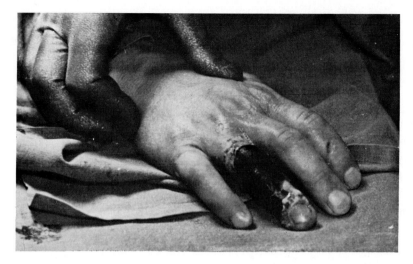

**Fig. 6-9.** *A degloved finger.* The gangrenous result of replacing skin that was avulsed when a ring caught on an obstruction. Split-skin grafting subsequently was attempted, but it failed and amputation had to be performed.

treatment of choice for the average physician is amputation of the finger at the level of the metacarpophalangeal joint. This may seem to be radical treatment for a finger which has full voluntary movement, but the methods of supplying skin cover are so unsatisfactory that after several months of treatment the resultant disability is often so great that amputation has to be performed. The reason for this unsatisfactory state of affairs is that the blood supply of the joints and tendons is largely destroyed. The ischemia of these moving parts is such that fibrosis occurs and, even if skin cover can be provided, it will only be over a stiffened finger in which the joint capsules are completely fibrosed.

Even the skin cover that can be provided is unsatisfactory. If split-skin grafts are used, they must be put on a virtually avascular bed, their "take" is poor, and there is considerable scarring beneath them. If an abdominal tube pedicle is constructed, the problem of adequate blood supply is still present, since the digital arteries have been destroyed. The blood supply that can grow in from the skin circumference at the base of the finger is not sufficient to support the full length of a tube of skin and subcutaneous tissues. The distal portion of the tube will have a very poor blood supply, and the tips of such fingers frequently break down.

Many occupations require the support supplied to grasp by the proximal phalanx of the ring finger; some surgeons therefore attempt to save this bone by covering it with skin grafts or local flaps. Such treatment demands skilled judgment and is not for the occasional surgeon.

## Degloved thumb

Amputation for an isolated degloved finger is the elective treatment. For a degloved thumb, it is the wrong treatment. The thumb is vital for opposition, and even if it is stiff, it can still function very efficiently. The thumb has only two phalanges, and the portion that is degloved is usually shorter than that on a finger.

TREATMENT. If the thumb is completely denuded, the patient should be admitted to a hospital, and the thumb should be surrounded by a pectoral tube pedicle.

If portions of subcutaneous tissues still remain or if immediate hospital care cannot be arranged, a strip of split-skin graft should be cut from the flexor aspect of the forearm of the same extremity. The graft should be wrapped in a spiral fashion around the thumb and anchored in place by several sutures. The sutures at the base and tip of the thumb should be left long, so that tie-over sutures can be placed on top of the compression dressing.

AFTERCARE. Movement should be encouraged after it is obvious that the graft has taken. This usually means that movement can be commenced in ten to fourteen days. Even if these grafts do take, frequently the skin does not stand up to the insults of heavy work, and tube pedicle replacement has to be undertaken at a later date.

## SKIN FLAPS

Skin loss on the hand or digits should usually be replaced by a split-skin graft. In certain areas, however, a skin flap can be used to give good coverage over sites that need the protection of skin and subcutaneous tissues. Split-skin grafts should not be placed over exposed tendons, exposed joints, or bone surfaces, because these grafts are unlikely to survive in such areas. If they did survive, their subsequent adherence and contraction would interfere with the function of the hand.

Flaps can be raised either locally within the hand or in more distant sites to which the hand can be moved for attachment of the flap. Flaps from a distance are not indicated in the care of small areas of skin loss and demand full inpatient management.

Local flaps are excellent coverage for small areas of loss because they carry into the site tissues that are characteristic of the hand both in texture and nerve supply. Several different types of flaps can be used, but all share one vital requirement; whatever type is employed, the flap must lie in its new site without any tension on its margins or base. Neglect of this basic requirement is the most common cause of total failure or unsatisfactory results (Fig. 6-10). Additional requirements in planning a flap are that it should be based proximally and that its length should never be more than twice its width. It would be better if the proportions were 1:1. In recent years a number of ingenious local flaps have been advocated for this type of work, but disasters have occurred when physicians who attempted these methods either ignored the fine technical details of the methods or lacked the judgment of the original author. *The use of flaps is sometimes essential; their planning, execution, and management is always difficult.*

The local flaps commonly employed within the hand are rotation, transposition, advancement, crossfinger, and thenar. Each flap is described in the chapter on the wound for which it is the most appropriate treatment.

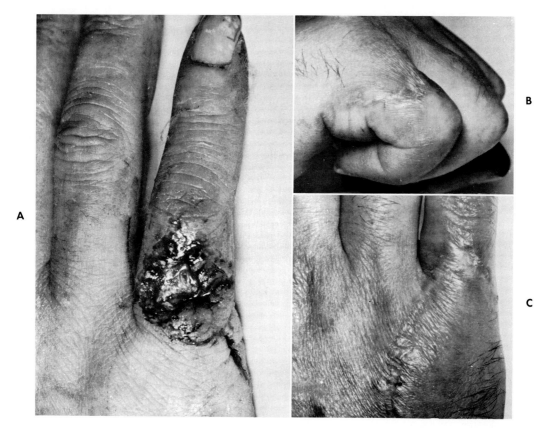

**Fig. 6-10.** *Rotation flap.* Rotation flaps from the dorsum of the hand can be used to cover defects on the dorsum of the proximal phalanx. **A,** In this case the cut extensor tendon was repaired before the flap was rotated. It can be seen in **B** that full function returned but that the skin is very tight in flexion. **C,** Reason for the tightness; the flap used was not large enough to provide an adequate skin cover. (From Flatt, Adrian E.: J. Bone Joint Surg. **37-B:**117, 1955.)

## Rotation flaps

Rotation of a flap of skin implies employing its inherent elasticity, and these flaps are therefore more commonly used in complex wounds on the dorsum of the hand or fingers, particularly in those involving a joint. It is important to realize that the line of rotation is the radius of a circle and that its length stretches from the point of the flap next to the defect to the farthest point on the base of the flap. The loose skin on the dorsum of the hand is deceptive. It is tight when a fist is made, and, when the flap is planned, the arc of the incision used to release the flap must be large in order to allow the flap to lie in its new site without tension.

ANESTHESIA. It is usually possible to plan the arc of the incision necessary to release the rotation flap before the hand is anesthetized. If this can be done, the appropriate area on the dorsum can be infiltrated with 2% lidocaine. It is well to infiltrate some distance beyond the line of the actual incision, because the nearby skin will have to be undermined with scissors to help in the movement of rotation. If the line of incision is not known, it is advisable to block a generous area with anesthetic agent. The flexor aspect of the forearm should not be infiltrated at this stage of the operation, since it is not certain that a skin graft will be required to close the secondary defect created by the rotation of the flap.

**OPERATIVE TECHNIQUE.** After the anesthetic has taken effect, the general skin preparation and local wound toilet can be done. It is a wise precaution to prepare the whole of the forearm under full sterile conditions, so that, if a split-skin graft is needed, the donor site will have been prepared. When the area is being covered with sterile towels prior to operating, care must be taken to arrange the towels so that the whole of the forearm will be easily available should a split-skin graft be needed. The sides of the wound must be trimmed by a minimal amount, but their edges must be at right angles to the skin surface to allow good apposition of the edges of the flap. Full débridement must be carried out in the depths of the wound, and any primary treatment necessary to repair damaged tendons or fractured bones must be completed.

The flap must be designed so that it is based proximally and thereby retains a reasonable venous return. Flaps that are based laterally may survive, but flaps based distally will swell from venous congestion. The swelling may be of sufficient degree actually to endanger the blood supply of the flap. Before permanently placing the flap, it is best to make the incision the length judged to allow for the rotation and then try placing the flap in position. Usually the distal part of the flap will be found to be under too much tension, and further relaxation produced by extending the incision will be necessary (Fig. 6-10).

The flap should be handled very delicately and not crushed along the skin edge with large-toothed forceps. It can be handled best by grasping a small portion of the subcutaneous fat in nontoothed forceps or by using small skin hooks. When the flap is ready for placing, the recipient area must be inspected for bleeding. No hemorrhage can be allowed in an area on which a flap is to rest. A considerable amount of time may have to be spent to ensure that the recipient area is dry. If the flap is to cover a joint, the skin of the flap must lie loosely over the joint to allow for the increased tension that will occur when the joint is flexed.

Only after the flap has been correctly placed without tension can attention be given to closure of the secondary defect produced by the rotation. Until the flap is correctly placed, no thought can be given to the raw surface left in the rotation area. To be influenced by the size of the raw area will mean that the flap will be sutured in place under tension. It may subsequently break down during the healing process, and the last state will be worse than the first. If the area from which the flap rotated can be closed without tension, this should be done. If closure is impossible without tension, a split-skin graft must be cut from the flexor aspect of the forearm on the injured side and then sutured into place.

When the flap is placed, it is wise to insert several interrupted fine nylon sutures spaced widely apart around the periphery of the flap. After these sutures have been placed, it can be determined whether the flap will be seated without tension and whether a split-skin graft will be needed to cover the secondary defect. If it appears that a skin graft is going to be necessary, local infiltration of the flexor aspect of the forearm should be carried out at once. The remaining sutures needed around the edge of the flap can be placed while the anesthetic is taking effect.

If a graft is used, the sutures that hold it in place should be cut with one end long, so that they may be tied over the dressings.

**DRESSINGS.** Drains should not be used. The suture lines should be covered with Telfa and a few layers of dry sponges. On top of this should be placed a considerable amount of fluffed-up sponges or Dacron batting. When this dressing is held in place by a stretchable bandage, an even, mild compression is applied to the area of the flap.

When a skin graft has been used, the grafted area should be covered with a piece of Telfa and some pieces of saline- or mineral oil–dampened cotton ball. The long ends of the sutures should be tied over these dressings to supply an even pressure to the graft. The rest of the area of the flap should be covered by Telfa, dry sponges, and fluffed-up sponges or Dacron batting. The dressing should be held in place by a mild compression force supplied by a stretchable bandage.

**AFTERCARE.** There should be no hurry to take out the sutures, and although the dressings should be changed at three- to four-day intervals, there is no need to remove even half the sutures before the twelfth day. When all sutures have been removed, the patient must be warned to make only very gentle movements with the injured finger or injured hand until the healing under the flap has been completed. It is wise to insist on a sling during the early healing phase. The hand and forearm must be elevated for the first forty-eight hours. To allow the limb to be dependent at this time will only compound any circulatory problems that may already exist.

Full healing normally takes about six weeks.

## Transposition flaps

Compound wounds of the palm of the hand need primary skin cover to protect the exposed tendons and bones in the floor of the wound. The palmar skin is inelastic, and therefore rotation flaps cannot be used.

When the wound is over a vital area, it may be possible to use a transposition flap that allows good skin to cover the primary defect and produces the secondary defect over an area of lesser importance.

This is not an easy operation to perform, and for the inexperienced it is wiser to refer the patient or place a split-skin graft over the area as a temporary measure until the patient can be transferred.

# 7 · INJURIES TO THE NAIL

**Avulsion injuries**
  Partial avulsion
  Complete avulsion

**Cutting injuries**

**Grinding injuries**

**Crushing injuries**
  Subungual hematoma
  Nail damage

**Disability**

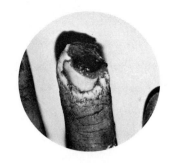

**Nail injury**

**T**he nail is an epidermal appendage, a modification of the stratum lucidum. It is therefore modified skin and when there has been loss of a nail or its bed, it should be treated by skin replacement. It is wrong to treat such injuries conservatively with dressings.

If a raw nail bed is left to granulate, it will gradually heal with scar tissue, which will cause a distorted and sensitive digital tip (Fig. 7-1). Throughout this prolonged healing process, the digit will be tender, painful, and a great hindrance during attempts to work. If, however, a split-skin graft is used as immediate treatment, the finger will rapidly lose its excessive sensitivity because of the protection provided by the skin graft. If the graft is sewed into place, the patient can usually continue to work throughout treatment (Fig. 7-5).

Patients often present with a partial avulsion of the nail and request that the removal be completed. It is wrong to do this. The nail should be replaced. The nail serves as a rigid backing for the pulp and terminal phalanx of the finger. This rigidity not only provides dorsal protection for the finger tip but, in addition, gives support to the pulp of the finger tip so that the nerve ends react immediately to sensory stimuli on the palmar aspect. Complete avulsion of the nail therefore leaves a tender, unprotected dorsal aspect of the finger and a palmar aspect that has lost some degree of its sensory discrimination.

Three main types of injury occur to the nail area: avulsion, cutting, and crushing.

## AVULSION INJURIES

The nail bed is a relatively strong layer of tissue separating the nail from the underlying bone. When a nail is avulsed, the nail bed remains attached to the periosteum of the distal phalanx. The root or growing part of the nail consists of part of the lunula or half-moon and the area proximal to it beneath the dorsal cuticle, nail fold, and skin.

Different degrees of avulsion can occur, and the nail itself can be cut to a vary-

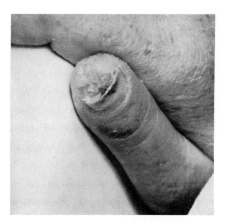

**Fig. 7-1.** *Nail bed injury left to granulate.* Conservative treatment that allows a raw nail bed to granulate is bad treatment. The area will heal with an irregular sensitive scar. (From Flatt, Adrian E.: Br. J. Plast. Surg. **8:**34, 1955.)

ing degree without avulsion having occurred. In cuts of the nail without disturbance of the deeper layers, no treatment other than adhesive strapping is needed to hold the nail together. Growth of the nail will slowly cover any injury that occurred to the nail bed.

## Partial avulsion

Avulsion of the nail can occur from the proximal or distal ends or even from the side (Fig. 7-2). Usually it is sprung up and out from beneath the onychal fold or cuticle with its edge lying on top of the dorsal skin. It must be left attached to its bed and trimmed at its periphery until the protruding edge can be tucked back beneath its usual border. Peripheral trimming of the nail is important, since attempts to force the lateral or proximal edges beneath their skin folds may well lead to chronic low-grade infection in these areas. After the edges have been trimmed sufficiently to allow the nail to be easily replaced, it can be held in place by a small padded adhesive dressing. Such replacement of a nail is really a form of splinting of the distal phalanx, and only very rarely will the nail reattach to its bed. Usually after about two weeks the nail bed is sufficiently healed for the nail to be removed, and the finger tip can then be left unprotected while the new nail grows.

A new nail grows at about 1 mm a week and takes at least six months to grow from its root to the finger tip, and care should be taken to prevent small vertical adhesions from forming in the region of the lunula between the skin and the cuticle overlying the nail bed area. If these vertical epithelial septa are allowed to develop, the new nail will grow down on either side of the obstruction and a split will be created (Fig. 7-3). The adhesions that cause this distortion can be prevented from consolidating by occasionally passing a probe or orange stick proximally beneath the dorsal skin during the first month after the nail avulsion. The tip of the probe

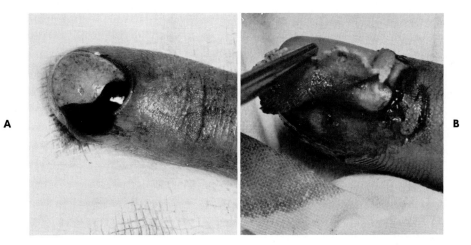

**Fig. 7-2.** *Partial avulsion of the nail.* In both cases the damage beneath the nail is more extensive than would appear on superficial examination. (**B** from Flatt, Adrian E.: Br. J. Plast. Surg. **8**:34, 1955.)

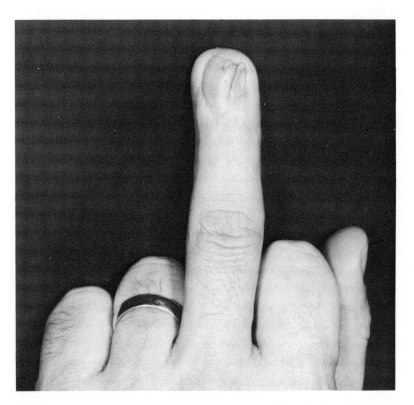

**Fig. 7-3.** *Split nail.* A vertical epithelial septum may join the cuticle and dorsal skin to the nail bed after a dorsal injury. The new nail will then split and grow down either side of the obstruction.

should be passed in an upward direction and swept laterally beneath the dorsal skin so that the skin is tented up by the tip of the probe. If the tip is passed downward against the upper surface of the distal phalanx, there is danger of disruption to the nail root and growing edge of the new nail.

## Complete avulsion

If the nail has been completely avulsed from its bed, some form of dressing must be applied to the raw bed. A petrolatum gauze or fine mesh dressing is usually applied, but experience shows that these frequently stick to the bed and are extremely painful to remove later because the nail bed is very generously supplied with nerve endings. A small piece of rubber glove cut to fit the raw area and smeared with an antibiotic ointment makes an excellent nonadherent layer between nail bed and outer dressings. These can be held in place by strapping or a Tubegauz bandage. After about a week the dressing can be changed to some form of dry dressing. During the third week the nail bed has usually hardened sufficiently to allow all dressings to be left off.

If the avulsion process has raised a flap of nail bed, this flap should be sutured in place with nonabsorbable sutures, which should be removed in about ten days. The dressings should be similar to those used for a simple avulsion.

Injuries that destroy or avulse the nail and portions of the nail bed cannot be treated by simple dressings, since actual epithelial loss has occurred. The epithelial loss must be replaced, and the replacement method depends on whether the injury was of a cutting or crushing type.

## CUTTING INJURIES

Most cutting injuries are of the tidy sliced type, but occasionally these wounds are produced by grinding injuries or other similar untidy means.

It is important to realize that these are injuries of the dorsum of the terminal phalanx and that they do not involve the palmar pulp of the fingertip. In fingers where pulp loss has occurred, even though there may be associated nail damage, treatment is directed to restoring the fingertip profile by supplying pulp volume and finger tip skin. The injury to the nail becomes a secondary consideration. Such treatment is discussed under pulp loss (Chapter 8).

If there is partial or complete loss of the nail and its bed, the treatment of choice is to apply a thin split-skin graft to the wound. When, in addition, there has been loss of actual fingertip skin, a graft of varying thickness should be cut so that the thick portion is applied to the pressure-bearing area and the thin portion to the nail bed area (Fig. 7-4).

**OPERATIVE TECHNIQUE.** An estimate must be made of the size of the graft needed (Fig. 7-5). This need only be a rough guess; rarely is a graft larger than 3 cm² needed to treat a single finger. A large enough area from which to cut the graft must be cleansed on the upper part of the flexor aspect of the forearm of the injured limb. This cleansing should be done before the routine preoperative toilet of the injured finger to avoid contamination of the clean donor site.

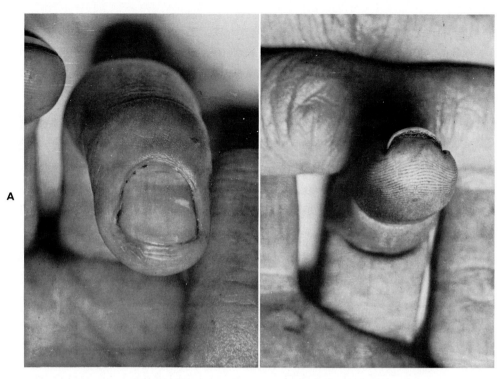

**Fig. 7-4.** *Split-skin grafting of nail bed injuries.* Two illustrations of the results obtainable when a split-skin graft of varying thickness is placed so that the thicker portion replaces the area of skin loss and the thinner portion covers the nail bed area. (**B** from Flatt, Adrian E.: Br. J. Plast. Surg. **8:**34, 1955.)

A square block about twice the size of the required graft must then be outlined on the forearm (Fig. 4-6). A 2% lidocaine solution is used, and, after the sides of the square have been outlined, the area of skin within it is undermined and infiltrated with the local anesthetic. The metacarpal block can then be placed in the finger, and, by the time this has been done, the donor area for the graft will be anesthetized.

The area needed is so small that it is unnecessary to use any of the various machines that are available for cutting grafts. A razor blade, large scalpel, or skin-grafting knife should be used to cut the necessary split-skin graft. If a graft of varying thickness is needed, the cutting edge should be allowed to come gradually nearer the surface as cutting proceeds. By this means a very thin portion of skin will be cut at one end of the graft. After the graft has been cut, it should be stored in a saline-moistened sponge. The donor site should be dressed with petrolatum gauze, several layers of sponges, and a gentle compressive bandage, which should be carefully applied so that all of the donor site and its dressings are completely covered. It is a wise precaution to seal the upper and lower edges of the bandage to the arm with adhesive tape.

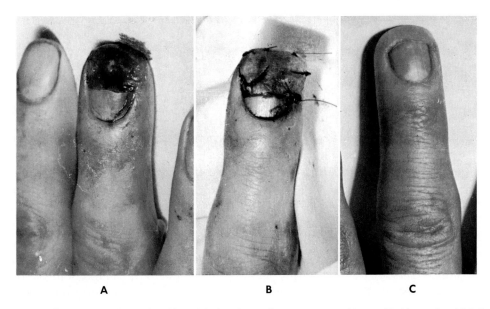

A                              B                              C

**Fig. 7-5.** *Split-skin grafting of nail bed injuries.* Immediate treatment with a split-skin graft, which is sewed into place, will produce perfect healing. Usually the patient can continue to work throughout treatment. In **B** note how the excess graft is distributed equally around the periphery of the wound. **C** shows how the thin skin graft becomes incorporated into the nail bed. (From Flatt, Adrian E.: Br. J. Plast. Surg. **8:**34, 1955.)

After the donor site has been sealed off by dressings, the final cleansing of the finger tip should be done. Surgical toilet of the wound area should include excision of any obviously dead tissue and ragged tags of skin around the edges of the wound. If the proximal portion of the nail is present, it should be cut back about 3 or 4 mm to make a suitable bed on which the graft can be placed. Usually the graft is cut larger than the necessary area, but this is no hindrance to good surgery. The graft should be laid in place virtually as if it were a patch and with its extra portions distributed equally around the periphery (Fig. 7-5).

If there has been actual loss of skin of the fingertip distal to the nail, then the thicker portion of the graft should be placed over this raw finger tip and the thinner part over the nail bed. Sutures should then be passed through the graft and the skin of the finger, with one end of the suture left long for tying over the graft dressings. The graft can be anchored in place over the nail by passing sutures through holes bored into the nail with the point of a No. 11 scalpel blade. Needles can be forced through the nail without boring preliminary holes, but this is unnecessarily traumatic, and there is a risk that the needle may break within the tissues.

## GRINDING INJURIES

The increasing use of portable high-speed grinding wheels in industry in recent years has caused a parallel increase in the incidence of grinding wounds of the dorsum of the terminal phalanx. These injuries occur when the wheel slips and cuts away a varying amount of dorsal tissue from the finger tip. In essence, these wounds are friction burns and they must be looked at from the point of view of a burn when assessing the prognosis, particularly since there is often quite a degree of full-thickness skin loss. The bottom of the wounds is frequently ingrained with minute pieces from the grinding wheel.

The operation must be designed to clean up the dorsum of the finger and remove all the ingrained dirt. Wholesale excision of the dorsal area is not justified, since it may remove so much of the subcutaneous tissues that the graft will have difficulty in taking. It is wise to use a split-skin graft of medium thickness in these areas so that a compromise can be reached between the certainty of the graft surviving and a durable protection being provided for the dorsum of the finger. No great harm will come to the fingertip if small particles from the grinding wheel remain behind and act as a tattoo in the depths of the new skin graft. Eventually, they will be covered by the nail and will be practically invisible.

**DRESSINGS.** Dressings consist of a small compression dressing of Telfa and some small pieces of cut-up sponges held in place by the tie-over ends of the sutures that anchor the graft in place. These dressings should have an outer protective cover of Tubegauz bandage. With this treatment the vast majority of patients can return to work the day of injury. The only discomfort that they are likely to feel is from the donor site of the skin graft.

**AFTERCARE.** The fingertip should be dressed on the fourth day so that blood and serum that has soaked into the dressings can be removed and the state of the graft assessed. The long ends of the sutures can be cut short, and similar dressings can be reapplied. If the Tubegauz bandage is put on firmly, it will hold the dressings securely in place. Thereafter, the dressings can be changed at two- to three-day intervals until the sutures are removed in about eight to ten days. Dressings should be left off just as soon as the graft has thoroughly taken and in a normal case should not be needed after the fourteenth to sixteenth day. The donor site need not be inspected for fourteen days. At this time the site is usually healed, and all of the dressings can be removed. Occasionally, however, epithelization may be slow, and the area will need protection for an additional few days.

Skin grafts take well in the area of the nail bed, and it is very unusual for a graft to fail. If, however, a graft has failed, it should be replaced immediately by a similar type of graft after the debris of the previous graft has been cleared away.

## CRUSHING INJURIES

Crushing injuries vary greatly in severity. Minor degrees of injury merely produce a subungual hematoma, but the more severe injuries can produce gross disruption of all the tissues of the finger tip. Avulsion of the nail is usually of secondary importance compared to the rest of the damage done by a crushing force, and the major part of treatment should be directed to the crush injury rather than to the nail damage.

## Subungual hematoma

Subungual hematomas are usually produced by a blow on the finger from a hammer or some similar object and cause an early acute extravasation of blood between the fingernail and phalanx. The blood causes a purple or dark blue area that is exquisitely tender because of the extremely high tension produced between these two rigid structures. Immediate elevation of the hand is good first aid and so is immersion in ice cold water for 20 to 30 minutes. But the treatment of choice is to trephine the nail and evacuate the hematoma (Fig. 7-6).

Although it is more elegant and impressive to do the decompression with an expensive trephine or the point of a scalpel blade, the patient is most impressed by the additional pain caused by the pressure applied to the boring tool. It is much better to heat a straightened paper clip even with a match and to apply the hot end directly over the center of the area of the nail that shows the discoloration from the hematoma. When the hot end of the paper clip passes through the nail, the heat is immediately dissipated throughout the liquid hematoma (Fig. 7-6). The blood will well out from the subungual region, and there will be instantaneous relief of pain. Very occasionally a large subungual hematoma will have loculated, and more than one area will have to be drained by this means.

## Nail damage

In most crush injuries the nail is usually only partially avulsed from the finger tip. Even if it has been completely detached but is still available, it should be kept. The problem in such crush injuries is the distortion of the fingertip and the nail bed. Subsequent swelling will further increase the distortion during the first week.

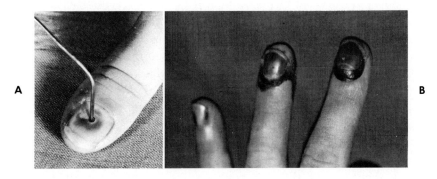

**Fig. 7-6.** *Subungual hematoma.* The exquisite pain caused by the pressure within a subungual hematoma is relieved by trephining the nail. **A,** A heated paper clip will readily release the hematoma. **B,** If left too long the blood will clot and trephining will not help, as can be seen in the long fingernail. The ring fingernail was successfully decompressed.

If the nail is in place, it serves as the best possible splint against which the tissues can be molded by a compression dressing.

Frequently the nail bed has been split or lacerated; it must be meticulously repaired before the nail is used as a splint, otherwise the edges of the wounds will separate when the dressing is applied. If the nail folds on its side have also been damaged, they should be repaired first, since by doing this the wounds of the nail bed will be correctly lined up. The nail bed should be repaired with very fine absorbable sutures of 6-0 or 7-0 catgut, and the edges must be precisely aligned if the new nail is to grow over without distortion.

Crush injuries to the nail are very painful, and analgesics must be given in adequate doses. Cooling of the fingertip and even enveloping it in ice bags frequently helps control the constant throbbing.

### Associated phalanx fracture

Crush injuries frequently split or even shatter the terminal portion of the distal phalanx into several splinters. Fractures may occur even when the hematoma does not appear very large (Fig. 13-25). Although these injuries are painful for several days, they are not disabling and need no specific treatment. Occasionally the phalanx may be fractured completely across its midshaft into two large fragments. In such cases it is wiser to impale the distal phalanx with a fine Kirschner wire and properly immobilize the fracture by passing the wire into the body of the proximal phalanx.

### Injuries with the nail attached

OPERATIVE PROCEDURE. The details of care of crush injuries are described on pp. 181 to 183. Because of the dangers of infection developing in damaged tissues, great care must be taken during the wound toilet. A particular search must be made beneath the detached portion of the nail for foreign material or blood clot, which could form a nidus of infection after the nail has been replaced. After the crush injury of the finger pulp has been treated, the nail should be trimmed around the periphery and replaced. Occasionally it helps to anchor the nail in place by passing a few sutures through holes drilled around its edges. A maximum of two sutures per side is sufficient, and they should not be tied tightly.

DRESSINGS. If the nail has been replaced, the best dressing is a small pad over the nail to absorb serum held in place by adhesive tape. This dressing can be changed as frequently as necessary. If a skin graft has been used, it should be dressed appropriately.

AFTERCARE. As soon as the edema caused by the crushing injury has subsided, the aftercare is the same as for any other nail wound. However, since crushing injuries cause much more discomfort than the neater slicing injuries, the majority of patients should not work for several days or until the discomfort is minimal.

### Injuries with the nail detached

OPERATIVE PROCEDURE. If the detached nail is available, it should be thoroughly scrubbed in soap and water, trimmed around the edges, and replaced in a manner similar to that described for nails which had remained attached. If there has been loss of nail bed as well as avulsion of the nail, the epithelial loss will have to be treated by skin grafting.

   **DRESSINGS**. See under Injuries with the nail attached.

   **AFTERCARE**. See under Injuries with the nail attached.

## DISABILITY

   Except in patients who have sustained crush injuries, there is no reason why there should be any degree of permanent disability resulting from nail injuries. The nail will grow over the area of skin graft and will readily incorporate the new skin into the nail bed. Very occasionally, complaints are heard concerning the appearance of the nail or of lack of adherence of the nail bed. These are cosmetic rather than functional disabilities, and only rarely do they actively hinder a patient's ability to carry on work.

# 8 · PULP LOSS

**The fingers**
  Distal phalanx injury
  Proximal and middle phalanx injury

**The thumb**
  Distal phalanx injury
  Proximal phalanx injury

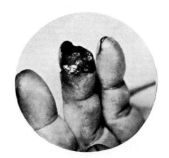

**Pulp loss**

Loss of the tactile skin and its underlying pulp on the palmar side of the finger is a common and potentially crippling injury. In the distal phalanx the major part of the nail and bony phalanx will be unharmed. In the middle and proximal phalanges the flexor tendons and the digital neurovascular bundles will be largely intact.

Many methods of repair have been recommended, varying from shortening of the finger, the use of split- or full-thickness skin grafts, to the use of local flaps such as palmar or cross-finger or even flaps from the chest or abdomen. Published opinions differ as to the effective return of sensibility in grafts or flaps, but I believe the most useful and durable fingers are produced by the use of local flaps.

## THE FINGERS
## Distal phalanx injury

If a finger with injury to the distal phalanx is looked at in profile, it can be seen that the plump, rounded end of the finger tip is missing because of loss of the terminal skin and pulp. However, the rigid support supplied by the nail and bone is still intact, since the injury tapers the finger from the region of the distal interphalangeal joint to the tip. Because the nail and bone are largely intact, this injury is not a partial amputation.

If the patient's occupation demands a full-length finger with normal padding and the best possible sensibility at its tip, a full-thickness flap should be taken from the palmar skin of the injured hand. The skin of the hand contains the appropriate nerve endings for sensibility and the correct proportions of subcutaneous tissues. If, however, there is no pressing need for a full-length finger, then a properly performed amputation using local skin flaps will give an excellent functional result. To cover a finger tip that has lost its pulp with a split-skin graft is useless. It can never have proper sensibility, and, because the cushioning of the fatty pulp is missing, it will be repeatedly damaged.

Many say that it is wrong to "mutilate" the palm of the hand by using it as a site for a flap, and they advocate the use of an abdominal flap. However, if the operation is properly performed, it leaves no noticeable defect on the palm, and the donor site is not a handicap to the patient. The use of abdominal skin leaves a discolored, protuberant, insensitive patch of skin on the fingertip, and the patient is considerably handicapped during the healing stage when the arm is strapped to the side. An additional point that must be remembered is that the fat beneath the abdominal skin is storage fat, and, even though it may be moved to the fingertip quite successfully, it will always retain its metabolic storage characteristics. If, therefore, the patient gains weight subsequent to treatment and excess fat is deposited on his abdomen, it will also be deposited in his fingertip. The fingertip will keep pace with the protruding abdomen (Fig. 3-2). The purpose of the operation is to replace the missing pulp of the terminal phalanx with a similar type of subcutaneous tissue. A lump of fat cannot be placed as a free graft in the finger. It has to be supported by a blood supply brought in by a pedicle. The palmar skin pedicle not only carries the necessary blood supply for the fat but in addition provides the correct type of skin for the fingertip.

In an ideal case, in which the major part of both the nail and bone is intact, a virtually normal fingertip can be produced. The greater the loss of bone, the less likely it is that the flap will give a reasonable fingertip. If the major part of both the phalanx and nail bed is destroyed, it is useless to do a flap operation, since the two rigid structures that could give any support to the fat and the skin are absent and a flabby fingertip will be the result.

The thenar flap operation is most suitable for the young working adult. It can be successfully used in children's hands, but in the elderly or arthritic hand there is a distinct possibility of joint stiffness occurring during the two-week immobilization period. The use of this operation in correctly selected cases will produce a better functioning finger in one month than can be achieved in a longer period of time by any other method. Improperly done, the operation can cripple the hand.

There are several variations in the way in which this operation can be performed. Some raise two flaps in an H plan and produce a closed epithelial system during the healing phase. Others go in the opposite direction and only partially close the donor site and do not apply a skin graft to the unclosed area. I believe that the raw flap donor site should be closed in such an important area and prefer to use a skin graft rather than the technically more difficult two-flap H procedure.

### Operation

**OPERATIVE TECHNIQUE.** The vital point in this operation is the correct selection of the donor site for the flap. If each finger is flexed in turn so that it touches the palm, it can be seen that a very small area of skin is covered in the region of the thenar eminence (Fig. 8-1). The actual sites of contact will vary with different individuals, but this general area is the correct donor site. There is a natural deviation of the flexed fingers, and to force a finger or fingers into an unnatural position, such as trying to make the flexed small finger lie parallel with the ulnar border of

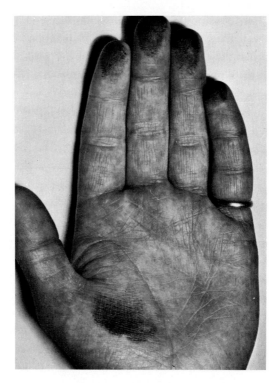

**Fig. 8-1.** *The donor site for a thenar flap.* If the fingertips are covered in ink and individually pressed onto the palm, a relatively small area on the thenar eminence will be ink stained. The size of the contact area will vary with different individuals, but this general area is the correct donor site. (From Flatt, Adrian E.: J. Bone Joint Surg. **39-B:**80, 1957.)

the hand, will produce so much tension on the flap that it will pull away, infection will result, and the operation will fail (Fig. 8-2).

After the general cleansing of the hand and forearm, the injured fingertip should be blotted with a dry sponge and then flexed into the palm so that the tip leaves a bloody imprint on the palmar skin. It is at this site that the flap must be raised. The fingertip should then be covered with a rubber finger cot, and cleansing of the rest of the forearm and hand should be completed.

**ANESTHESIA.** A local anesthetic of 2% lidocaine is then injected into an area 5 cm$^2$ on the upper part of the flexor aspect of the forearm, which will act as a donor site for a split-skin graft (Fig. 4-6). The general area from which the flap is to be raised is infiltrated, and a metacarpal block is done at the base of the injured finger.

A split-skin graft of medium thickness is then cut from the forearm with a razor blade or hand-held knife and stored in a saline-dampened sponge. The donor site should be dressed immediately with Telfa, saline-dampened sponges, and a stretchable bandage. Once the donor site is sealed from outside contamination, the finger cot is removed and the injured fingertip cleansed. The edges and depths of the wound should be trimmed of any obviously devitalized tissue, and any prominent

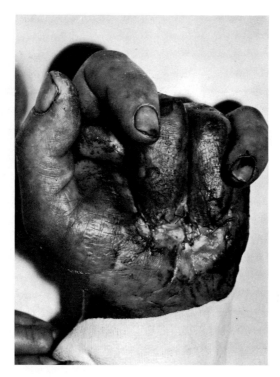

**Fig. 8-2.** *The donor site for a thenar flap.* In this case the correct donor site was not used. The ring and long fingers were forced toward a donor site in the center of the palm. The flaps have failed because of the tension caused by the unnatural position of the fingers. Note how the small finger is pointing in its correct direction, toward the base of the thenar eminence. (From Flatt, Adrian E.: J. Bone Joint Surg. **39-B:**80, 1957.)

bleeding vessels should be caught in mosquito hemostats. It is better not to bury catgut sutures in the wound, and the hemostats should therefore be left on as long as possible and then twisted off.

### Raising the palmar flap

The site of the flap will dictate the amount of flexion of the finger joints. The best position is one with medium flexion of all three joints. If the finger is tightly flexed at all joints, the donor site will be too distal. If the distal interphalangeal joint is extended, there is a tendency for the flap to bend back on itself and obliterate its own blood supply. It is better to have a patient voluntarily flex the finger, since by doing so he will hold all three finger joints in a position of comfort. If flexion is done passively, there is a tendency to force the joints into positions of extreme flexion that would become very uncomfortable during the immobilization. In middle-aged and elderly patients such extreme positions may cause some degree of permanent stiffness in the finger.

With the ideal position of flexion in mind, the finger should be flexed into the palm so as to localize accurately the donor site for the flap. The contact area may be

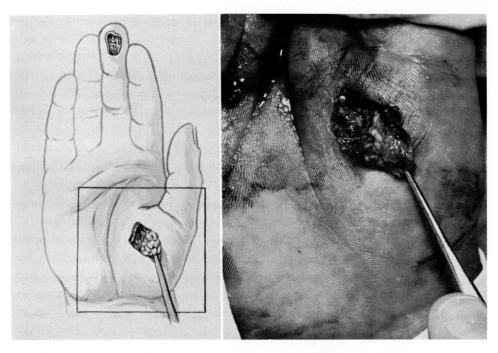

**Fig. 8-3.** *The thenar flap.* The flap is designed to be based proximally, and its end is cut with square corners to give the maximum blood supply to the corners. The forceps are turning the flap backward to show that about two thirds of the subcutaneous fat is carried with the flap and the remainder is left as a base for the split-skin graft that will be sewed into the donor site. (From Flatt, Adrian E.: J. Bone Joint Surg. **39-B:**80, 1957.)

outlined with an applicator stick dipped into methylene blue. Such an ink is hardly necessary since the patient's own blood makes a readily available substitute.

The flap must be based proximally, its length should not be more than twice its width, the end should be square, and at least two thirds of the thickness of the subcutaneous fat should be carried on the flap, the remaining fat being left as a bed for the graft (Fig. 8-3). The incision should be made with a No. 15 scalpel blade, but the flap should be raised by dissecting beneath it with small blunt-nosed scissors. Too enthusiastic dissection in this area with sharp instruments could possibly damage the motor branch of the median nerve—a tragedy that is difficult to explain away.

Raising the flap creates an area of skin loss in the palm. This area cannot be completely closed by suturing the edges of the donor site together. Attempts to close the wound by such suturing produce gross scarring in the palm and may severely restrict abduction movements of the thumb. The area of skin loss will have to be replaced by the split-skin graft that has been previously cut. The graft should be held in place by interrupted sutures of No. 5-0 nylon. In order for the graft to be sewed into place, the flap has to be turned back on its base so that the raw surface is upward. The graft is usually larger than the area to be replaced, and it should be distributed evenly around the periphery of the wound. At the base of the pedicle

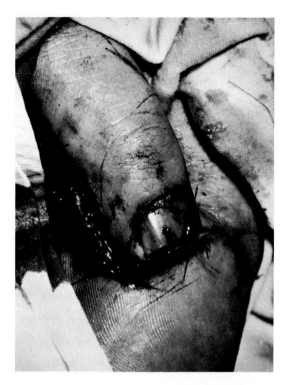

**Fig. 8-4.** *Attaching the thenar flap to the finger.* The flap is sutured to the fingertip at the distal edge of the nail. The nail should be cut back about 2 to 3 mm to leave the bed exposed, and a few holes should be drilled in the nail with a scalpel point so that the sutures may be easily passed. There is no need to suture the sides of the flap; indeed, to do so might interfere with the blood supply of the flap by stretching the skin and constricting the vessels. Note how the flap is at a 90-degree angle to the surface of the palm. (From Flatt, Adrian E.: J. Bone Joint Surg. **39-B:**80, 1957.)

the graft can be turned up onto the fatty surface so as to give some protection to the base of the pedicle during the healing period.

The flap is attached to the fingertip only at the distal edge of the nail bed. The nail should be cut back about 2 to 3 mm to leave the bed exposed, and several holes should be drilled in the nail with the point of a No. 11 scalpel blade. A firm attachment can be obtained for the flap by passing sutures through these holes (Fig. 8-4). No attempt should be made to suture the sides of the flap to the sides of the finger defect. A perfectly adequate blood supply will grow in from the edge of the nail bed, and, if sutures are put into the side of the flap, they will tend to stretch it so tightly in a transverse direction that the vessels running longitudinally could be obliterated.

**DRESSINGS.** Joining the flap to the finger in this manner leaves raw surfaces on most of the fingertip and the proximal part of the flap. These raw areas should be protected by a small wedge-shaped dressing of petrolatum gauze placed between the palmar surface of the finger and the split-skin graft on the palm. It should be packed in reasonably firmly so as to supply some pressure to the surface of the split-skin graft to ensure its take.

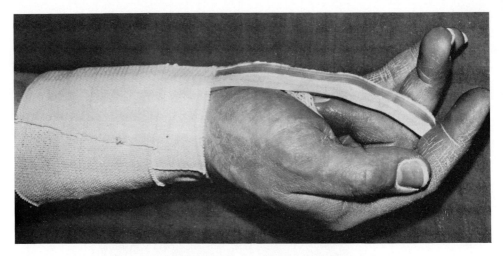

**Fig. 8-5.** *Immobilization following a thenar flap procedure.* The finger can be easily immobilized in the correct position by molding a padded aluminum splint over the finger and both sides of the forearm. The splint can be held in place by adhesive tape around the forearm. (From Flatt, Adrian E.: J. Bone Joint Surg. **39-B:**80, 1957.)

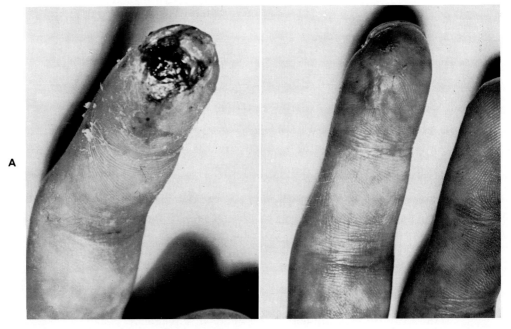

**Fig. 8-6.** *Detaching the thenar flap.* A flap should normally be detached after fourteen days. In this case the flap was detached after seven days, and only the portion of the flap near the nail bed had sufficient blood supply to survive, **A.** The remainder of the area was allowed to heal by granulations and a thin tender scar resulted, **B.** (From Flatt, Adrian E.: J. Bone Joint Surg. **39-B:**80, 1957.)

The finger should be immobilized by a long malleable aluminum splint padded with foam rubber on its contact surface. The splint should pass over the flexed finger and be molded over its contours and then passed proximal to both surfaces of the wrist. It can be held in position by an adhesive bandage passed around the wrist and forearm (Fig. 8-5). The finger must be carefully positioned so that there is neither too great tension nor too much compression on the flap. Ideally the base of the flap should be kept at about right angles to the surface of the palmar skin. The best position for immobilization of the finger is shown in Fig. 8-5.

**AFTERCARE.** The raw surfaces of the finger and flap will weep, and the exudate will soon begin to smell. Dressings should be renewed every three to four days, and this changing can be done easily from the side of the finger without disturbing the splint. Despite the discharge, healing proceeds rapidly, and the flap can be safely detached after fourteen days. The length of time that the flap is attached is important. Experience has shown that attachment for two weeks is quite sufficient to allow a satisfactory blood supply to grow into the flap from the finger. To separate the flap earlier than this will inevitably lead to loss of most of the flap (Fig. 8-6). To leave it attached for a longer period will not improve the blood supply and will invite a stiff finger (Fig. 8-7).

### Detaching the flap

For the flap to be detached, the base should be infiltrated with 2% lidocaine local anesthetic, and it should be cut cleanly across at the level where it bends at a

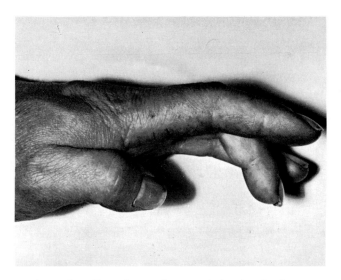

**Fig. 8-7.** *Detaching the thenar flap.* There is no advantage in leaving the flap attached for longer than two weeks, since an adequate blood supply is established during this time. In this case the finger was held in flexion for a longer period of time, and permanent contracture resulted. (From Flatt, Adrian E.: J. Bone Joint Surg. **39-B:**80, 1957.)

90-degree angle to the palmar skin. The palmar defect is readily closed if a few interrupted sutures are passed through the split-skin graft at the site of the detachment of the pedicle. A small adhesive dressing is usually sufficient protection for this area.

Any obviously dirty granulations on the flap's raw or deep surface should be trimmed, and any portion of the split-skin graft that has taken near the base should be removed. The raw area of the fingertip should also be cleansed of any obviously necrotic fat and dirty granulations. The skin edges of both the flap and finger area should be trimmed to 90-degree angles to the surface to allow proper seating of the flap and to get good skin apposition. Only a few millimeters of skin edge should be removed. It will usually seem that the flap is too long and that it sticks out too prominently from the fingertip. These factors are, however, advantages, since they create a properly curved surface for the fingertip when the flap is sutured to the proximal edge of the finger wound. The flap should be sutured all around its three sides with No. 5-0 nylon sutures. No drains should be placed beneath it.

**DRESSINGS.** The fingertip should be dressed with a small piece of Telfa and an equivalent-sized piece of dry-sponge dressing, and these two dressings should then be held in place by a Tubegauz bandage.

The donor site for the split-skin graft should now have its dressings removed. It will usually be perfectly healed and will require no further coverage. If, however, there are still small unhealed areas, then Telfa or small adhesive dressings should be used according to the size of the unhealed area.

**AFTERCARE.** Active movements of the hand and particularly of the finger that has been immobilized should now be encouraged, but, because of the palmar defect, it is unwise to allow the patient to return immediately to heavy work.

The sutures in the fingers and the palm should be removed seven to ten days after separation of the flap. At this time the fingertip is ugly and irregular, but over the next few weeks the flap will settle in very rapidly to produce a well-padded fingertip that will rapidly regain normal finger sensation.

### Disability

The patient who suffers a pulp loss of one of his fingertips and who does not have the type of surgery described will certainly be left with a marked and permanent disability. The disability will be pronounced even if the wound is closed with a split-skin graft. Any operation that does not replace the lost pulp and skin with similar pulp and skin from the hand can produce only an inferior result in comparison with the thenar flap procedure. If, however, a thenar flap is correctly used to provide the necessary skin and padding for the finger, there will be absolutely no permanent disability.

While the patient who has the finger skin-grafted can frequently return to work the same day, the thenar flap procedure will keep a patient from work for as long as a month. Many insurance companies do not care to cover this operation because of the length of time off work and because of the bad, but undeserved, reputation

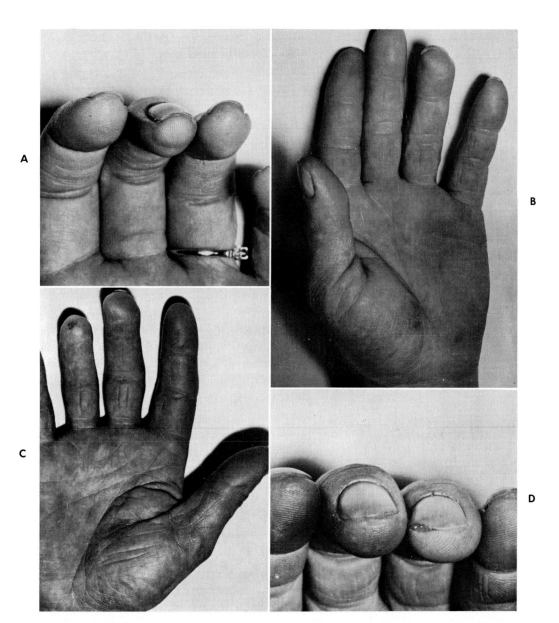

**Fig. 8-8.** *Replacement of pulp loss by a thenar flap.* Four illustrations of the type of result that can be obtained by the use of a thenar flap. **A** and **B,** Results obtained in the long finger. **C** and **D,** Results obtained in the ring finger. (From Flatt, Adrian E.: J. Bone Joint Surg. **37-B:**117, 1955.)

that the operation has acquired. However, there can be no doubt that if the patient accepts the fact that he may not be able to return to work for a month, he should be offered the benefit of an operation that will provide him with a virtually normal finger (Fig. 8-8).

Several other useful procedures that utilize local tissue to provide good pulp and skin cover for the fingertip have been described. The successful planning and execution of these operations demands a higher degree of judgment and surgical skill than is needed in employing the thenar flap. Others may disagree with this view, and some appropriate references to these more difficult procedures are included at the back of the book.

## Proximal and middle phalanx injury

Loss of skin and subcutaneous tissues on the palmar aspect of the proximal part of the finger frequently leaves the flexor tendons and bones exposed. Such extensive loss of tissue cannot be properly replaced by a split-skin graft. Full-thickness skin with its subcutaneous tissues is needed to provide a sufficiently well-padded area on the working surface of the hand. Skin with its subcutaneous tissues can only be moved to a new site on a vascular pedicle. If such skin is to be used, it must therefore remain attached to its donor site throughout the period of healing.

Many areas are available as donor sites, but by far the most suitable is the finger next to that which has been wounded. If the chest or abdomen is used as a donor site, the skin is of poor quality, and there are great problems in maintaining the correct position of immobilization. Cross-arm flaps can also be used, but the attachment of one arm to the other handicaps the patient so greatly that he is unable even to scratch himself whenever or wherever he desires.

Cross-finger flaps can be raised from the dorsum and side of an adjacent finger and placed into the defect on the wounded finger without tension. The defect created by raising the flap is covered by a split-skin graft.

The dorsal skin of masculine fingers is often hair bearing; however, this is not a contraindication to the use of this skin. Frequently many of the hairs will die after the transposition of the flap, and any hair that survives can be shaved or be permanently removed by electrolysis.

### Operation

This procedure is not one for a novice. Some experience is needed to obtain a successful result.

**OPERATIVE TECHNIQUE.** The selection of the donor site is the most important step in the operation. There is a choice of donor sites for the ring and long fingers, but there cannot be a choice for the border fingers. For a defect on the ring finger, it is usually better to choose the long finger as the donor, because the area of skin available on the small finger is frequently restricted.

The flap can be planned with its base lateral, proximal, or distal. A lateral base is usually by far the most satisfactory. Because of the problems of venous drainage, a flap based distally should not be used unless it is absolutely essential. The proportions of the flap should be the standard 1:2, width to length. Often in flaps based laterally these proportions are reversed so that the width of the base is twice the length of the flap. Such reversal gives an excellent blood supply to the flap.

If possible, the flap should be planned to leave in place the skin over the proximal interphalangeal joint. If the defect is so large that the skin over the joint cannot be left in situ, there should be no hesitation in including it in the flap. The whole area can be satisfactorily replaced by a split-skin graft.

ANESTHESIA. The wounded and donor fingers should both be given metacarpal blocks with 2% lidocaine. An additional area about 8 cm² on the upper part of the flexor aspect of the same forearm should also be infiltrated with 2% lidocaine (Fig. 4-6). This area will serve as the donor site for the split-skin graft needed to cover the defect created by raising the flap.

While the local anesthetic is taking effect, the forearm should be thoroughly cleansed. The entire hand is covered with sterile towels, which may be placed over the wound dressings. The upper arm should also be toweled off so that a thick split-skin graft can be cut from the anesthetized area. The graft can be cut with a razor blade or hand-held knife and should be stored in a saline-dampened sponge. The amount of skin needed can be judged by looking at the size of the dorsum of the donor finger. The donor site should be immediately dressed with Telfa, saline-dampened sponges, and a stretchable bandage.

After the skin-graft donor site has been dressed, the wounded finger can be satisfactorily cleansed since the anesthetic will have taken effect. Thorough débridement must be carried out, and the skin edges of the wound must be excised to give a straight edge. It may be necessary to enlarge the defect to properly accommodate the flap. It is important not to create a longitudinal scar on the palmar aspect of the finger, and the flap should be carried to the neutral or midlateral line of the finger.

When the size of the skin defect has been established, an accurate pattern should be cut out of some semirigid material, leaving sufficient base on the pattern for the pedicle to be drawn on the donor finger (Fig. 8-9). A useful material is the sterile tinfoil used to package petrolatum gauze or scalpel blades. The flap is designed to be based on a pedicle that is adjacent to the wounded finger. When the dorsal skin is lifted up and turned over on its base, the raw undersurface of the flap will be in contact with the raw area of the wound (Fig. 8-9).

The pattern should be laid on the donor finger so that the edge of the flap will be on the lateral neutral border of the finger. This border is defined by a line joining the apices of the creases at the proximal and distal interphalangeal creases (Fig. 15-12, p. 292). When the pattern has been accurately placed, it should be outlined with an ink such as methylene blue. It is wise to draw the outline slightly larger than the pattern to avoid risk of tension on the flap when it is sutured into place. The two corners should be drawn slightly rounded rather than as neat right angles. The blood supply of such rounded corners is good, and they are more easily sutured into the wound than 90-degree corners.

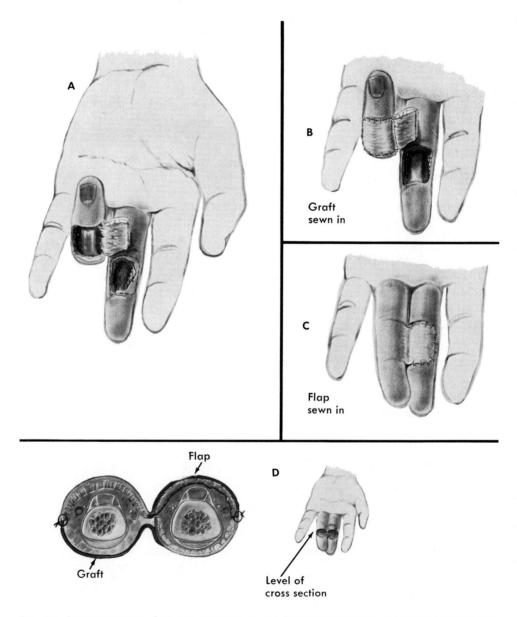

**Fig. 8-9.** *Cross-finger flap.* Skin and pulp loss on the flexor aspect of the proximal or middle pha-langes is best replaced by skin from the dorsum of an adjacent finger. **A,** Flap raised on the dorsum of the ring finger suitable to replace the defect outlined on the long finger. **B,** The raw area created by raising the flap has been covered by a split-skin graft. **C,** The flap is sutured into the defect along three sides. **D,** A cross-sectional drawing to show how no sutures are placed in either the flap or graft along the junctional area between the two fingers.

### Raising the flap

The three sides of the flap should then be cut with a No. 15 scalpel. Both skin and subcutaneous tissues should be cut through, but care must be taken to avoid cutting into the tendon or the peritendinous tissues. The far edge of the flap should be raised with skin hooks, and the plane of cleavage between the deep surface of the subcutaneous tissues and the paratenon should be found. Dissection with scissors opening parallel to the surface of the skin easily separates the two layers of tissues (Fig. 8-9). This dissection is carried down to the lateral side of the finger to a plane just dorsal to the digital neurovascular bundle. This bundle is protected by a layer of fibrous tissue passing from the deep surface of the dermis to the peritendinous tissues. These fibers will have to be cut to give sufficient mobility to the base of the flap.

The flap should be tested repeatedly against the area in which it is to be seated. As soon as it lies in place without tension, dissection around the base can be stopped. The flap should now be covered with a moist sponge and left while the donor site is grafted. If there are any large spurting vessels, these will have to be clamped. Oozing areas may be left, since they will dry up during the time the skin graft is being sutured into the donor site.

### Placing the skin graft

The donor site must be completely dry before the graft is sutured into place. Bleeding vessels should be caught in hemostats and twisted off (Fig. 4-1). If catgut is used to ligate a vessel, the graft will not take at the site of the foreign body. Pressure with moist sponges will help control any oozing. If dry sponges are used, they will prolong the bleeding by tearing off the blood clot as it forms in the mesh of the sponge.

When the field is dry, the graft should be sutured into the defect. One end of the sutures should be left long so that they can be tied over a dressing to maintain an even pressure on the graft. Sutures can be placed on three sides of the defect, but no sutures should be passed through the base of the flap. The graft should be left long at this site so that it can be pressed down into the groove between the adjacent fingers after the flap has been sewed into place. The dressings should not be tied on until after the flap has been sutured into place.

### Placing the flap

The flap should be sutured in place with interrupted sutures of fine monofilament nylon. The two corners should be placed first and sufficient sutures placed around the three sides to hold the edges of the flap and skin wound accurately together. Sometimes the flap will tend to tent over the depths of the skin wound. It is unwise to place any quilting sutures in the middle of the flap to hold it down because this could cause serious disturbance of the blood supply. It is also unwise to place a drain beneath the flap because of the risk of introducing infection and because the drain may cause a pressure necrosis of part of the flap. A carefully built-up dressing is quite sufficient to overcome this tenting and to obliterate the dead space.

After the flap has been sutured in place, the skin graft should be placed deep in the cleft between the fingers (Fig. 8-9). It should cover any raw surface on the base of the pedicle and then should come up the side of the wounded finger so that the graft covers the edge of the wound across which the pedicle is lying.

**DRESSINGS.** Two areas must be dressed. On the dorsum of the hand a small piece of Telfa that has been cut to the appropriate size should be placed on the graft. A dressing of moistened cotton wool pledgets is then built up over the graft and in the cleft between the fingers. The fingers must not be forced apart by this dressing, since such forcing apart will stretch the pedicle and jeopardize the blood supply of the flap. After the dressing has been built up sufficiently, a piece of gauze sponge is placed on top and the long sutures tied over to maintain constant mild pressure on the grafted area.

When the graft dressing is tied in place, the hand should be turned over and a similar but less bulky dressing made to fit the area of the flap. This dressing is not held in place by ties. The two fingers must then be slightly flexed and placed on a padded metal splint broad enough to accommodate the two fingers. The splint should cross the wrist and lie on the flexor aspect of the forearm, holding the wrist joint in the functional position. The fingers should be lightly bandaged onto the splint, and the forearm should rest in a sling. The patient must be warned to keep the hand at rest in the sling throughout the time the flap is attached. However, he should be encouraged to do shoulder and elbow exercises every day.

**AFTERCARE.** There will be a small amount of exudate from the area of the base of the pedicle. However, if the skin graft has been correctly placed, there will be no raw surfaces, and the amount of exudate will be minimal.

The dressings over the graft and the flap should be changed on the fourth postoperative day. The ties holding the dressing in place over the graft can be cut short since they will not be required for future dressings. If both the graft and the flap are healing well, the dressings should be replaced with Telfa and dry sponges cut to the appropriate size. They can then be left undisturbed until the pedicle is separated.

If a hematoma is present under either the graft or the flap, it must be removed either by cutting a small hole in the graft or by removing a suture from the side of the graft or flap. Holes must not be cut in the flap for drainage purposes. After the hematoma has been evacuated. Telfa and dry-sponge dressings are cut so that slight pressure can be applied when the bandages are replaced.

The fingers must be immobilized for two weeks. After this time the blood supply will have grown into the flap from the sides of the wound sufficiently well to support the skin and subcutaneous tissues when the base is severed.

### Detaching the flap

The pedicle should be cut across two weeks after the time of operation. Although it is possible to separate it a day or two earlier, especially if the base is broader than the length of the flap, there is no advantage in earlier separation since there is no risk of stiffness of the fingers when they are held in the functional position for such a short length of time.

Using 2% lidocaine, both fingers should be anesthetized by a metacarpal block after the dressings have been removed. When the anesthetic has taken effect, the fingers should be cleansed and the pedicle cut. The exact line of separation of the pedicle is determined by the line of the fourth and unsutured side of the wound. The pedicle should be cut across on this line with a sharp scalpel. After the fingers have been separated, it is advisable to cleanse the web space between them because an appreciable amount of exudate and epithelial debris usually collects at this site.

The sutures should now be removed from both the flap and the skin graft. The fourth side of the original wound has usually become somewhat mushy during the two weeks of immobilization. The edge should be trimmed before the cut edge of the flap is sutured in place. Interrupted fine monofilament nylon sutures should be used. The base of the flap is usually sticking out from the side of the donor finger with the graft on its upper surface. This flap must be returned to the donor finger in such a manner that its cut edge lies along the line of the neutral border of the finger. The amount of flap and/or graft that has to be excised will depend upon the length of the pedicle. The graft can be cut across on the line of the neutral border and the flap turned in to meet it. Sutures can be passed through the graft provided that they are passed relatively deeply.

**DRESSINGS.** Each finger should be individually dressed with the minimum amount of dressings. Splints are not necessary for the fingers. If it is likely that the patient will not obey instructions to keep the fingers relatively still, then bulky dressings will be an efficient means of allowing only minimal movement. After the fingers have been dressed, the original dressings covering the skin graft donor site should be removed from the forearm. The area is usually healed, and no further dressings are necessary. If the site is not fully healed, similar dressings should be applied until healing is complete.

**AFTERCARE.** The fingers should be kept relatively still until the sutures are removed after ten to fourteen days. As soon as the wounds are healed, there is no need for dressings, and active use of the hand should be encouraged.

The patient should be warned about the immediate lack of sensibility in the transposed flap and the consequent risk of damage to the skin. Sensibility will return to the flap to a greater degree than it would return to a split-skin graft, but it will be many months before the recovery is complete.

The skin graft on the dorsum of the donor finger may tend to contract during the first few months after surgery. This contraction can be counteracted if the patient frequently massages the grafted area with lanolin or similar substance.

## THE THUMB

Pulp loss from the distal or proximal phalanx of the thumb is uncommon. The importance of the thumb is so great that full-thickness cover for the loss in either area must be provided. Local flaps from adjacent areas can supply the necessary skin

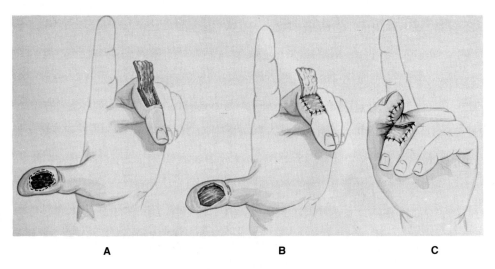

| A | B | C |

**Fig. 8-10.** *Thumb: distal phalanx pulp loss.* Skin and pulp loss from the distal phalanx of the thumb is replaced by a flap raised from the dorsum of the long finger. **A,** Flap raised from the dorsum of the middle phalanx of the long finger; the amount of tissue to be excised from the edges of the skin wound has been outlined. **B,** The area of skin loss created by mobilizing the flap has been closed by a split-skin graft, and the edges of the wound have been excised. **C,** The flap is rotated, and the end and distal portions of the sides are sutured into the thumb wound.

and subcutaneous tissues. Loss from the distal phalanx should be replaced by a flap raised from the dorsum of the middle phalanx of the long finger. Loss from the proximal phalanx is repaired by a flap raised from the tissues on the radial side of the metacarpal of the index finger.

### Distal phalanx injury

The long finger is selected as the donor site for two reasons: first because it is wise to avoid using the index finger as a donor site and second because the thumb rests naturally against the radial side of the long finger. The dorsum of the middle phalanx of this finger is usually both wide and long enough to supply sufficient skin to cover any loss on the flexor aspect of the distal phalanx. The flap is based proximally, and its distal end is slightly rotated so that it can be sewed to the thumb. The exact site and line of reflection of this flap needs careful selection. Fig. 8-10 illustrates a flap designed parallel with the sides of the donor finger, but on occasion it may be better to plan a more obliquely lying flap to ensure proper coverage without kinking the root of the flap.

The detailed steps of the procedure are similar to those of the cross-finger flaps used in the fingers and described on p. 142. Occasionally it may be necessary to encroach on the skin covering either, or both, of the interphalangeal joints in order to obtain sufficient skin for the thumb. Because of the importance of the thumb, this transgression is justified. Only a relatively small encroachment can be tolerated, and great care must be taken to supply good skin over the joint areas. The split-skin

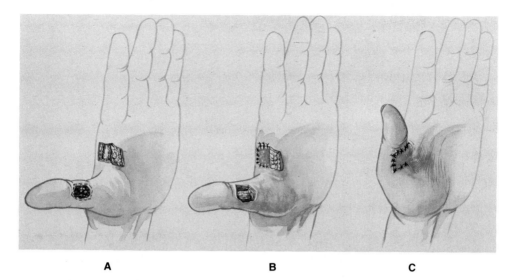

**A**          **B**          **C**

**Fig. 8-11.** *Thumb: proximal phalanx tissue loss.* Skin and subcutaneous tissue loss on the flexor surface of the proximal phalanx can be replaced by a flap raised from the tissues over the index metacarpal. **A,** Line of excision of the edges of the thumb wound; the flap is raised to fill this defect. **B,** The thumb wound edges have been trimmed and a split-skin graft sewed into the raw area created by raising the flap. **C,** The flap is sutured into the defect along three sides.

graft must always be sewed into place. Postoperative immobilization is sometimes difficult. It is hard to devise efficient metallic splints, and the best support is supplied by molded light plaster-of-paris splints. The base of the flap should be severed at fourteen days.

## Proximal phalanx injury

Tissue loss over the flexor aspect of the proximal phalanx can be covered by skin and subcutaneous tissue raised from the ulnar side of the cleft between the thumb and the index finger (Fig. 8-11). The skin and subcutaneous tissues on the radial side of the index metacarpal are mobilized on a flap. The hinge or base of the flap is placed on the palmar aspect of the side of the index metacarpal. The size of the flap needed must be accurately measured by making a pattern of the thumb defect.

The principles of the operation are the same as those used for cross-finger flaps and are described on p. 142. Postoperative immobilization is not difficult, and simple dressings are usually sufficient. The flap may be detached from its base after fourteen days.

AFTERCARE. Both distal and proximal phalangeal flaps are subject to the same immediate lack of sensation as a cross-finger flap. The patient must be particularly warned to protect the transposed skin during the period of sensory recovery.

# 9 · AMPUTATIONS

**Factors influencing level of amputation**

**Amputations of the fingers**
    Partial amputation
        Distal phalanx injuries
        Middle and proximal phalanx injuries
    Complete amputation

**The severed fingertip**

**Amputations of the thumb**

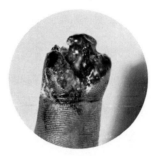 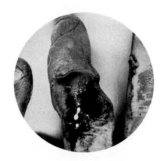

**Complete amputation**        **Partial amputation**

**D**uring the primary care of patients with traumatic amputations the preservation of length is of fundamental importance. If, at the end of surgery, the amputation stump looks untidy but has obtained good skin cover and preserved even an extra 0.5 cm of effective length, then the correct primary treatment has been given. A sense of tidiness is a liability when treating these injuries. There is no need to follow the recommended ideal levels of elective amputations. It is the patient's privilege to subsequently decide if the stump is not cosmetically or functionally acceptable.

Such dogmatic advice invites controversy, but in the case of the thumb the importance of length is so fundamental that the advice is good. The decisive factor in determining the length of an injured finger must be the patient's occupation. Amputations cannot be adequately cared for until a careful history has been taken to show how each digit is used in the patient's work. Apart from the patient's occupation, the level of amputation is influenced by which finger has been injured, the degree of damage, and whether the patient is a child or adult.

The aim of primary care of amputation of digits is to maintain as much length as possible consistent with good skin coverage. When the maintenance of length is all important, bone should not be sacrificed to obtain skin flaps, because skin grafting can provide adequate cover for the stump.

There has been a recent revival of the traditional "do nothing" approach to these

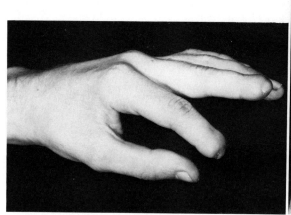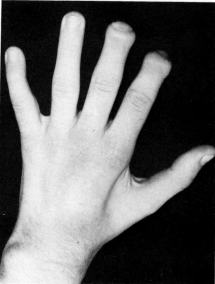

**Fig. 9-1.** *Fingertip amputations.* The "do nothing but a dressing" advocates sometimes have too great a faith in the power of healing. This boy's index and long fingers did eventually heal, but the resultant scarring has produced permanent deformity of the nails.

injuries. The proponents of the dressing-only technique maintain that the regenerative capacity of the fingertip is unique and remarkable and that therefore to dress the raw area with a flap or a skin graft is unnecessary. I am unconvinced. I have seen too many painful puckered fingertips to believe that this is a routinely successful method of treatment.

It is probable that areas up to about 1 cm² may heal satisfactorily, but larger areas lead to so many secondary contractures that significant deformity can result. The patient shown in Fig. 9-1 had the tip amputations of his index and long fingers treated by a "do nothing" proponent. He came with a "do something" plea for restoration of his fingertips and fingernails. It could not be done. The treatment had been incorrectly used in fingers that had lost too much bony length, and there was no support for the growing nails that curved in response to the scarring.

Ultimately, the majority of patients are grateful for the retention of stump length. At the time of surgery, it may take some persuasion to overcome the common attitude of "just cut it off back a bit, Doc." This attitude tends to be encouraged by the policy of some insurance companies to assess compensation by joint levels rather than by restoration of function.

## FACTORS INFLUENCING LEVEL OF AMPUTATION
### Occupation

Finger length may be of such importance to the patient's occupation that it will override the normal indications for amputation. Total amputation of a digit would be disastrous to a violinist, but a surgeon could adapt to such a loss. Amputation of the distal portions of several fingers can be equally crippling to patients with various occupations.

Administrators and some desk workers do not need fingers or even hands to earn their living. However, the appearance of the hand is often important, and the retention of fingers that may become totally stiff is quite justified in some instances.

Between these two extremes lie the manual laborers. Usually the man who performs heavy work with his hands is not unduly concerned about their appearance. Stiff fingers would be a nuisance and even a liability in his work, and amputation is therefore the treatment of choice for some patients.

## Digit injured
### The thumb

The thumb is the fundamental digit for the function of opposition, and all possible length must be preserved. Pinch is most easily and accurately carried out against the radial fingers, and preservation of length of the index and long fingers is therefore of great importance.

### The index finger

The index finger is principally used in opposition to the thumb in fine pincer movements needed to pick up a small object. Length of the index finger is therefore important. If the amputation has been proximal to the insertion of the flexor superficialis muscle, the remaining stump is too short for accurate pincer movements and the long finger will be used instead.

Amputation of the remaining stump of the index finger may be carried out as a secondary procedure but should not be done at the primary operation. Many patients will learn to use the long finger for pincer grasp but will still use the stump of the index finger for a variety of pinch and grasp functions (Fig. 9-2).

If either of the border fingers (index finger or small finger) has to be amputated at the level of the metacarpophalangeal joint, a problem arises concerning the bulky metacarpal head. In laborers, especially, the head of the metacarpal should not be amputated. When the head is left in place, adequate breadth is still maintained in the palm of the hand (Fig. 9-3). In all other patients it is also best to leave the metacarpal head in place at the time of primary surgery. Beveling of the outer side of the head is advisable to reduce the prominence on the borders of the hand. Many persons in light occupations also find the head of the amputated digit a useful portion of the hand and do not welcome a reamputation on an oblique plane through the metacarpal shaft. For those who do wish it, such an operation can be easily performed as a secondary procedure (Fig. 9-4).

### The ulnar three fingers

The ring and long fingers are less important than the other digits, and severe injuries of one or the other can be treated by amputation. The level of amputation

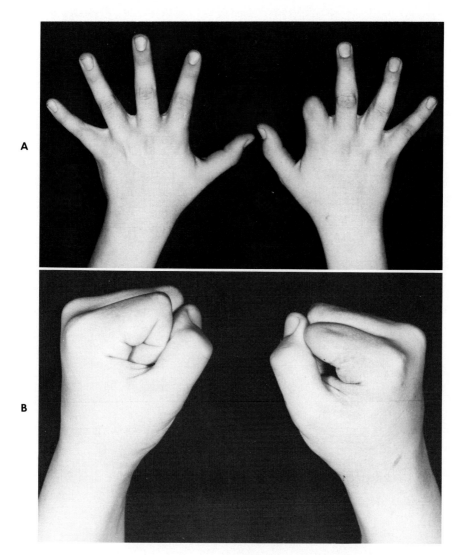

**Fig. 9-2.** *Index amputation.* **A,** When most of the proximal phalanx can be saved, the patient should be allowed to try using it. **B,** This boy uses his index stump in grasp and does not wish to be deprived of it.

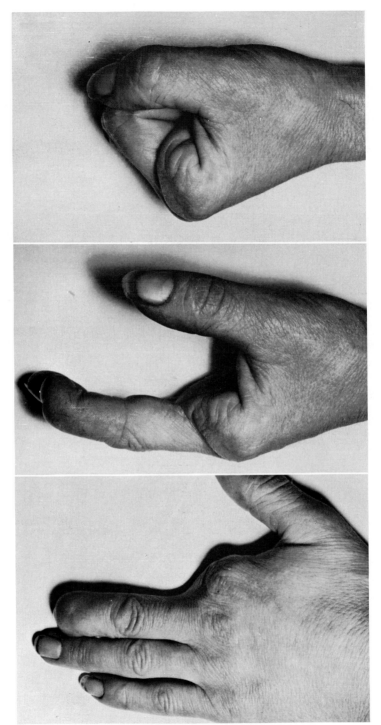

**Fig. 9-3.** *Amputation through the metacarpophalangeal joint.* Removal of the head of the metacarpal is not essential in these cases. This patient has worked for thirty-eight years in heavy industry and is thankful for the breadth of his palm.

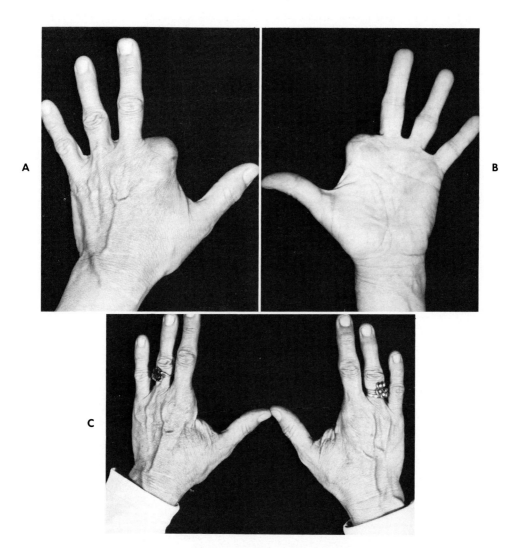

**Fig. 9-4.** *Index finger ablation.* **A** and **B,** This lady lost both her index fingers in a punch press. She returned to work but found the "knobs" a hindrance. **C,** Both metacarpals were amputated obliquely through their shafts. She states she can use her hands more easily and "nobody notices" the absence of her fingers.

on the long and ring fingers is unimportant if the index and small fingers are normal. Any length of stump will be of functional value provided that the finger joints are normal. The small finger is treated with scant respect by compensation schemes, yet it is of great importance in all forms of power grip. It cannot be amputated without causing appreciable loss of stability of grip, and preservation of its length is always desirable. The military recognizes the value of the digits. In a recent report on amputations in helicopter pilots it is recorded that "valuation of fingers in order of importance—thumb, index, small, long and ring—was considered."*

**Several fingers**

If several fingers have been damaged, the most conservative treatment is the best, and every attempt must be made to preserve length at the time of the primary operation (Fig. 9-5). The patient must be warned that it is possible that reamputation may be necessary later but that such a decision cannot be taken at the time of primary operation because of the impossibility of deciding how much functional recovery will subsequently take place.

---

*Humbert, P. V.: Evaluation and disposition of Army helicopter aviators with finger amputations, Aviat. Space Environ. Med. **48:**949-952, 1977.

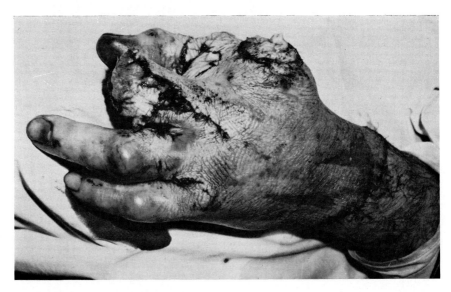

**Fig. 9-5.** *Preservation of length in amputations.* In the primary care of traumatic amputations neatness must give way to the preservation of length. In this case the index finger had to be sacrificed and a small portion of its palmar skin used to close the defect. Because the index finger was missing, it was vital to conserve length of the long finger. The use of local flaps produced a ragged looking closure but a reasonable length of finger.

## Degree of damage

In partial amputations, the bone is severed, but the distal portion remains attached by a soft tissue hinge. Many partially amputated fingertips will clearly survive, and their treatment is replacement. Occasionally the amputation is complete in everything but name. The skin bridge is so thin or so narrow that it cannot carry the neurovascular bundle necessary to support the distal end. In this type of amputation it is wise to cut the skin bridge, preserve the fingertip, and treat the wound as a complete amputation.

The techniques of microsurgical repair have become so efficient that many attempts are being made to replant amputated digits and limbs. This surgery is done in specialized centers, and the decision as to whether such an operation is possible must rest with the surgeons trained in these special techniques. Clean guillotine type amputations of several digits or across the hand may be suitable, whereas extensive crushing of the amputated part or heavy soil contamination is a contraindication to replantation. The primary physician's responsibility is to contact the replantation center staff, discuss the details of the injury, and, if a decision is made to attempt replantation, arrange rapid and suitable transportation both for the patient and the amputated part. The technical details of replantation are discussed in Chapter 16.

It is the badly damaged finger of doubtful viability that presents many problems in selecting the correct treatment. Any finger in which both palmar neurovascular bundles have been destroyed proximally cannot survive, and amputation must be carried out at or proximal to the level of the division of the nerves and vessels. Amputation should be considered for a finger in which one digital bundle has been destroyed and both flexor and extensor tendons damaged. When this degree of damage is combined with a fracture of the proximal or middle phalanx, then amputation is probably the best treatment. If both neurovascular bundles are intact despite other extensive damage, the patient must be offered the choice of amputation or preservation of the finger. It must be made clear that if he elects to keep the finger, he will be retaining a rigid digit that might be a liability to him in his occupation.

A finger with extensive skin loss frequently has other associated soft tissue damage and may need to be amputated. Amputation is even more likely to be needed if the skin loss is circumferential. If the soft tissue damage was caused by a crushing injury, the prognosis for the finger is poor. The inevitable necrosis and further tissue death following a severe crush injury will almost certainly condemn the finger, and it is best to remove it as primary treatment.

## Amputation of children's fingers

The healing powers of children are enormous, and attempts to preserve length that would be doomed to failure in an adult frequently succeed in a child's finger. Partially amputated fingers will almost invariably survive provided that the wound was not produced by a crushing injury. In complete amputations very little trimming of bone should be done, and no worries need be caused by leaving the epiphysis at the base of the phalanges. It is very unlikely that the skin growth at the tip of the amputation stump will not keep pace with the epiphysis. But if the growth of bone begins to stretch the skin of the fingertip, there will be plenty of time to plan secondary procedures.

## AMPUTATIONS OF THE FINGERS
### Partial amputation

Many wounds through the fingertip leave the distal portion of the finger attached by a small bridge of skin. The usual inclination is to complete the amputation immediately by snipping the remaining skin bridge with scissors. Such behavior is prodigal and should be avoided.

Careful clinical examination will often show that the distal portion is viable. If the circulation in the fingertip appears good, it will usually be found that the digital nerve has remained intact and the sensibility of the distal portion is also satisfactory. The state of the blood supply is best examined by very gently squeezing the distal portion and wiping its cut surface with a moist sponge to remove most of its blood content. If, after releasing the pressure, there is a ready return of color and the cut surface begins to ooze, the blood supply is satisfactory. The sensibility of the distal portion can be tested by a pinprick.

If both the circulation and nerve supply are good, the length of the finger should be preserved by suturing the distal portion back into place. If the blood supply to the tip is nonexistent, the amputation must be completed by cutting the remaining skin bridge. However, if the blood supply is good but the response to pinprick testing is poor, the tip should be sutured back into place in anticipation that a satisfactory nerve supply will develop at a later date.

The level at which the partial amputation has taken place is of great importance (Fig. 9-6). There is a considerable amount of tissue in a finger, and if this is to be supported by a single vascular bundle, the conditions must be ideal. If a single neurovascular bundle is neatly cut across at the base of a finger and no other damage done, the blood supply will usually be sufficient to support the finger if the patient is young. In elderly patients it is unlikely that the finger would survive.

Wounds through the distal phalanx involve only the pulp and the terminal bone, and the adequacy of their blood supply is no great problem. In more proximal wounds the flexor and extensor tendons must almost inevitably be damaged in addition to the bone and neurovascular bundles. Such extensive damage implies that very little function would be retained even if the finger did survive.

In general it can be said that fingers wounded distal to the level of the insertion of the flexor digitorum superficialis muscle in which the bone and the tendons are involved will survive if the wound is sutured.

Wounds of the proximal phalanx that involve both the tendons and bone jeopardize the function of the finger so much that, even if it survived replacement, it would be a useless finger. Complete amputation should be considered in such cases.

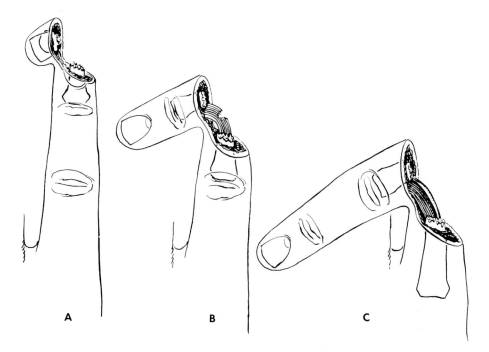

**Fig. 9-6.** *Partial amputation of the finger.* The finger can be injured at any level, but the injuries can be classified into three groups dependent on which bone of the finger is damaged. The more proximal the damage, the less likely it is that the single undamaged digital artery and its veins can support the finger. **A,** In distal phalanx amputations survival is almost certain. **B,** In amputations through the middle phalanx survival is probable. **C,** It is doubtful that a finger amputated through the proximal phalanx will survive.

### Distal phalanx injuries

The finger should be anesthetized by a 2% lidocaine metacarpal block. When cleansing the area of the wound, great care should be taken not to put additional strain on the skin bridge that attaches the distal portion to the main body of the finger.

When the loose portion is sutured in place, the nail is often a very useful landmark to ensure that the correct position has been obtained; the whorls on the fingertips can also be used as localizers. Interrupted sutures should be inserted around the periphery of the wound until it is closed (Fig. 9-7).

If the nail is attached to its bed, several sutures should be passed through holes drilled in the nail with a No. 11 scalpel blade. When the nail has been only partially avulsed, it should be replaced and anchored with sutures passed through it and the nail bed. Such replacement of the nail will give good protection to the dorsum of the fingertip during healing (Fig. 9-8). If the nail has been totally avulsed, the sutures will have to be passed through the nail bed and are likely to tear out unless great care is taken.

Frequently the terminal phalanx is fractured or cut across. No attempt need

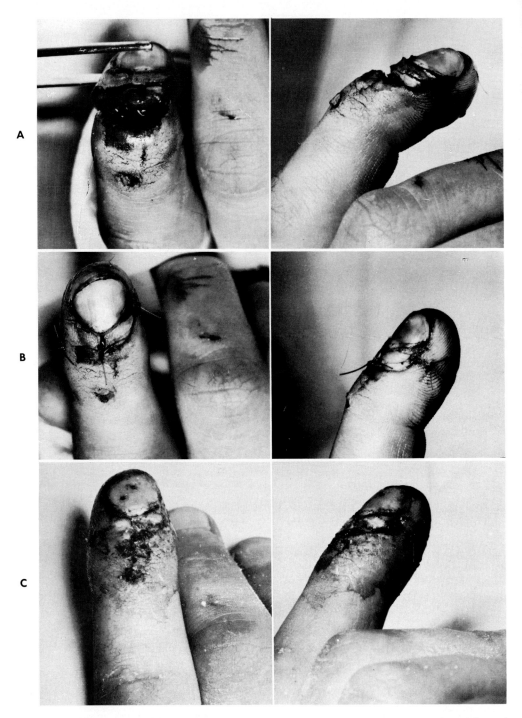

**Fig. 9-7.** *Partial amputation of the distal phalanx.* This series of photographs shows how a fingertip that is almost completely avulsed will survive after it is sutured back into place. **A,** The finger before treatment. **B,** Sutures in place; note how a suture has been passed through the nail. **C,** Survival of the fingertip three weeks after the original injury.

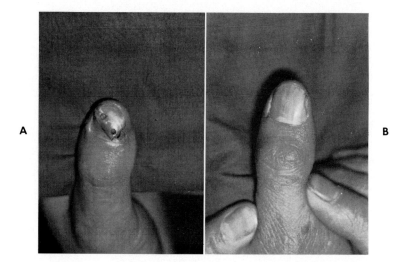

**Fig. 9-8.** *Partial avulsion of the nail of the distal phalanx.* When a partial amputation has partially avulsed the nail, it should be replaced, and sutures should be passed through it to hold both the nail and amputated tissues in place. **A,** The nail still attached and giving protection to the fingertip. **B,** The new nail that has grown up normally to displace the old nail. If the old nail had been removed, the new nail might well have been distorted.

be made to treat the fracture itself; if a correct soft tissue reposition is made, the bone ends will be brought together sufficiently well to allow union to proceed (Fig. 9-9). Even if the fracture does not unite, it is no great handicap, and only very rarely will any functional difficulties develop.

**DRESSINGS.** The finger should be kept as cool as possible by using the minimum of dressings. This cooling cuts down the metabolic rate and can on occasions make the difference between success and failure in this type of treatment. A piece of Telfa and a small piece of sponge dressing held in place by adhesive tape will usually be sufficient dressing for such injuries.

**AFTERCARE.** After operation, the hand must be kept elevated to about shoulder height for a day or two so as to aid the circulation by preventing the venous congestion that would occur in a dependent limb. There is usually a considerable seepage of serum from these injuries, and the dressings will need to be changed about every forty-eight hours.

Between the sixth and tenth days the color of the finger may be very depressing when it is dressed. Along the margin of the wound the thickened keratin of the palmar surface of the finger becomes whitened and rather soggy. The areas around the dorsum and the sides tend to become blackened and may even appear mummified. This change is caused by the death and separation of the superficial layers of keratin; however, beneath them the epithelium is alive. This darkened layer can be safely removed with forceps and scissors just as soon as it is ready to separate. The sutures can be removed after about ten to twelve days, by which time the finger-

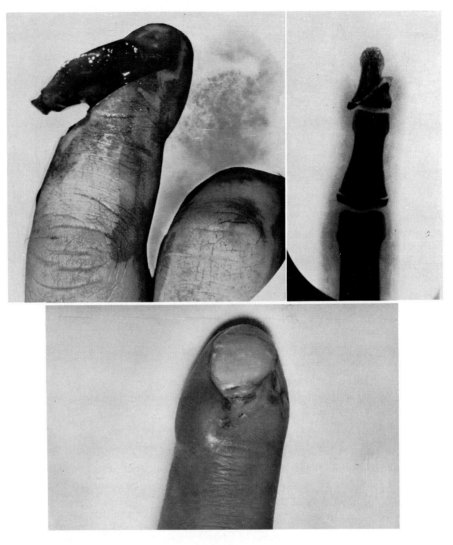

**Fig. 9-9.** *Partial amputation with phalangeal injury.* In cases in which the distal phalanx is fractured or cut across, the bone damage should be ignored and the soft tissues carefully sutured in place. In the finger shown it can be seen that the fingertip survived and that, although the bone was completely transected, the finger healed without significant distortion. (From Flatt, Adrian E.: J. Bone Joint Surg. **37-B:**117, 1955.)

tip can be left unprotected. The healed area is not yet secure and should certainly not be used for strenuous work or soaked in water for long periods of time.

### Disability

Full recovery from distal phalanx injuries usually takes a month from the time of wounding. Patients whose occupations involve heavy work will have to be away from work at least until the sutures are removed. After this time they will need to

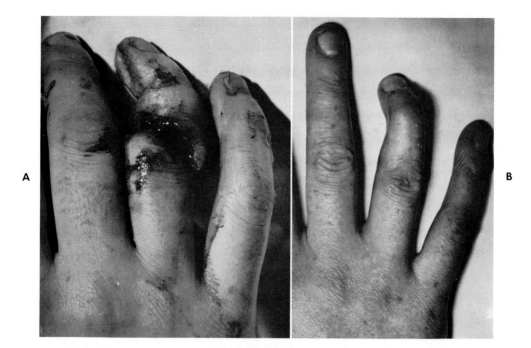

**Fig. 9-10.** *Partial amputation of the middle phalanx.* Uneven edges of these wounds need not be trimmed if the skin is viable. Careful suturing with interrupted fine nylon sutures will give a good result. **B,** Excellent skin healing but some distortion of the finger produced by concurrent injuries to the tendons.

protect the finger with some form of splint if they are to return to work.* Patients with light occupations may return to work the day after injury.

There is no permanent disability from this injury unless the nerve supply is totally destroyed. If the nerve supply has been destroyed, there will be atrophy of the pulp, and this will interfere with skilled work requiring use of the fingertip. The disability for a manual laborer is minimal.

### Middle and proximal phalanx injuries

The finger should be anesthetized by a 2% lidocaine metacarpal block, and the wound should be very carefully cleansed. In these more proximal wounds, there is danger of hemorrhage from the digital vessels. When the ends of the vessels are found they should be caught in mosquito hemostats and eventually twisted off (Fig. 4-1). There should be the minimum of trimming of the skin edges; uneven edges are acceptable if, by leaving them, more viable skin is retained. The skin wound must be carefully closed with interrupted sutures (Fig. 9-10).

---

*An excellent light splint can be made by coating three to four layers of Tubegauz bandage with water glass (sodium silicate). The splint hardens in twenty-four hours and can be removed with scissors or by soaking in warm water. I am indebted to Dr. Erroll Rawson of Seattle, Washington, for this information.

Fractures through these phalanges usually do well if reduction is maintained by internal fixation inserted at the time of primary surgery. Details of internal fixation can be found on p. 239. Internal fixation is particularly suitable for treating this type of injury because the surface of the fracture can be seen, and the wire can be introduced exactly in the center of the cross section of the fracture.

### Disability

Prognosis must be guarded in these cases. The main disability is caused by the damage to the bone and tendons. Bone union in the proximal and middle phalanges is relatively slow, and the finger may not be fit for even moderate work for a month from the time of injury. Mobilization of the joints will take several weeks. The tendons may be so damaged that they become adherent, and secondary tendolysis may have to be attempted.

DRESSINGS. See under Distal phalanx injuries, p. 161.

AFTERCARE. See under Distal phalanx injuries, p. 161.

## Complete amputation

The immediate aim of treatment of a freshly amputated finger stump is to provide skin cover with the maximum possible length of the finger. There are two fundamentally different ways of providing such skin cover: a skin graft can be sewed into place, or flaps can be mobilized to close over the raw stump. Each method has its protagonists, but neither should be used to the exclusion of the other. Frequently the amputation is of a slicing nature and automatically provides a dorsal-, lateral-, or palmar-based flap.

Problems arise when the amputation is of the clean-cut transverse type. If grafts are used, it must be appreciated that the grafts will become adherent by scarring onto the raw bone of the phalanx. This anchoring of the skin to the rigid underlying bone removes any potential mobility of the graft and therefore makes it more liable to damage by future trauma. In digits in which the preservation of length is vital, a thick split-skin graft should be used. If the amputated portion has been saved and is in good condition, full-thickness skin can be cut from it and used as the graft (Fig. 9-11).

If skin flaps are used, it is inevitable that some length of bone must be sacrificed in order to get a full-thickness cover of skin. This slight shortening is usually outweighed by the great advantages offered by immediate full-thickness cover with skin carrying normal finger-skin sensory powers. This type of amputation is frequently useful in patients in the semi-skilled and unskilled occupation groups.

In amputations through the middle phalanx, it is possible that after bone trimming less than half the length of the phalanx may be left. Should this be so, it would be wise to consider reamputation to the proximal joint as a primary measure. The flexion power of such short stumps is often restricted, and they may protrude during gripping or fist making.

In amputations through the proximal phalanx, even a short length of stump

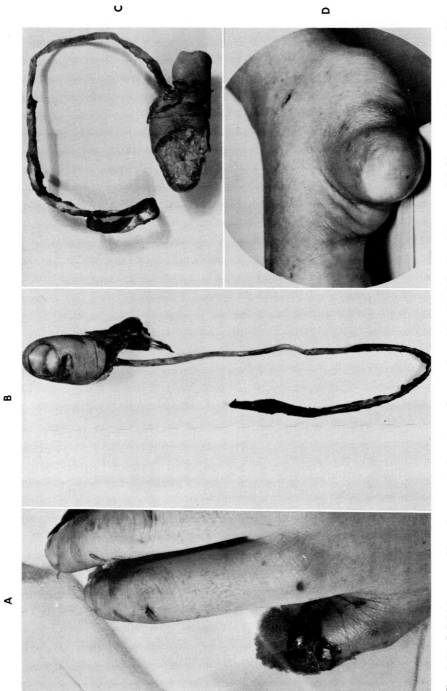

**Fig. 9-11.** *Full-thickness grafting of an amputation stump.* Preservation of length of the thumb is essential. The amputation stump should not be shortened to provide flaps for closure. **A,** The original injury at the level of the interphalangeal joint. In this case the patient brought her avulsed thumb, **B,** with her. **C,** Use of the skin of the distal phalanx to provide a full-thickness skin graft. **D,** Satisfactory result obtained.

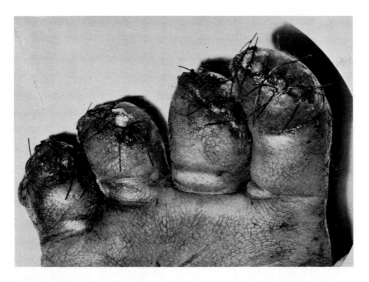

**Fig. 9-12.** *Multiple amputations.* When several fingers are amputated, even short lengths of the proximal phalanx should be preserved. In this case all available skin was used, and as a result the suture lines lay unevenly across the ends of the stumps. Since length is vital in these cases, the position of the suture lines is unimportant.

should be preserved at primary treatment (Fig. 9-12). The intrinsic muscles are usually able to flex such stumps quite satisfactorily, and they should not, therefore, be sacrificed.

Whatever treatment method is used, the flexor and extensor tendons that appear in the edge of the wound should not be sutured together. The tendons should be pulled down, cut off, and allowed to retract. Contaminated, dirty, or ragged tendons must not be allowed to retract into the clean proximal tissues; the site of their sections must be proximal to any potentially infected area. After they are cut, they will take up a position appropriate to the tone of their proximal muscle bellies, and there will be no interference with flexion and extension of the remaining stump. If, however, the tendons are sutured together over the end of the raw bone at the amputation site, they will become adherent to the bone and to each other, thereby destroying the delicate balance of movement between the flexor and extensor mechanisms of the hand.

### Operation
#### *Use of split-skin grafts*

The proximal part of the flexor aspect of the forearm on the injured side should be cleansed and an area 8 cm² injected and undermined with 2% lidocaine anesthetic (Fig. 4-6). The area around the base of the finger should then be surgically cleansed, and a metacarpal block should be induced with 2% lidocaine.

After the finger has been anesthetized, the skin graft should be taken; it can be cut with a grafting knife or a razor blade. A piece of skin approximately 3 cm² of the

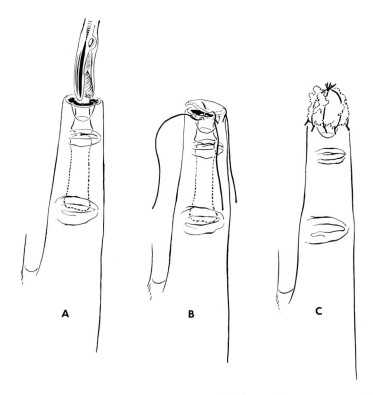

**Fig. 9-13.** *Split-skin grafting of an amputation stump.* **A,** It is usually necessary to nibble off protruding bone until the bone end lies a few millimeters below the level of the soft tissues. **B,** The graft must be sewed onto the end of the stump and one end of each suture left long. **C,** The long ends of the sutures are tied over the fluffed-up dressing to maintain an even pressure on the graft.

thick split-skin variety is best. The donor site should then be dressed with Telfa and dampened sponges held in place by a stretchable bandage. The skin graft should be stored in a saline-dampened sponge.

The hand and wounded finger should now be cleansed and a careful inspection made of the tissues at the amputation site. Any devitalized area must be removed, and the edges of the skin wound should be trimmed so that the graft will lie evenly upon them. It will usually be necessary to nibble off small pieces of protruding bone from the stump end with bone rongeurs (Fig. 9-13). It is advisable to cut back a few millimeters proximal to the level of the soft tissues in the hope that they will fall inward and tend to cover the raw bone end. Any bleeding vessels should be clamped with mosquito forceps and twisted off. Catgut must not be buried beneath the skin graft, because at the burial sites the graft cannot take. Cold compresses may help to stop any generalized oozing. However, a very slow ooze should not prevent one from putting the graft in place. The graft should be sewed into the defect, using interrupted sutures spaced evenly. If there is appreciable oozing of blood on the fingertip, a few very small drainage holes can be stabbed through the graft to prevent the formation of a hematoma. One end of each suture should be left long so that the dressings can be tied into place over the graft (Fig. 4-8).

DRESSINGS. A piece of Telfa should be cut to the size of the grafted area and placed with the plastic surface next to the graft. Pieces of wet cotton ball or small pieces of gauze dressings should then be built up over the end of the finger stump and held in place by tying the long ends of the sutures together (Fig. 4-8). The whole finger and its dressings should then be covered with a Tubegauz bandage.

AFTERCARE. On the fourth day the sutures should be cut so as to leave several long ends. All the dressings should be removed and the graft inspected. Usually the graft is completely successful and will already be showing pink areas of vascularization. Dressings similar to those which were removed should be used, and they should be tied into place with the long ends of the sutures.

Occasionally small blisters may be seen on the surface; these should be punctured. If the graft has failed completely, it must be removed. The finger should be dressed for a day or two until clean granulations are present before regrafting.

The dressings may now be left intact for another six to eight days. From about this time the graft will be well seated and the sutures can be removed. No protection will be needed for the fingertip except for a light covering when the patient is working. At this stage a skin graft is not ready to be plunged into hot detergent solutions while washing dishes. It will need at least another seven to ten days of consolidation before it is able to withstand such treatment.

### Use of full-thickness grafts

As a general rule, full-thickness skin grafts are not used to graft potentially dirty traumatic sites. Such grafts do not take as easily as split-skin grafts, and their use creates the difficulty of having to close their donor site.

Occasionally the amputated portion will be brought in with the patient. If it is in good condition, it would be wasteful to throw it away. A sufficiently large full-thickness graft can almost invariably be cut from the palmar aspect of the amputated portion (Fig. 9-11). If the fingertip has been completely avulsed by a crushing injury, it should not be sewn back nor should it be used as a donor site for a skin graft (Fig. 10-3, p. 185).

When taking the graft, great care must be exercised that all the fat is removed from the deep surface. If any fat is left, it forms an absolute barrier to the penetration of tissue fluids or granulation tissue, and the graft above it will die. The graft must be carefully sewed into place after meticulous care has been taken to obtain a bloodless recipient area.

About ten days after the operation, the graft will look dead, with peeling blackened areas on its surface. Such an appearance is very similar to that of the distal portion of a partial amputation stump, and for the same reason. The deeper dermal elements are living, but the more superficial epithelial and keratin layers are dying and being cast off. When these blackened areas are shed, they may leave what appears to be raw surface beneath them. The "raw" area is dermis, and, if it is protected from infection by adequate dressings, it will rapidly become epithelized on its surface.

### Use of skin flaps

Whatever type of flap is used to close the amputation stump, it is almost inevitable that the bone will have to be trimmed. This cutting back of the bone must be done with care, and the bone end must be neatly rounded off. The bony spicules produced by the trimming must be removed from the wound. If they are left in the tissues, they may be absorbed uneventfully, but sometimes they provoke a foreign-body-like reaction with resultant scarring. Sometimes the larger pieces may become actual sequestra and be a constant source of trouble until they are removed.

When the amputation stump is examined, the larger portions of skin should be thought of in terms of potential flaps for coverage of the fingertip. Ragged pieces that are clearly too small or nonviable should be discarded. The use of a little ingenuity with the viable flaps produced by the original trauma will often show that there is sufficient skin for closure of the amputation stump with only the minimum excision of bone. These flaps can be based anywhere around the circumference of the finger, but for purposes of description they are broadly classified as lateral, palmar, or dorsal.

If the amputation is a clean transverse cut across the finger, no flaps will be available for coverage. For the occasional inexperienced operator the best type of closure that allows preservation of maximum length is known as the fish-mouth closure. Equal-length dorsal and palmar flaps are fashioned, and the suture line runs transversely across the tip of the finger. The experienced hand surgeon may elect to close the defect with one or the other of the neurovascular island pedicle flaps that have been described (p. 175). These procedures should only be employed by surgeons with considerable experience and sound judgment.

**OPERATIVE PROCEDURES COMMON TO ALL FLAPS.** Before the area around the base of the finger is cleansed, the finger should be given a thorough preliminary washing to allow a metacarpal block to be carried out with 2% lidocaine. Nylon sutures, No. 5-0, should be used for skin sutures, and only the very finest catgut should be used for ligatures on vessels whose bleeding cannot be stopped by twisting off. After the anesthetic has taken effect, the stump can be properly cleansed and the tissues inspected. Any obviously dead, dirty, or devitalized tissues must be removed, including any ragged skin flaps that are not viable. The edges of the viable skin flaps should be trimmed at right angles to the skin surface.

If an amputation is through a joint, the condyles should be shaped and trimmed, particularly on the lateral sides, so as to prevent a bulbous end. It is advisable to excise the articular cartilage so that the subcutaneous tissues will gain a firm attachment to the bone. If the cartilage is left in place, the same attachment will eventually occur after the cartilage has degenerated. During this degeneration, it is possible that pieces of cartilage will detach and act as sequestra. These pieces will be extruded through a sinus in the stump and may cause a persistent discharge.

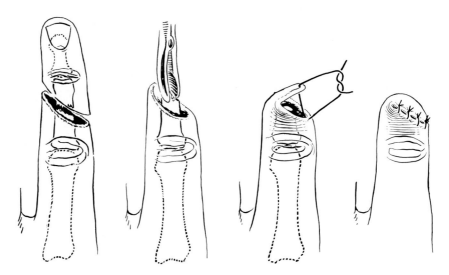

**Fig. 9-14.** *Flaps used in closing amputation sites—the lateral-based flap.* This flap can be used successfully when the amputation passes through the middle or proximal phalanx. A "dog ear" will be produced at the base of the flap.

When the ends of long flexor and extensor tendons are exposed in the amputation stump, they should be pulled down and cut off proximal to any contaminated area before allowing them to spring back into the more proximal portion of the hand.

In all except clean transverse amputations, the viable flaps should be rotated around the stump to see whether closure is possible. Usually the bone will have to be cut back to allow closure without tension. There should be enough skin available to allow some closure without tension and some eversion of the edges when the sutures are placed. Care should be taken not to excise too much fat from the deep surface of a flap in order not to interfere with the blood supply of the tip of the flap. If there is too much tension when the flap is stretched across the bone, it is better to excise a little more bone than fat and thereby make a more mobile fingertip that is not under tension. If the fat is cut away, the deep surface of the flap will adhere to the bone, and the skin will become tethered at this point. The flap will then be subject to just as much trauma as a skin graft, and little advantage will be gained by using the flap.

Often the rotation of a flap will create a "dog ear" or irregular protruding triangle of skin near its base. This "dog ear" should not be trimmed if there is any risk of interfering with the blood supply of the flap (Figs. 9-14 and 9-15). These "dog ears" usually settle down in a few months, but if they are persistently troublesome, a secondary trimming can be carried out several months after the primary operation when the stump is fully healed and a good blood supply has been established.

**DRESSINGS COMMON TO ALL FLAPS.** In all complete amputations the finger end should be capped with a small square of moistened Telfa. This should be covered

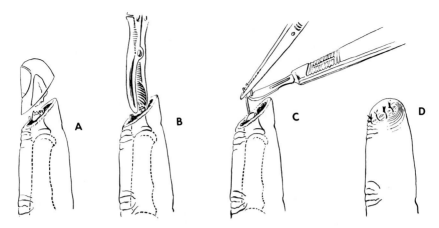

**Fig. 9-15.** *Flaps used in closing amputation sites—the palmar flap.* This flap is used when skin is available. In **B** the protruding bone is being cut back, and in **C** the digital nerves cut cleanly off after being pulled down. Note in **D** the "dog ear" that forms at the base of the flap.

with a very small amount of sponge gauze dressing. These dressings should be held in place with a Tubegauz bandage (Fig. 3-11).

**AFTERCARE COMMON TO ALL FLAPS.** Since no drains are used in complete amputations and virtually no oozing occurs, the dressings can be left undisturbed for at least a week. Any time after this the dressings can be changed and alternate sutures removed. If all goes well, the remaining sutures should be removed in forty-eight hours. They should certainly all be removed by the fourteenth day. When the sutures have been removed, there is no need for any further dressings. Patients should be warned that the superficial keratin layers will gradually be shed from the surface of the flaps.

Many patients will wish to wear some form of leather or plastic finger cot over the amputation stump. This protection can be encouraged for about the first three weeks. After this length of time the protection of the digit becomes a habit that is detrimental to good functioning of the hand.

*Dorsal flaps*

If dorsal flaps of skin are present, the nail and nail bed must have been amputated, and it is probable that the amputation passes through the middle phalanx. Despite the fact that dorsal skin is thinner and has less sensory discrimination than palmar skin, it is still quite adequate cover for an amputation stump. The bony phalanx should be trimmed back until the skin edges can be closed without tension. By using lateral or palmar flaps in addition to the dorsal flap, the amount of bone that has to be excised can be reduced. Using such flaps will place the suture lines over the end of the stump. Provided that the flaps are carefully sutured together without undue tension, the resultant scar is no handicap.

### Lateral and palmar flaps

Flaps that originally lie in the long length of the finger can be safely rotated 90 degrees and used as transverse coverage for the raw area. In amputations through the middle and proximal phalanges, these flaps give good coverage, and there are no difficult technical problems in their use (Figs. 9-14 and 9-15). If fat is to be removed from the deep surface of the flap, it should be done in a tapering fashion so that fat is present around the base of the flap but very thin at its tip. If other flaps of skin are present or can be easily made around the periphery, they should be utilized. By using them, addition length can generally be saved.

In amputations through the distal phalanx, considerable trouble is caused by the presence of the root of the nail. If the nail has been transected distal to the nail root area, it is advisable to suture the edge of the flap to the nail bed by passing the stitches through holes drilled in the nail with a No. 11 scalpel blade. If the area of the nail root has already been damaged, there should be no hesitation in cutting back the skin edge proximal to the nail root and totally excising the area. The lateral or palmar flap should then be sutured to the new dorsal skin edge (Figs. 9-14 to 9-16).

Excision of the nail root is one of the most difficult procedures in all of surgery. It is impossible to see the actual cells of the nail root, and the area of potential growth can only be guessed. The entire area decided on should be excised in one block. Piecemeal dissection and scratching about in the general area of the nail root will lead to seeding of nail root cells and the subsequent growth of nail spicules in aberrant areas. Frequently this nail spur will grow out from the site of union of the amputation flaps. The only cure for such troublesome nail fragments is excision. The patient should be warned of the technical difficulties and advised that repeated attempts at excision may be necessary.

### Equal-length flaps or fish-mouth closure

Equal-length flaps can be fashioned from a clean transverse amputation stump, either from the two sides or from the dorsal and palmar surfaces.

Lateral flaps can be used when the nail root is still intact, and it is important to preserve as much length as possible. The vertical scar down the fingertip is occasionally troublesome. Trouble occurs more usually, however, when the nail attempts to grow distally over the site of union of the lateral flaps with the nail bed. This T-shaped area of scar is usually irregular in level, and the nail does not adhere easily. As a result, the nail is frequently subject to trauma, and, because of pocketing of dirt in the irregular nail bed area, it is likely to get infected.

Equal-length palmar and dorsal flaps can be used when the amputation is through the proximal or middle phalanx or the proximal portion of the distal phalanx (Fig. 9-17). The line of suture is halfway between and parallel with the palmar and dorsal surfaces. The scar is therefore in a better position than the equal lateral flaps, since the feeling portion of the palmar surface of the finger stump is unscarred.

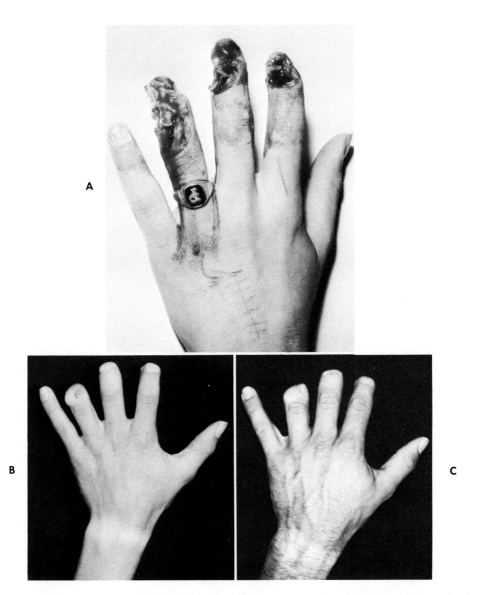

**Fig. 9-16.** *Palmar and lateral based flaps.* **A,** This patient scooped out the dorsum of the ends of his index, long, and ring fingers with a power tool. The index and long fingers were closed with palmar flaps and the ring finger with a flap based on its radial side. **B,** One year later the flaps are a little bulky, particularly in the ring finger. **C,** Ten years after injury the flaps have settled in, and he has a satisfactory hand.

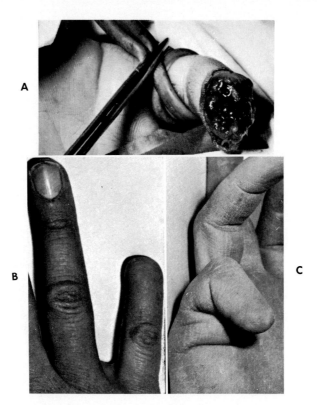

**Fig. 9-17.** *Fish-mouth closure.* In this case equal-length flaps were fashioned from the dorsal and palmar aspects of the finger. In **A** note the incorrect use of a rubber catheter as a tourniquet around the finger (see also Fig. 15-5, p. 280). (From Flatt, Adrian E.: J. Bone Joint Surg. **37-B:**117, 1955.)

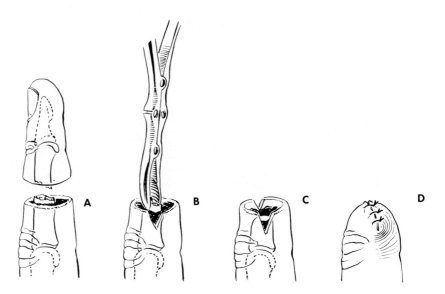

**Fig. 9-18.** *Flaps used in closing amputation sites—the fish-mouth closure.* Equal-length dorsal and palmar flaps are made by excising a narrow wedge-shaped area on the lateral sides of the finger, **C.** The tip of the bone has to be cut back to allow closure.

The incisions on the sides of the stump can be made equally well either with scissors or a sharp scalpel. In order to allow good closure, a V-shaped wedge of skin will have to be excised on opposite sides of the finger. For dorsal and palmar flaps the wedges are cut from the true lateral sides (Fig. 9-18). For lateral flaps the wedges have to be cut from the vertical midline of the finger on the dorsal and palmar surfaces.

Very little fat need be excised, and the bone should be nibbled back little by little until closure of the flaps is possible.

### Flaps and a graft

Occasionally a finger will be left with a viable flap that will cover the majority of the raw amputation stump but in which there is no hope of obtaining further local skin without cutting back the bone. If it is vital to maintain length, it is possible to sew the flap into place and to apply a thick split-skin graft to the remaining raw area. This combination of treatments is far from ideal but in special circumstances can be justified. Wherever possible, the flap should be rotated so that the palmar half of the finger stump is covered by flap skin. This rotation is advisable even if it means producing a "dog-ear" at the base of the flap and slightly increasing the area of raw surface left to be grafted. When this combination of treatment is used, both dressings and aftercare should be the same as if skin grafts had been applied.

Two methods using small triangular flaps separated from the surrounding skin and moved on soft tissue pedicles have been popularized in recent years. Both are

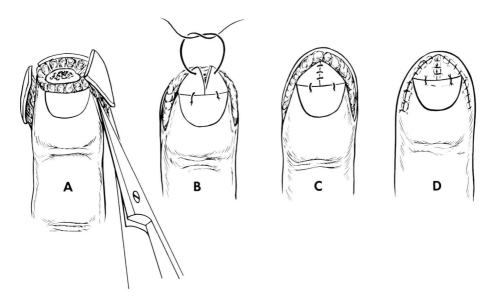

**Fig. 9-19.** *The Kutler method.* **A,** Two triangular flaps are mobilized on the sides of the fingers by dividing just enough pulp to allow them to be brought together in the midline. **B,** The flaps are sutured together. **C,** Some of the pulp has to be excised to allow the palmar skin to be brought up to the flaps. **D,** Final closure. (Modified from Fisher, R. H.: J. Bone Joint Surg. **49-A:**317, 1967.)

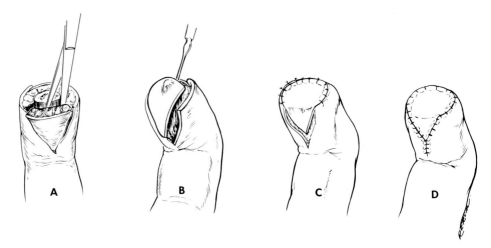

**Fig. 9-20.** *The Kleinert method.* **A,** The distally based triangular flap is developed by cutting only through the full thickness of the skin; on its deep surface it is separated from periosteum and flexor tendon sheath. **B,** The flap is mobilized sufficiently to bring its base up to the edge of the nail bed. **C,** It is sutured to the circumference of the fingertip. **D,** The V incision on the palmar aspect of the finger is closed by converting it to a **Y.** (Modified from Atasoy, E., Ioakanidis, E., Kasdan, M. L., et al.: J. Bone Joint Surg. **52:**921, 1970.)

excellent operations in the hands of their originators or other equally well versed in the subtlety of using these tiny flaps. The occasional and inexperienced operator will do his patient a disservice if he attempts these procedures. A brief description is included here so that a judgment may be made whether the patient would benefit from the full-thickness coverage that could be provided by these procedures.

The Kutler method develops a triangular flap on either side of the finger as in a fish-mouth procedure but moves these triangles on a neurovascular pedicle developed from the deep tissues. The triangles are moved to and sutured over the end of the finger. The wounds can then be closed without skin grafts (Fig. 9-19). When this method is used for an amputation as proximal as the middle third of the nail bed, long-term follow-up shows that the nail may curve over palmarward in a manner similar to that shown in Fig. 9-1.

The method developed by Kleinert and his associates mobilizes a simple palmar flap based distally and carried on a similar neurovascular pedicle derived from the deep tissues. The flap is moved distally over the end of the finger and the wounds closed in a V-Y fashion (Fig. 9-20).

Both procedures provide full-thickness innervated skin to the fingertip with minimal loss of length. The constraints on the indications and the problems of execution are fully described in the original papers.

### Disability

There is virtually no occupation to which a patient with a single amputated digit cannot return the day after injury. Unfortunately this idea is not generally accepted by the average patient. Even if the stump has been closed by a skin graft, there is no contraindication to returning to work if the graft has been properly sewed into place. The patient who does not return to work after surgery should certainly have done so by the time the last sutures are removed. Once the flaps have healed, there should be very little hypersensitivity of the tip—neuromas of the digital nerves are not common if the nerves have been cut cleanly across.

The permanent disability rating can be established only in relation to the performance of the patient's occupation. There is no constant relationship between length of finger lost and functional ability lost. Percentage disability ratings vary so much from state to state that no accurate guide can be given.

## THE SEVERED FINGERTIP

From time to time one hears of somebody who has a neighbor who knows somebody whose finger has been successfully sewn back after complete amputation. Attempts to arrange an introduction to the proud patient are usually unsuccessful, as are routine reattachments of amputated digits. Survival has been recorded in cases in which suitable microvascular techniques were employed; these techniques involve a type of surgery that is not performed in an emergency room.

If a very small portion of the tip of the digit has been cleanly severed, it may be treated as a free graft and sutured in place. The essentials of treatment are early and very accurate replacement of the fingertip, which must be kept cool both before and after surgery. If the tip has been amputated by a crushing injury, it is useless to sew it back; a split-skin graft is the treatment of choice (Fig. 10-3).

## AMPUTATIONS OF THE THUMB

The thumb is of such vital importance that it must never be amputated unless the situation is hopeless. Clinical judgment must be used, but it is useless to suture in place a thumb that has had all of its blood supply destroyed.

Partial amputations of the thumb usually survive satisfactorily. The final function is usually good because the thumb is short and the anatomy of its tendons is relatively uncomplicated. Complete amputations must be provided with skin cover. If the manner of amputation has not left any available skin flaps, maximum length should be preserved by using skin grafts rather than flaps fashioned after the further shortening of the bone.

The details of operative treatment of partial and complete amputations of the thumb are identical with partial and complete amputations of the finger. (See pp. 158 to 164 for partial amputation and pp. 164 to 177 for complete amputation of the finger.)

# 10 · CRUSH INJURIES

Crush injuries of the hand

The crushed finger

The crushed fingertip

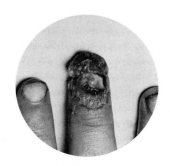

Crush injury

## CRUSH INJURIES OF THE HAND

**C**rush injuries are always serious. Although the epithelium may appear to be intact, the pressure has affected the deeper tissues, small vessel damage is often severe, and necrosis may subsequently occur.

### General remarks

Crush injuries of a single digit can be successfully treated in the outpatient department. Possibly two or even three digits can be cared for in this manner, but any crush injury causing greater damage is a major problem and deserves full inpatient hospital treatment.

Because the crushing force is distributed throughout the tissues, there is depth to the injury, and the deep cells are just as severely involved as the more superficial cells. The crushed tissues do not have any effective surface drainage, and they tend to remain edematous. The edema will involve the muscles, tendon sheaths, fascial spaces, and even the joints. Unless the fluid is rapidly removed by effective treatment, it will clot, become organized, and eventually form dense scar tissue. Pressure from the edema and direct damage to the vein walls will cause obstruction and even total obliteration of the venous return. This damming up of the venous return from already damaged cells frequently proves too much for their survival, and areas of necrosis subsequently develop. This process may take several days, and it is therefore extremely difficult to define the full area of injury on the day the wound occurs.

Skin wounds are usually produced by outward explosion of the compressed tissues rather than by direct injury to the epithelium (Fig. 10-1, *A*). The raised internal pressure causes the soft tissues to extrude through the skin wound. Even though a wound is relatively short, its length bears no relationship to the extent of the underlying damage. A guide to the likely sites of damage is provided by the line of the skin

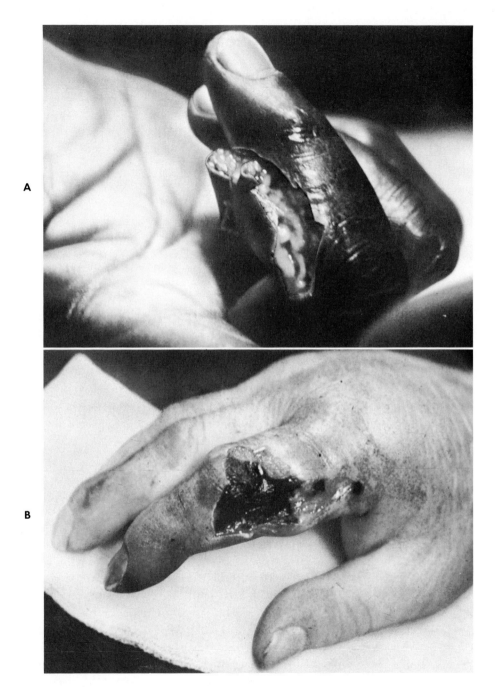

**Fig. 10-1.** *Crush injury.* **A,** This finger was squashed between two railroad cars. The internal pressure became so great the finger "exploded." Tendon, bone, and neurovascular damage was so extensive amputation was performed. **B,** A heavy blow crushed the dorsum of this finger one week before this photograph was taken. The full extent of the damage is now revealed.

wound, which is commonly at right angles to the direction of the crushing force. Wounds caused by blows from blunt instruments are localized crush injuries. In these injuries the skin wound is a direct result of the contusion and is not produced by the pent-up pressures within the tissues.

Crushing injuries are probably the most difficult to treat of all types of injuries to the hand. The difficulty lies in assessing the extent of the damage and in predicting what the state of the tissues will be a few days after the injury. Since the prognosis is uncertain, it is best if the patient regards the primary treatment as an elaborate dressing and understands that the full extent of the injury will not be apparent for three to four days (Fig. 10-1, *B*).

An easy solution when only one finger is involved is amputation, and, because it is so easy, it is wrong. In certain cases in which there has been total destruction of all blood supply of a digit, no alternative to amputation exists, but in all other cases very careful assessment must be made before a decision to amputate is made. Amputation is strongly indicated if the crush injury of the finger is complicated by fractures associated with tendon and nerve damage (Fig. 10-1, *A*). If several digits are involved, every effort must be made to save as much length as possible at the first operation.

During the primary treatment of a crush injury, wholesale excision of skin and deep tissues is not justified, but it is equally bad to leave behind hopelessly damaged tissues, since infection readily develops in such dead or devitalized areas. The decision regarding viability is based on a combination of inspection, experience, and sheer luck. It is impossible to be dogmatic about the potential survival of tissues that are bruised, contaminated, and covered with blood. However, a test using the tourniquet can be of great help in predicting the viability of damaged skin and even deeper tissues.

## Tourniquet "blush" test

The tourniquet "blush" test is used after the preliminary débridement has been carried out. This primary débridement is carried out with the tourniquet inflated, and during this time all old blood clot, foreign bodies, and obviously dead or hopelessly damaged skin and deeper tissues should be removed. Any tissue that may possibly survive is left attached, a moist sponge is held lightly over the wound, and the tourniquet is released. After three to four minutes the wound is inspected. In those areas of the skin with a good blood supply, a reactive hyperemia will be occurring and the tourniquet "blush" will be developing. In some areas the damage may be borderline, and the return of blood will be slower than in the blushing areas. Patience will be rewarded by the disclosure of a greater area of tissue viability than is apparent when the sponge is first removed. There will be no return of blood in completely devitalized tissues, no matter how long one waits. Even though this test is of greatest value in determining the state of the skin, it is also of use in deciding how much deeper tissue can be salvaged and how much must be sacrificed. Although the blush does not occur in these tissues, brisk bleeding from questionable areas shows that they will survive, and any areas that do not show at least capillary oozing must be excised.

It must be remembered that this test demonstrates the presence of the arterial supply only. The state of the more important venous return is not assessed. Later thrombosis in damaged veins may kill tissues by venous engorgement despite an active arterial supply.

## THE CRUSHED FINGER

OPERATIVE TREATMENT. After a thorough preliminary cleansing, the digit must be anesthetized with a metacarpal block of 2% lidocaine. Any other adjacent wounds should also be anesthetized by a local injection. A tourniquet should be in place but should not be inflated at the beginning of the operation. Preliminary toilet of the wound should be done with wet sponges and plenty of sterile saline solution. As blood clot is washed away, bleeding may be started from injured vessels, which should be caught in mosquito hemostats. After all major bleeding has been stopped, the cuff should be inflated and detailed toilet of the wound carried out.

Before the deeper parts of the wound can be adequately inspected, it may be necessary to enlarge the skin wound. There should be no hesitation in extending the line of the wound along a natural skin crease if by so doing one can more easily inspect the deeper tissues. It is quite wrong to put in retractors and to pull heavily on the edges of the wound, since this only further damages tissues that are already in a very precarious state.

After all of the obviously dead and devitalized tissue has been removed, the tourniquet "blush" test should be carried out. When this test is completed, the remaining areas of dead tissue will have been demonstrated and should be excised. After this has been done, the hemostats that were put onto bleeding vessels in the early stage of the operation can be twisted off, since intravascular clotting will prevent any further bleeding. If any vessels should bleed, the hemostats must be replaced. To tie off the vessels with catgut would bury foreign material in the depths of a wound that is already in a poor state to resist infection.

After the general débridement has been completed, the skin wound should be examined before the deeper structures such as nerves and tendons are inspected. Ragged skin edges should be trimmed back a few millimeters so that a reasonably vertical edge is available for suturing. Even small, proximally based flaps should be preserved, since they can subsequently be rotated into defects if they are viable. Occasionally the palmar skin is avulsed and raised from the deeper tissues with very little evidence of damage on its surface. It is wise to incise these raised areas, clean out the hematoma that will be found, and inspect the underlying dermis. If the dermis shows areas of disruption and extensive bruising, these should be excised.

Nerves that appear bruised and slightly damaged, but are in continuity, should be left untouched. If nerves have been completely severed, their ends are usually ragged and are therefore unsuitable for primary repair. However, a side-to-side anastomosis with a fine black silk suture should be done. Subsequent formal repair will be made considerably easier by this anastomosis.

Tendons are frequently damaged, but they are rarely completely severed. Any small ragged tags should be excised, but, provided that the main bulk of the tendon is in continuity, more detailed treatment is not justified. Tendons frequently seem to have astonishing powers of repair, and very little additional operative treatment should be carried out other than surgical toilet. If the flexor tendons are severed, no attempt should be made to anastomose them, but it is wise to prevent retraction of the proximal tendon end by anchoring it in place with a single wire suture. The extensor tendons are also better left as they are. Final repair of tendons can be done later under proper conditions.

Fractures are frequent in crush injuries and add to the problem of total care. There is no bone to spare in the hand, in the sense that the bones are no larger or stronger than their function demands. Any completely loose bone fragments must be removed, but any pieces that have retained a blood supply through soft tissue attachments should be replaced in as normal a position as possible. When the skin cylinder of the finger is closed by suturing and the finger placed on a splint in the functional position, the soft tissues will mold the bone fragments into approximately the correct position. In general more elaborate attempts at reduction and the use of internal fixation are not justified because of the additional trauma that they inflict on the crushed tissues.

When all of the tissues of the wound have been treated, the problem of surface repair must be faced. Because further swelling of the crushed areas is inevitable, all skin sutures must be put in relatively loosely. In the linear wounds interrupted sutures of monofilament No. 5-0 nylon should be used. Any viable skin flaps that remain should be replaced or rotated into a suitable position. Any damaged bone or tendon that is exposed in the wound should be covered with subcutaneous tissue and skin. Frequently skin flaps can be rotated into position to provide such necessary cover.

After suturing as much of the wound as possible without tension and after using any flaps to the best advantage, there may still be raw areas lacking skin cover. It would be wrong to attempt to close such areas by dragging the skin edges together with tight sutures. Additional flap coverage over the palmar aspect of the finger can be obtained after releasing incisions have been made along the neutral border of the finger. Some experienced surgeons do this. Most should not because skilled judgment is needed and ill-conceived releasing incisions may interfere with the surviving blood supply and lead to further skin loss. If one is in doubt, the remaining raw areas, which are, in fact, areas of skin loss, should be dressed with a split-skin graft. This graft should be taken (under local anesthesia) from the flexor aspect of the same forearm but should not be cut until gloves and the towels around the donor site have been changed. These precautions are necessary to prevent the donor site from becoming infected.

The graft should be of relatively thin split skin, and it must be held in position by sutures placed around the margins of the wound. Care should be taken to make sure that the graft will cover the irregular surface of the deep tissues. If it is allowed to tent over deep areas, hematoma will form beneath it, and the graft will die.

DRESSINGS. The area of the wound should be covered with a layer of Telfa and a considerable amount of Dacron batting or fluffed-up sponges placed over the injury and the hand itself. These dressings must not be wrapped circumferentially around the digit or hand; swelling is inevitable, and a tourniquet type dressing could cause disaster. When skin grafts have been used, small pieces of cotton ball soaked in saline solution should be carefully placed over the grafted area. The cotton balls should be separated from the graft by a layer of petrolatum gauze and held in place by tying together the long ends of the skin graft sutures. The dressings used should be voluminous and, in general, should cover the whole hand except in very minor wounds. They should be held in place by a stretchable bandage. The fingertips must be left exposed.

The principle in the application of the bandage is that it should compress. It is *not* applied as a pressure bandage. This distinction may seem academic rather than practical, but too much pressure can cause great damage by further interfering with the already imperiled venous return. On the other hand, too little compression will fail to obliterate dead spaces or to supply enough additional support to control capillary oozing.

If only one finger has been crushed, it can be rested on a padded malleable aluminum splint. Frequently the hand is so generally sore for the first few days that the patient will appreciate having the whole hand rested in a bandage such as is illustrated in Fig. 3-8, p. 52. If the injury affects more than one finger, a functional splint will almost certainly be needed.

AFTERCARE. The crushed area will be painful because of the tension within the tissues and the direct trauma to the sensory nerve endings. Analgesics must be given in adequate dosages.

The hand must be supported in a sling, and the exposed fingertips must be inspected frequently during the first two days to make sure that the circulatory return is good. Dressings should be changed after about forty-eight hours because by this time they will be bloodstained and will serve as a perfect culture medium for local bacteria if they are not removed. After changing the dressings, the fluffed-up sponges and compression bandage should be reapplied and retained in place until the sutures are removed. Because of the edema in the tissues, sutures should be retained longer than is customary, and they should not be taken out before at least ten days have elapsed. Even at this time it may be necessary to begin by taking out alternate sutures. If all sutures are removed at one time, it is possible that the wound will split open. When the epithelium appears thoroughly healed, it is safe to release the hand from its dressings and to commence very gentle active exercises. The patient must be warned that he has suffered a serious injury, that the return of function will be slow, and that the edema may persist for many weeks.

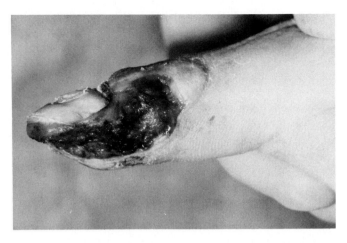

**Fig. 10-2.** *Skin loss in crush injury.* Ten days after this fingertip was crushed the area of skin loss is ready for split-skin grafting. One week after the injury obviously dead tissue was removed and moist dressings applied to prepare the bed of the skin graft.

## THE CRUSHED FINGERTIP

Crush injuries of the fingertip frequently occur in young children whose fingertips get caught in doors being closed. A comminuted fracture of the distal phalanx may be sustained, but more commonly there is a general disruption of the soft tissues in the area at the tip of the finger.

Children's fingers show remarkable powers of recovery, and conservative treatment only is indicated for these injuries. No attempt need be made to try to gather the tiny comminuted fragments into an accurately reconstituted terminal phalanx. If the soft tissues are correctly molded into the shape of a fingertip, the bone fragments usually return to an acceptable position. The lacerated and partially avulsed skin and subcutaneous tissues should be sutured in place with a few very fine sutures. I usually prefer 6-0 catgut for children and more often than not use the same suture material in adults. A Telfa dressing with a small section of sponge and Tubegauz coverage is sufficient to mold the swollen fingertip into its previous general shape. During the period of primary treatment, the nail should be retained so that it can act as a splint against which the swollen tip can be molded. If a subungual hematoma is present, it must be drained by trephining a hole in the nail. If the pressure of the hematoma is allowed to persist, it may lead to necrosis of the nail bed and even the terminal phalanx. The child's parents must be warned that the nail will eventually fall off and will be replaced by new nail.

Occasionally the damage to the skin and its circulation has been so great that a portion of the fingertip will die (Fig. 10-2). Directly after the area of loss has declared itself, it should be debrided and moist dressings applied for a few days. As soon as the granulations are healthy, a split-skin graft should be applied.

Optimism about these injuries is warranted, but it can be carried to unreason-

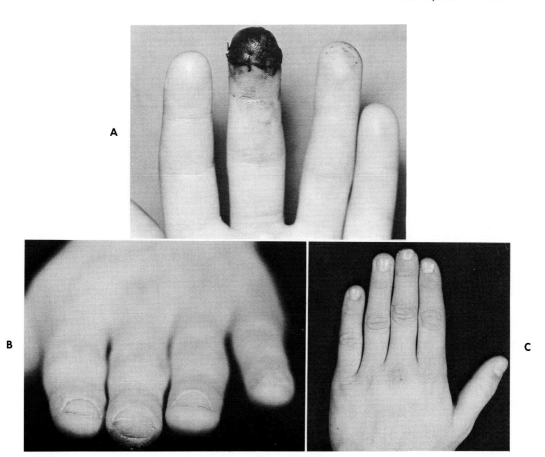

**Fig. 10-3.** *Crushed fingertip.* **A,** This boy's fingertip was avulsed in a school accident. The end was retrieved and replaced; ten days later it is obviously dead. **B,** The tip was removed, the end cleaned and allowed to granulate for four days and then covered with a thick split-thickness skin graft. This would have been a wiser primary treatment. **C,** Despite the amputation the long finger is still entitled to its correct name.

able lengths. A totally avulsed fingertip that has been crushed off has been so badly injured throughout its tissues that it cannot reasonably be expected to live (Fig. 10-3). In such circumstances the best primary treatment is to dress the amputation stump with a split-skin graft. The skin of the amputated portion should not be used as the donor site because it has already been badly damaged.

Crush injuries of the palm and wrist can cause massive disruption of the carpal rows and the intercarpal ligaments. This destruction of the proximal transverse arch shows clinically as a midline separation between the two pairs of radial and ulnar fingers. In addition there is usually a rotational deformity to the ring and small fingers. A swollen hand showing these physical signs is in serious trouble and should be referred to a specialist capable of reconstituting the essential bony arches of the hand.

# 11 · TENDON INJURIES

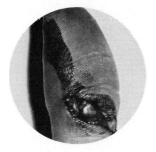
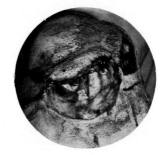

**Tendon injury**                    **Tendon injury**

Injuries to the tendons of the hand are serious and should not generally be treated in the outpatient department. Flexor tendons absolutely must not be repaired in an office or outpatient operating room, and only certain extensor tendon injuries can be safely treated in this manner.

Considerable damage is frequently caused by ill-advised digging for the proximal ends of cut tendons. Because of the tone in muscle, it is inevitable that some retraction will occur. The amount of retraction is influenced by several factors, and a careful history must be taken of the position and functional activity of the hand at the time of injury. If, for instance, the hand was lying passively palm upward and a sharp edge cut across the fingers, it is not likely that the proximal end of the flexor tendon will retract to any great extent. If, however, the injury was caused by a bottle breaking while being held firmly in the hand, the proximal end of the tendon is likely to be retracted far from the site of injury.

A flexor tendon can retract to a considerable degree even if it is cut distal to the origin of the lumbrical muscle. The extensor tendons, however, are joined to each

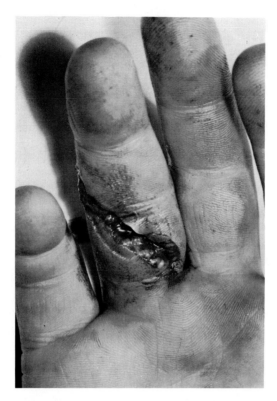

**Fig. 11-1.** *Lacerating wound damaging the flexor tendons.* A lacerating wound of a finger may damage a considerable length of tendon in the longitudinal direction. A wound such as this must be thoroughly explored before it is sutured.

other by cross ties on the dorsum of the hand and can only retract to an appreciable degree if they are cut at the level of the wrist.

In untidy or lacerated wounds the tendons are quite frequently damaged in a longitudinal direction rather than in a transverse direction (Fig. 11-1). These injuries appear serious, and the tendons are frequently stripped up for an appreciable distance so that ragged strands are lying around the wound. The reparative powers of tendons are good, and, if only à third of their cross section is in continuity after the ragged strands have been removed and a general débridement is carried out, a good prognosis can be made. If the damage is in an area covered by a tendon sheath, it is advisable to cut back the sheath on either side of the damaged area until about 0.5 cm of normal tendon is exposed.

Tendons heal by a modification of the normal repair process. About two weeks after a cut tendon has been sutured, the fibroblastic structures begin to reorganize into parallel strands so that the form and shape of the tendon can be created before more fibrous consolidation occurs. Three weeks after operation the healing is sufficiently strong to allow gentle, active movements. There is good evidence to show that active movements started after the third week have a favorable effect on the ultimate strength of the repair. Strong healing, allowing full use of the tendon, will be completed by the end of six weeks.

## TENDON INJURIES IN CHILDREN

Tendon injuries are frequently missed because of the great difficulty in performing a proper examination. Patience, ingenuity, guile, and even bribery may be needed to obtain a complete survey of a child's damaged hand. The hands should never be the first parts examined. Eventually after noting the postures of both hands the normal hand should be inspected: passive and active movements obtained and then passive movements of the injured hand. It is probable that active movements of the injured hand will never be forthcoming, and the diagnosis of tendon damage will have to be made by comparison and exclusion.

Gentle pressure on a fingertip often gives valuable information on tendon continuity, since the differences between adjacent fingers or when compared with the normal hand are often marked. For flexor tendons it is often helpful to squeeze the flexor mass in the forearm on the ulnar side at the junction of the middle and distal third. Intact tendons will produce a flexion excursion of 1 to 2 cm.

Immobilization of the hand of a child after tendon repair is virtually impossible. Unfortunately, early or delayed separation of tendon repairs is quite common, since children cannot and will not carry out careful guarded movements. Luckily, permanent joint stiffness in children is very uncommon, and it is best to use a plaster cast that immobilizes all the fingers, damaged or not, and holds both the wrist and elbow in flexion, the former being at about 30 degrees and the latter at nearly 90 degrees of flexion.

## INJURIES TO THE FLEXOR TENDONS

The flexor tendons can be damaged by either closed or open injuries. The common closed injury is avulsion of the profundus insertion when the finger is caught in the clothing of some athletic opponent. These injuries may not be very painful and are frequently ignored by the owner and missed by the physician. The key to diagnosis is the posture of the finger (Fig. 11-2). The extensor mechanism is unopposed as a result of the injury, and the distal interphalangeal joint will pass into hyperextension. If the diagnosis is made soon after injury, the tendon can be reattached by a surgeon experienced in treating flexor tendon injuries. The converse situation in which the profundus is intact but the superficialis is cut does not produce any recognizable characteristic resting posture.

Open injuries to the flexor tendons can occur at many different sites, but in none of these is one justified in attempting repair under local anesthesia in an outpatient operating room. In recent years there has been an increasing number of reports concerning the primary repair of flexor tendon injuries. The majority of these reports come from experienced surgeons whose skilled judgment allowed them to select patients who were considered suitable for such treatment. In addition, their technical skills enabled them to repair the cut tendons with the minimum

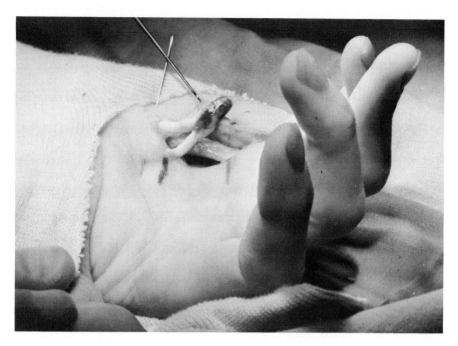

**Fig. 11-2.** *Avulsion of flexor profundus insertion.* Hyperextension of the distal interphalangeal joint shows that the extensor mechanism is unopposed and that the profundus tendon is not acting. This patient was first seen two weeks after injury; a considerable amount of granulation tissue has formed around the tendon end.

amount of additional trauma. The occasional operator would be wise to resist the temptation to suture the cut tendon ends. To do so would only add the additional trauma and edema of surgery to an area that is already so packed with vital anatomical structures that there is no room for even the minimum posttraumatic swelling. The inevitable result is slow healing, fibrosis, adhesions within the tendon sheaths, and gross limitation of function.

The area of the hand in which both the superficialis and profundus tendons lie tightly enclosed in a sheath is particularly prone to posttraumatic adhesions. This area lies between the distal palmar crease and the crease of the proximal interphalangeal joint and has been well called "no man's land." Suture of the skin wound is the only permissible surgery for these patients when only outpatient care is possible. Primary repair of both tendons is doomed to failure. More extensive procedures can be done at primary operation, but these involve selective excision of various structures and are quite unsuitable for outpatient surgery.

The areas of the hand proximal and distal to "no man's land" are areas of temptation. Although the tendons are not confined in such a rigid narrow cylinder as in the tendon sheath, they are lying in areas that do not allow much room for an inflammatory reaction. Under the proper conditions repair is possible in these areas, but, because extensive incisions and exploration are necessary, outpatient surgery is impossible.

Flexor tendon injuries cannot be surgically repaired in an emergency room. The skin wounds should be closed, a minimal dressing should be applied, and arrangement should be made for continuing care with proper hospital facilities.

## INJURIES TO THE EXTENSOR TENDONS

Injuries to the flexor tendons have such a deservedly poor reputation that extensor tendon injuries seem, in contrast, to be relatively simple to treat. This, unfortunately, is not true, and attempts to repair the complex extensor mechanism within the length of the finger are usually unsuccessful. The extensor tendons can be damaged by closed tearing or avulsion type injuries and by open wounds.

Even a relatively small wound on the dorsum of the finger can cause a severe injury to the extensor mechanism. The extensor tendons lie between skin and bone in a narrow space that contains no subcutaneous tissues. This lack of protective tissues means that adhesions readily occur between the tendons and the adjacent skin and bone. In the finger the edema that follows injury or surgical repair can cause such tension that there may be serious impairment to the blood supply of the dorsal skin.

Although the tendons are thin, they are usually intimately related to the dorsal capsules of the finger joints. A lacerated tendon over a finger joint, therefore, implies that the joint has been opened. Tendon repair should not be performed over an open joint; however, in the fingers there is no alternative, and the functional result can therefore be expected to be poor.

Extension of the middle and distal phalanges is accomplished by the intrinsic muscles joining together on the dorsum of the distal two phalanges. This very complicated mechanism responds very poorly to surgical repair, and frequently a badly damaged dorsum of the finger will eventually result in a virtually useless extensor mechanism, even after a very delicate repair has been carried out.

However, a poor surgical result does not necessarily mean that the patient is dissatisfied. Fig. 11-3 shows a printer's left long finger that was caught beneath a cogwheel of moving machinery. The extensor in the finger was virtually severed over the proximal interphalangeal joint region, and the capsule of this joint was also damaged. In addition, the tendon over the middle phalanx was damaged. The results obtained are poor if considered from the point of view of functional anatomy. However, this deformed finger did not prevent the man from returning to his original work with full pay.

## DORSUM AND PALM
### Injuries to the extensor tendons

When tendons are severed on the dorsum of the hand, often there is very little retraction of the proximal end of the tendon because of the cross connections between the tendons. These extensor tendons are flat and thin on cross section as they pass over the metacarpals. End-to-end suturing is technically very difficult, and an accurate and neat anastomosis is almost impossible to achieve. If a single

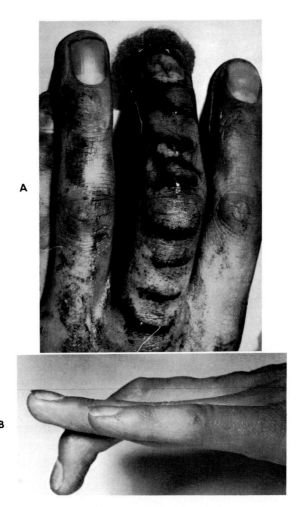

**Fig. 11-3.** *Tendon injury on the dorsum of the finger.* This finger of a printer was caught beneath a moving cogwheel. **A,** The extensor mechanism was damaged at two sites, and the proximal interphalangeal joint was entered. **B,** The anatomical result obtained was poor, but the patient was able to return to his occupation. (From Flatt, Adrian E.: J. Bone Joint Surg. **37-B:**117, 1955.)

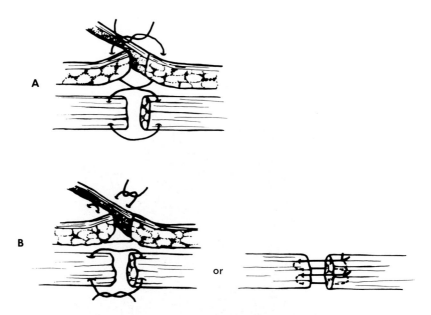

**Fig. 11-4.** *Extensor tendon repair.* **A,** When a single tendon has been cut through a small wound, a single figure-of-eight suture may be sufficient to close both wounds. **B,** In more extensive wounds it is better to close the skin separately with interrupted horizontal mattress sutures. The tendons should be repaired by one or more interrupted sutures.

tendon has been cut through a small wound, it is possible to close both with a figure-of-eight stitch (Fig. 11-4, *A*). If the wound is more than a small puncture wound, it is probably better to close it with interrupted skin sutures independently of the tendon repair (Fig. 11-4, *B*). The tendons can be joined with braided wire or synthetic monofilament sutures—even as large as 3-0 in adults. The criss cross technique is satisfactory, but several interrupted sutures can be used (Fig. 11-5).

The hand should be protected in a bulky dressing for about two weeks, but it is not necessary to splint the interphalangeal joints. In the third week following repair gradually increasing active range of motion exercises can be started.

**OPERATIVE TREATMENT.** Local anesthesia block with 2% lidocaine will be needed to allow adequate débridement of the wounded area. The points of entry for the infiltrating needles must be placed some centimeters away from the wound edge. The area must be thoroughly cleansed before the needles are inserted.

After the anesthetic has taken effect, the entire area must be thoroughly cleansed and the edges of the skin wound trimmed if necessary. Only after this toilet to the wound has been finished should the cut tendon or tendons be repaired. If the transection is clean and at right angles to the long line of the tendon, no trimming will be necessary. If the tendon ends are ragged, they must be cut cleanly across with a scalpel or sharp small scissors before they are anastomosed.

It is best to place the suture in the proximal end of the tendon first and to place the finger in extension so that the distal end is brought passively as near the prox-

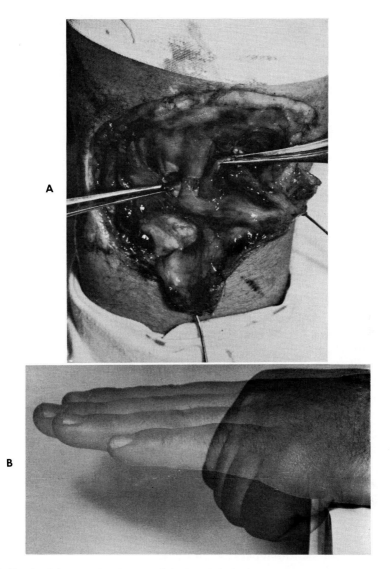

**Fig. 11-5.** *Tendon injury on the dorsum of the hand.* **A,** In this case one tendon has been partially severed and two have been cut across (their ends are held in forceps). **B,** These tendons were joined by end-to-end sutures of braided wire, and a reasonable result was obtained. (From Flatt, Adrian E.: J. Bone Joint Surg. **37-B:**117, 1955.)

imal end as possible. Often there is a gap between the tendon ends; this can be closed by pulling the proximal end distally and then transfixing the tendon at right angles with a long narrow Keith needle to hold it in its more distal position. This transfixion will not damage the tendon since the cross section of the needle is so small, but it will make the anastomosis considerably easier because it will not be necessary to maintain a constant traction on the proximal end. The needle is removed immediately after the anastomosis is complete. Dorsiflexion of the wrist will also help to relax some of the tension on the extensor tendons.

The wire sutures should be buried in the tendon ends by the Bunnell method (Fig. 4-9). Before the knot is tied, the ends of the tendons should be pushed together slightly so that when the knot is tied the area of junction is wrinkled and somewhat bulky. This bunching-up of the sutured area is necessary because, during the first few weeks after repair, the sutures tend to release the tension by cutting through the tendons so that the ultimate result will be a smooth junctional area.

After the knot is tied, the two ends of the wires should be passed through at least 3 cm of the proximal tendon and pulled tight so that the tendon is bunched up. If the wires are then cut off flush with the tendon surface, the cut ends will retract within the body of the tendon and leave a smooth gliding surface (Fig. 4-9). Such repairs of the tendons are easy to write about, but an indication of the technical difficulties involved is reflected in writings on the subject that invariably use drawings rather than photographs to illustrate the recommended technique (sic).

Ideally the suture line of the skin wound should not be directly over the site of tendon repair, but frequently this juxtaposition cannot be avoided. In these cases every attempt should be made to place a subcutaneous tissue barrier between the skin and tendon. If possible, some subcutaneous tissue should be mobilized and rotated on a pedicle carrying a blood supply so that it lies between the tendon repair and the skin. If this is impossible, interrupted catgut sutures should be used to make a separate closure layer between skin and tendon. The catgut sutures should be placed with their knots facing into the deep tissues (Fig. 4-2). The skin can be closed with interrupted nylon sutures or with a continuous wire suture if the wound is relatively straight.

**DRESSINGS.** A Telfa dressing should be placed on the wound, and a fluffed-up compression dressing will be needed to control any tendency for venous oozing.

Because of the cross connections of the tendons on the dorsum of the hand, immobilization of all the fingers and the wrist is necessary to protect a single injured finger. Immobilization in full extension is not necessary, and the hand can be rested on a cock-up plaster-of-paris splint that will immobilize the wrist and metacarpophalangeal joints in the functional position.

Occasionally there is such a loss of tendon tissue that the suture site is put under too great a strain if the functional position is used for immobilization. In such instances the hand should be placed in the functional position immediately after the tendon anastomosis to determine whether the strain is too great. If the cut ends tend to separate, the fingers must be immobilized in extension.

**AFTERCARE.** Splinting should be maintained for two weeks. In the third week following repair gradually increasing active range of motion exercises can be started, but heavy manual labor should be avoided for at least another two weeks.

If the fingers are immobilized in extension, the functional position has been abandoned, and this violation of the fundamental principle will cause trouble after the hand is released from the splinting. The flexor mechanism will have become extremely stiff, and it will take several extra weeks of active exercising before the function of the hand is fully restored.

Frequently, after these injuries are repaired, the involved finger may appear to have an extension lag for several weeks. Usually such a lag is taken up after six to eight weeks of active exercises.

## Compound injuries involving the extensor tendons

Because of the thinness of the dorsal skin and lack of subcutaneous tissues, compound injuries involving the skin, tendons, and metacarpal shafts are relatively common. Injuries involving these structures can all be treated at one operation, which can occasionally be carried out on an outpatient basis.

In cases in which a skin flap has been raised by the trauma, surgery can be carried out beneath it, and the flap can then be sutured back into place provided that it has been proved to be viable. Occasionally there will be small areas of loss of the dorsal skin. Use of a large rotation flap will replace the skin loss without any need for skin grafting. However, the amount of loss that can be compensated for is small, and the incisions needed to mobilize the flap must be large to overcome the tension which will be produced when a fist is made.

Fractures of the metacarpal shafts should be immobilized by internal splinting by transfixion with a single Kirschner wire (Figs. 13-12 and 13-13). The wire should be so placed that one end will be palpable beneath the skin of the hand and can later be reached by a small incision and withdrawn. The extensor tendons should be repaired by buried wire and the flap of the skin replaced. Usually a drain is not necessary and would serve only as a means of introducing infection into the repaired area.

## THE FINGERS
## Injuries to the extensor tendons
### At the metacarpophalangeal joint

The area of the metacarpophalangeal joint is the leading edge of the fist, and the extensor tendon is tightly stretched over this most prominent part of the clenched hand. The tissues restraining the tendon and attempting to keep it centralized over the head of the metacarpal are under considerable tension and may yield if the force becomes excessive. In teenagers and young adults the tendon may dislocate during wrestling or other violent activities, and in the elderly it may dislocate even when flicking the fingers (Fig. 11-6).

Penetrating wounds over the joint often cut the tendon; they are easily recognized by the characteristic drop-finger position and the patient's inability to raise the finger against gravity. Penetrating wounds caused by teeth are heavily infected; their care is discussed on pp. 303 to 306.

OPERATIVE TREATMENT. The operation should be done with the patient under 2% lidocaine local anesthesia. The anesthetic should be injected through puncture wounds made several centimeters away from the wound edge. There is frequently

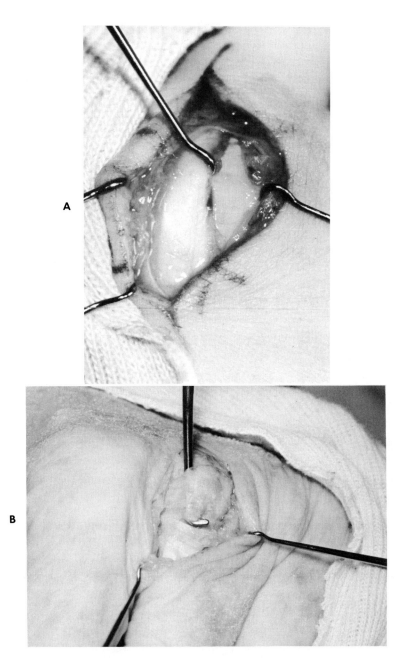

**Fig. 11-6.** *Dislocation of extensor tendon.* **A,** A 19-year-old gymnast felt a sudden pain when gripping the high bar. Two hooks are holding apart the tear in the transverse fibers adjacent to the extensor tendon. **B,** A 72-year-old man had removed a hair from his face and felt a sudden pain when flipping the hand. The blunt hook is passed beneath the transverse fibers from which the extensor tendon has pulled loose. (**B** from Kettelkamp, D. B., Flatt, A. E., and Moulds, R.: J. Bone Joint Surg. **53-A:** 229, 1971.)

actual skin loss in wounds in this area, and the amount of loss should be determined after débridement and excision of the skin edges have been completed.

Loss of skin over the joint can be replaced by rotation flaps raised from the relatively loose dorsal skin. This looseness is deceiving, and only small areas of skin can be replaced by this means. The flap must be generous in size, and great care must be taken to stop any hemorrhage from the deep surface of the flap before it is sutured in place. The technical problems of moving such a flap are discussed on pp. 119 to 121. The use of such a flap will allow full-thickness skin cover to be placed over the site of tendon suture and will thereby lessen the risk of adhesions. If a split-skin graft is used in such a situation it will probably survive, but the subsequent scarring will be gross, and there will be a severe limitation of function.

After the skin flap is mobilized and tests show that it will lie in its new position without tension, the cut tendon can be repaired.

The extensor tendon has a relatively large cross section at this site, and end-to-end suture with braided wire gives a good result. The hood of the joint formed by the fibers connecting the intrinsic muscles to the central tendon is frequently damaged. It is important to repair this if possible so that the normal balance is restored between the long extrinsic and the short intrinsic tendons. The cut edges should be joined by several very fine, plain catgut sutures.

DRESSINGS. A Telfa dressing should be placed over the suture line and a fluffed-up compression dressing carefully applied so that the rotation flap is subjected to even pressure. This pressure must not be so great as to obliterate the blood supply of the flap. It is wise to immobilize the hand on a functional splint. Although it is tempting to use less extensive splinting, it must be remembered that a large area of the dorsum has been disturbed by mobilization of the flap. This large area should be protected to allow good primary healing to occur.

AFTERCARE. It is a wise precaution to inspect the flap on the day following surgery. Occasionally a hematoma will occur, and unless it is drained the tension created by the swelling may interfere with the blood supply of the flap.

The skin sutures can be removed between the tenth and fourteenth days, but active movements should not be allowed until three full weeks after the operation.

## At the proximal interphalangeal joint

Sudden severe flexion force, closed crushing injuries, or direct blows over the joint can cause division of the central slip of the extensor tendon, but the lack of true extension is frequently missed. The pain and swelling is usually treated by rest or a splint in partial flexion; this keeps the ruptured ends apart and encourages further flexion by the unopposed flexor digitorum superficialis. The two lateral slips will gradually migrate down the sides of the fingers and thereby alter their relationship to the axis of the joint. Once they have passed from the extensor to the flexor side of the axis, their action reinforces that of the extrinsic flexors, and the finger rapidly becomes fixed in flexion at this joint. In contrast, the distal interphalangeal joint will be hyperextended by the action of the lateral bands (Fig. 11-7).

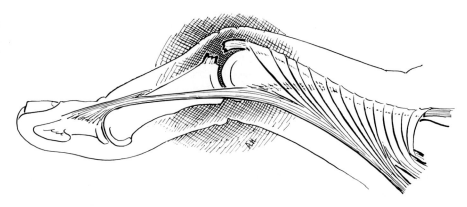

**Fig. 11-7.** *Boutonniere deformity.* When the attachment of the central slip of the extrinsic extensor tendon is destroyed, the two lateral slips will migrate down the sides of the finger until they lie below the axis of the proximal interphalangeal joint. Their action then reinforces that of the flexors of the finger and produces a flexion deformity of the proximal interphalangeal joint.

This posture is known in English as the "boutonniere deformity" and to the French as "le button-hole." If the injury has remained unrecognized and unsplinted, it may take several weeks to fully develop. However, in open, or extensive, injuries in the region of the joint it may occur immediately following the injury. A boutonniere deformity can occur as a complication of the method for reducing fractured metacarpal necks by pressure against the head of the proximal phalanx. This pressure can so obstruct the blood supply to the tendon that it will necrose and rupture when movements are allowed after the treatment of the fracture is complete.

### Treatment

X-ray films should always be taken of injuries in this region. If the x-ray film shows a chip fracture at the base of the middle phalanx, immediate operative replacement is the correct treatment. If the x-ray films do not show any bone damage, conservative treatment should be tried.

CONSERVATIVE METHOD. A light plaster splint is applied to the flexor aspect of the forearm on the injured side. From the distal end of this, an extension passes around the injured finger to hold it completely extended. If the proximal interphalangeal joint is held in full extension for three weeks, the severed tendon ends should heal together with very little added length. Unfortunately, in a significant number of cases the finger will revert to the boutonniere deformity after the plaster has been removed. Further immobilization is pointless, and operation should be advised.

OPERATIVE METHOD. Operations in this area demand very delicate surgery, and they should only be attempted when full hospital facilities are available. The objective is replacement of the avulsed bone chip or suturing of the cut tendon ends. This replacement may seem simple enough to do, but the technical difficulties presented by the delicacy of the tissues and their intimate relationship to each other are so great that good results are not common even in the hands of experienced surgeons. The occasional operator would be well advised to refer such patients to a more experienced colleague.

## At the insertion of the tendon

Closed avulsion of the insertion of the extensor mechanism into the base of the distal phalanx is one of the most common of all tendon injuries. The long flexor tendon will immediately pull the distal phalanx into a flexion deformity although the joint can still be passively extended to normal. The deformity is commonly known as either a "mallet," or a "baseball," finger.

The long and small fingers are most commonly affected, followed by the ring and then the index fingers. For those under about the age of 35 a significant force is needed to produce the injury. Over this age only a trivial force is needed, such as catching the finger when tucking the sheet under a mattress.

There are three types of injury. In one the central extensor tendon is severely stretched and the finger droops although there is still some active extension of the terminal joint. If the injury is more severe, the tendon will be ruptured or torn from its insertion, and the dorsal capsule will also be torn. All voluntary extension will be lost and there will be a 40 to 45-degree extensor lag. In the third kind of injury there is actual bony avulsion of the tendon insertion, and the degree of droop or extensor lag will depend on the associated tearing of the extensor mechanism and dorsal joint capsule.

In effect, the injury allows the extensor mechanism to concentrate all of its power at the proximal interphalangeal joint. If the injury is not repaired, the middle phalanx will rapidly become hyperextended at the proximal interphalangeal joint.

Crush injuries to the dorsum of the finger can occasionally be complicated by the late onset of a mallet finger. This deformity occurs because the blood supply to the distal portion of the tendon was damaged at the time of the original injury and is further restricted because of strangulation by the scar tissue formed during healing. The avascular tendon is unable to withstand the forces put through it, and it therefore ruptures. Because of the avascularity of the tendon, treatment of these delayed mallet fingers is difficult.

X-ray films of these injuries should always be taken. A lateral view of the joint will show whether or not there has been an avulsion fracture of the base of the phalanx. It is sensible to take an x-ray film of the whole finger; it costs the patient no more and may reveal hidden injury. A mallet finger that is produced by an end-on injury will force the distal joint into flexion but may also force the proximal interphalangeal joint into hyperextension (Fig. 11-8). The whole finger should be carefully examined for pain and tenderness in all three digital joints because avulsion flake fractures may have occurred on the flexor aspect of more proximal joints.

### *Treatment*

It is essential to restore the anatomical relationship on the dorsum of the finger. To reestablish continuity, the ruptured end of the long extensor tendon must be

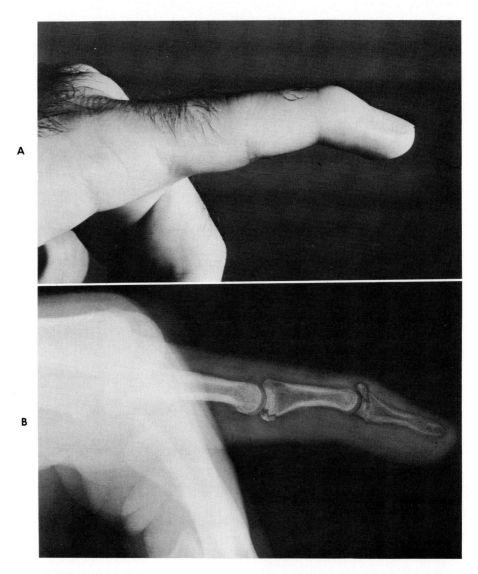

**Fig. 11-8.** *"Mallet finger."* **A,** This medical student produced what appeared to be a classical mal-let finger when he suffered an end-on injury to his little finger. In addition, he had some pain in the proximal interphalangeal joint. **B,** X-ray film of both joints shows avulsion fractures on the dorsum of the distal and the palmar aspect of the proximal interphalangeal joints. He must also have violently hyperextended the proximal interphalangeal joint.

brought back into place at the base of the distal phalanx by immobilizing the finger in a position of flexion at the proximal interphalangeal joint and hyperextension at the distal interphalangeal joint.

Holding the proximal interphalangeal joint in flexion will overcome the ten-dency for the extensor tendon to retract proximally. This flexing of the proximal interphalangeal joint will pull distally on the middle slip of the extensor tendon.

Pulling the middle slip distally will also pull the lateral slips in a distal direction, since they are joined together by cross ties. This distal pulling on the lateral slips will produce a passive lengthening of the extensor tendon and will help the approximation of the ruptured ends.

A finger can be immobilized in the correct position either by conservative or operative means. Conservative methods employ various forms of splinting and are more widely used. When used correctly they can be curative. The great advantage of splinting is that there is unlikely to be a limitation of flexion, which can frequently occur after operative treatment. I believe that the distal joint should be extended and the middle or proximal interphalangeal joint held flexed for the first three weeks. The splint can then be shortened and the distal joint held immobilized for a total of eight or even ten weeks.

The variety of shapes, sizes, and materials employed in splinting this lesion is enormous. The proponent of each type remains professionally or commercially convinced that his variety is the most suitable. The very existence of such a large number of appliances shows that none is markedly superior to any other. The key to their successful employment is experience and attention to fine detail in their use.

CONSERVATIVE METHOD. Whatever method is used, the joint must not be placed in full hyperextension. This position obliterates the blood supply over the dorsum of the joint, and I have seen necrosis of the dorsal skin and subsequent joint infection caused by this extreme position. If a splint is to be used, it is wise to consult a senior colleague who is experienced in its use and who has the time to explain the problems associated with the particular appliance selected.

Whatever method of external immobilization has been selected, the key to its success is keeping the joint from flexing throughout the immobilization period. The most dangerous time is when the splint is being adjusted or changed. The healing tendon must be protected by passively holding the joint fully extended while the changes are made (Fig. 11-9).

If there has been an avulsion fracture, lateral x-ray films will show whether there is adequate contact between the bone surfaces. The x-ray film must be read carefully to make sure the injury is not, in fact, an intra-articular fracture in which the lack of joint extension is a secondary result.

OPERATIVE METHOD. The indications for operative treatment are few and are largely economic in the sense that some manual occupations simply cannot be followed with a splint on the finger. The choice usually lies between two methods.

USE OF A KIRSCHNER WIRE. Because of the difficulties of applying a splint and making sure that it maintains the position necessary for good reduction of the avulsion, many operative methods have been devised, and in most of them some form of transfixion of the terminal joint with an intramedullary Kirschner wire is used. The insertion of the Kirschner wire is not easy, but this method in practiced hands is good and allows the rest of the injured hand to move freely. A special apparatus has been devised to guide it into place successfully.

Use of the wire violates the fundamental principle of treating a closed injury by

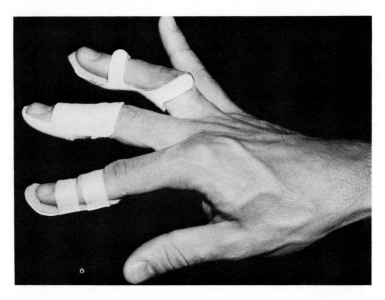

**Fig. 11-9.** *"Mallet finger."* A variety of splints can be used for this injury. The index carries a short splint that does not include the proximal interphalangeal joint. The long finger is treated in a commercially available splint that can be taken off for washing and then strapped on again. The ring finger has the proximal interphalangeal joint also immobilized. Note that none of these splints force the distal joint into hyperextension.

closed means. The insertion of the wire inevitably makes the lesion a compound one and creates the risk of introducing infection into the depths of the finger. Treatment with external immobilization should be tried in all cases unless the attending physician has considerable experience in Kirschner wire operative technique. The use of the wire should be restricted to those injuries for which a splint or cast either cannot be used or has been tried and proved to be inadequate.

The wire is introduced through the end of the finger using a power drill so that the operator's other hand is free to hold the finger in the corrected position. A 1.1 mm Kirschner wire is a suitable size, and after introduction it is cut off beneath the skin and a Band-Aid applied to the puncture wound. The wire is usually left in about six weeks, after which another month of night splinting is advisable.

DIRECT SUTURING OF THE RUPTURED TENDONS. If there is an open wound over the joint, operative repair of the tendon rupture is permissible. The wound usually allows a direct approach to the site of rupture, but it should be extended if there is an inadequate exposure. The tendon ends should be joined by a buried wire suture (Fig. 4-9) and the skin wound closed by interrupted nylon sutures.

Even after the tendon ends have been anastomosed, the site will have to be protected from strain for at least three weeks. The best way to do this is by transfixion with a Kirschner wire.

When there has been an avulsion fracture of the base of the phalanx, it is often extremely difficult to replace the fragment of bone in a satisfactory position. On occasions it may be wiser to excise the bone and reattach the tendon end to the periosteum of the dorsum of the phalanx (Fig. 11-10).

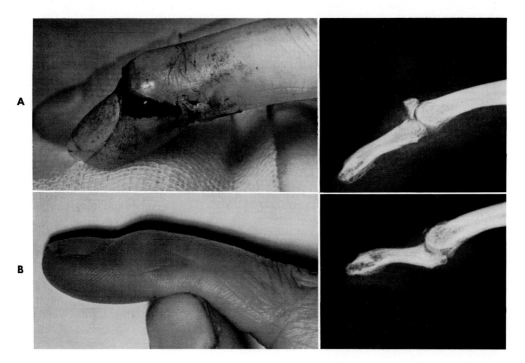

**Fig. 11-10.** *Compound mallet finger injury.* **A,** In this case it was found impossible to replace the small avulsed fragment of bone. It was excised and the extensor tendon reattached to the dorsum of the phalanx. **B,** The result obtained was not perfect; 20 degrees of extension were lacking, but the patient was satisfied with the result. (From Flatt, Adrian E.: J. Bone Joint Surg. **37-B:**117, 1955.)

There is a school of thought which holds that if x-ray films show that there has not been a fracture, conservative treatment cannot guarantee that the ruptured ends of the tendon have been placed sufficiently close together to ensure good healing. It follows from this thesis that an open exploratory operation is indicated. The incision should be made transversely across the dorsum of the distal interphalangeal joint and developed into two flaps by a short right-angled extension at each end of the main incision. Mobilization of the two flaps will show the area of tendon rupture. The ends should be joined by a buried wire suture and the skin wound closed by interrupted nylon sutures. There need be no hesitation in using a Kirschner wire to immobilize the joint for the necessary three weeks since the operation has already converted a closed wound into an open wound. This method of treatment is successful in experienced hands but is not to be recommended for routine use in outpatient surgery clinics for patients with newly inflicted wounds.

## Injuries to the flexor tendons

Because of the close proximity of the nerves and vessels to the tendons in the palm, a cut tendon implies damage to other structures, and a very thorough examination is necessary for any palmar wound. Even if it can be established that there is only tendon damage, one is not justified in repairing the lesion in an emergency operating room. Although the risk of adhesion formation is less than inside the finger, it is still significant, and cut tendons in the palm deserve high-quality repair under ideal conditions.

## THE THUMB: INJURIES TO THE FLEXOR AND EXTENSOR TENDONS

OPERATIVE TREATMENT. The tendons of the thumb on both the flexor and extensor surfaces do not have any attachments to surrounding structures and will therefore retract to a very marked extent if they are cut while under tension. The tone in these muscles is also sufficient to cause a considerable degree of retraction even when the thumb is at rest. If it is elected to search for the proximal end of the tendon, its extensive retraction will necessitate a large incision. On the extensor surface it is sometimes possible to palpate the actual cut end of the tendon in relatively thin patients. On the flexor aspect it is usually impossible to get any indication of the site of the cut end by palpation. Occasionally the proximal end of the tendon will curl on itself, and a lump can be felt. Usually, however, this lump is not felt until the inflammatory reaction has increased its size.

The long flexor tendon of the thumb lies in a sheath that tends to retain it in the best functional position. However, unlike the fingers, it is a solitary tendon, and primary repair is therefore attempted more frequently than in the fingers. Under ideal operating room conditions such surgery is justified. Emergency rooms and outpatient operating rooms in general are not suitable areas for such delicate and important surgery. It is foolish to operate on patients with such injuries without being prepared to make extensive incisions to search for the proximal tendon end. Such an operation cannot be properly done under local anesthesia.

At operation a sufficient amount of sheath must be removed proximal and distal to the site of suture so that binding within the sheath is avoided. Because of the length of travel of the tendon when the thumb is flexed, nearly three times as much sheath must be removed proximally as distally.

The flexor tendon lies deep in the thenar muscles and travels against the side of the first metacarpal. If it is cut in this region, it is almost inevitable that the periosteum will be damaged. If repair is done in this region, the tendon should be rerouted into the muscular and subcutaneous tissues to avoid adherence to the damaged periosteum.

The long extensor tendon of the thumb has a relatively large cross section throughout its course and over the phalanges is comparatively uncomplicated in comparison with the extensor mechanism of the fingers. These features make it amenable to immediate surgical repair if the proximal end can be brought distally without additional trauma.

If the extensor pollicis brevis tendon has been cut, the metacarpophalangeal joint will fall into flexion and the interphalangeal joint will hyperextend. The deformity is similar to the flexion and hyperextension of the middle and distal finger joints in a boutonniere deformity. The disability from this posture in the thumb is even greater than in a finger, and tendon continuity must be restored under proper surgical conditions.

If surgical repair is decided upon for either the flexor or extensor tendons, the ends should be joined by the buried wire technique of Bunnell (Fig. 4-9). Both tendons will have to be immobilized for three weeks in the functional position. In the case of the flexor tendon, tension on the suture will be relieved if the thumb is held in some degree of opposition and the wrist in neutral or a few degrees of flexion.

# 12 · JOINT INJURIES

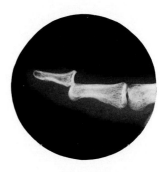

**Joint injury**

**A** *sprain* is an injury of a joint ligament or capsule.
  A *strain* is an injury of a muscle or tendon.

## SPRAINS

Sprains and dislocations are among the more common closed injuries of the hand. Simple severe sprains of the ligaments around a joint are uncommon. The injury that produces the symptoms of simple severe sprain is frequently a momentary dislocation which reduces itself immediately after the trauma.

The tissue damage caused by sprains is often quite extensive, and such injuries deserve better care than they are usually given. Recovery is always slow, and the patient should be warned that minor, but persistent, symptoms will be present for several months. It is even possible that there will be some degree of permanent functional disability.

Most sprains can be adequately treated by external immobilization of the injured part with adhesive tape. The application of the tape is an art that can be learned only by apprenticeship. A half hour spent with an experienced football trainer while he tapes his team for battle is more valuable than many hours spent trying to interpret textbooks and diagrams. Many of the techniques used by trainers are directly applicable to clinical medicine, and their opinions of the usefulness of various methods of taping is based upon tremendous experience.

Many physicians inject local anesthetics and even steroids into sprained areas. However, such treatment does little to help the natural process of healing, and the pain in the joint is not usually so acute as to demand anesthesia. The injections are sometimes given to enable the patient to return immediately to some form of competitive sport. However, the physician who gives such injections assumes a heavy responsibility, for when the area is anesthetized, there cannot be any warning pain if extra force is put on the joint and such force in an already weakened area can easily convert a simple injury into one considerably more serious. The superimposed trauma will require many more weeks of treatment than the original injury would have needed.

When tape is used, it is wise to paint the skin to minimize the risk of skin reaction. Tincture of benzoin is commonly used with good results, but tincture of rosin* appears to cause even fewer skin reactions.

## The wrist

Pain around the wrist from a "sprain" may be caused by an avulsion flake fracture; it is quite possibly due to a fracture of the carpal scaphoid or partial tearing of intercarpal ligaments and only rarely is it produced by a true sprain of the wrist ligaments. The diagnosis of sprain should never be made until bony injury has been excluded by clinical and radiological tests.

A flake avulsion fracture from the dorsum of a carpal bone is a frequently missed injury, and the patient is often dismissed as a malingerer. If the patient has fallen with the wrist into flexion and there is palpable point tenderness on the dorsum of the hand, several x-ray films must be taken to profile the dorsum of the carpus and show up any chip fracture (Fig. 12-1). The treatment of one of these small avulsion fractures is sympathy and calculated neglect. Simple strapping and "light duties" until symptoms subside are usually quite sufficient.

If a flake fracture is not suspected or detected, the pain should be regarded as due to a fractured scaphoid until this has been disproved. The majority of fractures of the scaphoid are caused by falls on the outstretched hand. It is just such accidents that are thought to cause sprains of the wrist. The signs and symptoms of both conditions are similar—painful limitation of wrist movements, no deformity of the joint, and tenderness on the radial side of the joint.

X-ray films of the wrist taken in three planes are essential. While the posteroanterior and lateral views are helpful, it is the oblique view that will show the bone in profile and probably reveal the fracture. However, films taken immediately after injury frequently do not show a fracture. Such lack of radiographic evidence must not be accepted as absolute. If a fracture is present, it will show up in films taken two to three weeks after the injury. The care of this fracture is discussed in the next chapter.

X-ray films of the carpal bones and wrist joint are hard to interpret, and many

---

*To make a stock bottle of tincture of rosin, dissolve 1 pound of rosin in 1 gallon of 85% to 90% alcohol.

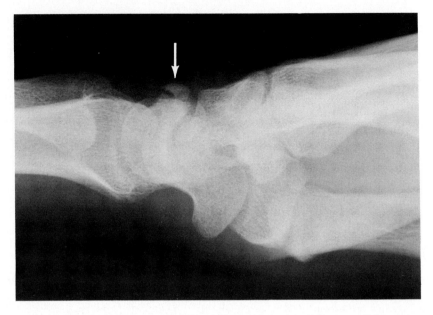

**Fig. 12-1.** *Carpal avulsion fracture.* In this injury a flake of bone has been torn off the dorsum of the triquetrum. These injuries may be missed unless several lateral x-ray films are taken. (From Flatt, A. E.: Postgrad. Med. **39**:17, Jan., 1966. © McGraw-Hill, Inc.)

intercarpal ligament injuries have been missed at the acute stage. Chronicity of symptoms leads to retrospective review of the films and the taking of additional views that show up the carpal dissociation. The most common tear is that of the scapholunate ligament and if intercarpal ligamentous disruption is suspected, expert help should be sought.

Symptoms of carpal tunnel syndrome can be caused by these wrist injuries and even by more distal injuries, which may cause a tenosynovitis. The patient will refer the symptoms to the injured area, and it is therefore easy to miss the superimposed median nerve compression.

## The thumb

Sprains of the thumb are common and crippling. Dr. Richard Kirkpatrick has published an excellent but pitiful account of his life with a sprained right thumb.* The metacarpophalangeal joint is usually affected, and it is uncommon for an injury to occur to the interphalangeal joint without the more proximal metacarpophalangeal joint also being involved. It is usually the ulnar collateral ligament that is affected, and the tear is variously called "gamekeeper's thumb," or "skipole thumb."

An injured thumb with pain and swelling around its joints must be subjected to a thorough clinical examination, even though the patient may protest at the inevitable

*J.A.M.A. **234**:1017, 1975.

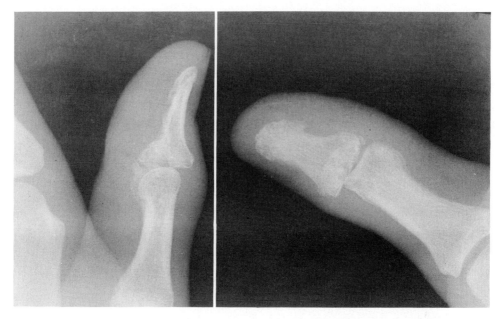

**Fig. 12-2.** *"Sprained thumb."* This injury was treated as a simple sprain for six weeks. An x-ray film was finally taken because of persistent pain, and the full extent of injury was disclosed: an intra-articular fracture and dislocation of the interphalangeal joint.

extra discomfort. The examination must include observation of the active and passive range of movements, which should be compared with those of the unaffected thumb. In all cases of suspected sprained thumb x-ray films should be taken in both lateral and anteroposterior planes (Fig. 12-2).

If clinical examination shows that there is a possibility of ligamentous rupture but the x-ray films do not show any fracture, then lateral strain films will have to be taken. Films of the unaffected side will be needed for comparison. Such complete examination is necessary because many patients with so-called sprained thumbs have, in fact, suffered a serious ligamentous injury with rupture of one of the lateral ligaments.

More often than not the strength of the ligament is greater than that of the bone to which it is attached, and the sprain will cause a small avulsion fracture from one of the bone attachments (Fig. 12-3). If this injury is not detected during the clinical examination, the joint will tend to lie open on the damaged side and the ligament will heal with lengthening. Such ligamentous lengthening will allow subluxation of the joint whenever the thumb is in use. This habitual subluxation can become a crippling deformity, particularly if the ligament is lengthened on the ulnar side of the joint, thereby destroying the integrity of the pinch mechanism.

If a tear of the ligament is probable, its integrity must be tested by lateral stress. If this force makes too much pain, a metacarpal local anesthetic block should be given so that the ligament can be properly tested.

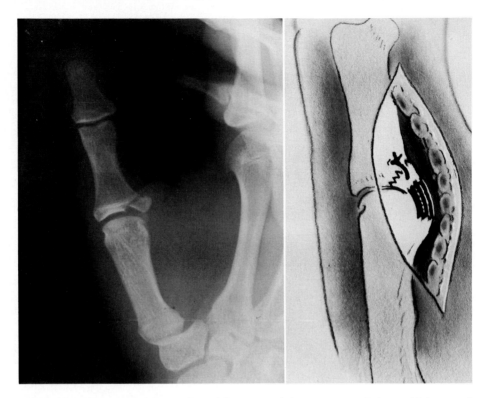

**Fig. 12-3.** *"Sprained thumb."* The collateral ligaments of the metacarpophalangeal joint are often stronger than the bone to which they are attached. Avulsion fractures must be treated by immediate replacement so that the integrity of the joint can be restored.

### Simple sprain

TREATMENT. If clinical examination reveals that the strength of the collateral ligaments of the joint is largely intact and that no fracture has occurred, adhesive strapping is the best treatment. An adhesive tape spica built up around the thenar eminence and the proximal phalanx will provide sufficient immobilization. The tape should be worn for at least three weeks and must be reapplied if it becomes too loose during this time. Active movement within the limitation imposed by the strapping should be encouraged throughout the period of treatment.

If there is any fear that taping might not be adequate protection, a plaster spica cast extending from the tip of the thumb to below the elbow should be applied. The metacarpophalangeal joint should be held in slight flexion and tension applied so as to relax the injured ligament. A month is the average length of time the cast should be worn.

### Ruptured ligament

TREATMENT. If the ligament has been shown to be ruptured but x-ray films do not show any fracture, operative repair is the treatment of choice. This surgery should not be attempted in an outpatient department.

Conservative treatment does not give as satisfactory a result as operative treatment. The best nonoperative treatment is the plaster cast immobilization described on p. 210. After the cast is removed, the thumb must be protected for an additional two weeks by adhesive strapping. Despite these measures, it is probable that the ligament will heal with an increase in its length, causing instability of the joint and chronic discomfort.

### Avulsion fracture

TREATMENT. An avulsion fracture is a serious injury. The bone chip is usually tilted and is frequently rotated so that no amount of closed manipulation can reduce it to its original position. Such fractures should be treated by open operation, which must not be performed in an outpatient operating room. After surgery has been performed, the thumb must be immobilized in a plaster cast for at least three weeks. After the cast has been removed, the thumb must be protected by adhesive strapping for an additional two weeks. The ultimate prognosis following such treatment is good, but the patient must be warned to expect some degree of stiffness and discomfort for many weeks following surgery.

## The fingers

Periarticular injury to any of the three joints of a finger is common and is usually associated with prolonged swelling and discomfort. The patient must be warned that these injuries can produce permanent disability and that recovery will be slow regardless of treatment given. The full range of movement will not be regained for several months, and it will probably take a similar period of time for the periarticular swelling to disappear. In severe sprains it is possible that the periarticular swelling will never completely disappear and that the range of movement will not return to its full extent.

"Sprained finger" is a common lay diagnosis for virtually any finger injury and must be tested by a thorough clinical examination, which must include a comparison of the stability of the injured joint with its counterpart on the opposite hand. If the injury occurred several hours before the patient is seen, it is usually too painful to tolerate a proper examination. The finger should be anesthetized by a metacarpal block so that a proper stress test of the ligament can be carried out. X-ray films must be taken to exclude the possibility of a flake fracture or avulsion chip from one of the bones forming the involved joint (Fig. 12-4).

### Simple sprain

TREATMENT. If it can be clearly shown that the injury is a true sprain and that the collateral ligaments of the joint are largely intact, then the joint should be protected by immobilization. In very mild sprains the finger can be buddy taped to a neighbor. For more severe injuries the finger must be placed in the functional position with all three joints in about 150 degrees of extension. It may be bandaged or strapped to a small malleable aluminum splint. A collodion splint made from several layers of bandage can be used, but it has many practical disadvantages when com-

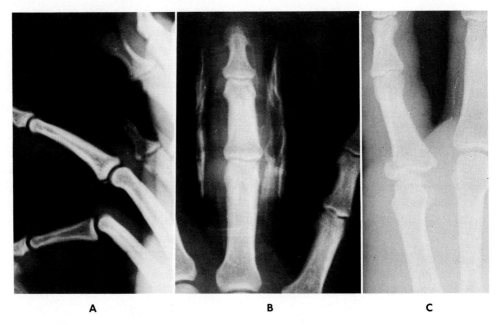

**Fig. 12-4.** *"Sprained fingers."* Three individuals injured a finger in a college football game. All were diagnosed on the bench as "sprains." **A,** A small avulsion fracture from the palmar side of the middle phalanx base; severe joint injury has been incurred. **B,** No bony damage can be seen, but clinically the radial collateral ligament of the proximal interphalangeal joint was totally unstable. **C,** A basal fracture of the small finger proximal phalanx. This is the least severe injury of the three joints. The articular surfaces are intact, and the finger will regain full function months before the other two.

pared with the metal splint. Once the correct position has been established and the metal splint appropriately bent, it can be removed for toilet purposes and then reapplied. When the interphalangeal joints are involved, the splint need not be longer than the length of the finger. When the metacarpophalangeal joint is injured, the metal splint will have to extend onto the flexor aspect of the forearm to give adequate protection to the joint.

In children it is almost impossible to ensure that splints will remain in the correct position. However, adequate immobilization can be obtained by strapping the injured finger to an adjacent digit. Since the joints of the fingers are not all on the same level, the tape will have to be applied with the fingers in the functional position. The parents must be warned of the problems involved in keeping the adjacent skin surfaces clean and in preventing the accumulation of too many foreign bodies between the fingers.

Regardless of the method of immobilization used, the splint should be removed during the third week. The actual day will depend upon the disappearance of the symptoms. Gentle active exercises should be started, but the hand should not be used for powerful gripping for at least a week.

**Ruptured ligament and avulsion fracture**

TREATMENT. Both ruptured ligament and avulsion fracture can be diagnosed by a thorough clinical examination, and both conditions can be properly treated only by surgical repair. Such surgery is delicate and difficult work. It cannot be successfully done in an outpatient operating room. It will often be difficult to persuade the patient to accept admission to a hospital for "only a sprain." But the results in patients in whom operation was refused are so poor that operation should be strongly advised.

# DISLOCATIONS

Dislocations can occur at the wrist joint or any of the joints of the fingers or thumb. The injury is caused by a hyperextension force, and in every case it is more common for the distal bone to lie on the dorsum of the more proximal bone.

Lay people frequently reduce dislocations soon after they have occurred. Lay people are frequently lucky, but a doctor who undertook such treatment without first determining the extent of the injury by x-ray examination would rapidly run out of luck. Sometimes x-ray films will not be available, and calculated risks will have to be taken to relieve pain. However, in the majority of patients reduction can wait until full information about the injury can be obtained from x-ray films so that the proper treatment can be planned.

Dislocations cannot occur unless there has been severe soft tissue damage. Consequently the joint needs efficient immobilization throughout the healing period. Immediate movement is contraindicated in dislocated joints. It is illogical to expect the mass of traumatized tissue around the joint to heal more rapidly and with less reaction when it is subjected to the additional insult of tearing of the healing tissues by early movement. The usual reaction will be further hemorrhage, more fibrosis, and a definite restriction in the range of the joint.

Occasionally, but rarely, the reverse reaction can occur, and a chronic stretching of the capsular structures will result. Such stretching usually follows repeated, relatively minor dislocations rather than a primary major dislocation. Stretching of the joint structures allows chronic subluxation to occur, with the inevitable aftermath of early degenerative arthritis of the joint.

Reduction of a dislocation within the hand is relatively easy. It is best accomplished by traction in the line of the limb accompanied by direct pressure over the joint. The metacarpophalangeal joint is the exception to this generalization and has a deservedly bad reputation for being irreducible. Anesthesia is frequently not necessary. Attempts to produce local anesthesia are often unsatisfactory and, in any case, do not relieve the more proximal muscle spasm.

## The wrist and palm

Dislocations of the wrist are uncommon. Dislocations through the carpal joints are frequently misdiagnosed as dislocations of the wrist joint. True intercarpal dislocations may or may not be associated with carpal fractures: they are rare and show great variety. The three commonest are anterior dislocation of the lunate, trans-

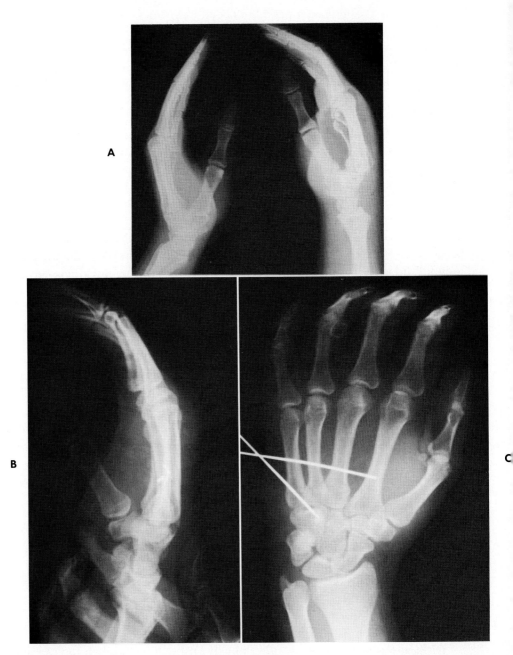

**Fig. 12-5.** *Carpometacarpal dislocation.* **A,** The normal hand is on the left; on the right the heads of the dislocated metacarpals are tilted into the palm and their bases protrude dorsally. The dislocations are hard to hold reduced by closed means, and temporary Kirschner wire fixation is often the best treatment. **B** and **C,** Two wires are necessary to maintain the reduction.

scaphoid-perilunar dislocation, and perilunar dislocation with scaphoid rotation. These are complicated injuries which deserve expert care. True dislocations through the wrist joint are more commonly posterior than anterior. They are often complicated by a fracture of the radius into the joint itself. X-ray films must always be taken.

TREATMENT. If there is no fracture, the wrist should be supported on a palmar cock-up splint in the position of function and the arm placed in a sling for seven to ten days. At the end of this time the splint may be removed, but the forearm and hand should still be supported with some form of elastic bandage. Immobilization should continue for at least three weeks to allow sufficient time for soft tissue healing. If the dislocation is accompanied by a fracture of the radius, treatment must be the same as for a fractured wrist.

Carpometacarpal joint dislocations are more common in the more mobile ring and little fingers. The metacarpals tend to tilt so that their heads protrude into the palm and their bases are prominent on the dorsum of the hand (Fig. 12-5).

These dislocations are inherently unstable and are best treated by temporary Kirschner wire fixation. These injuries are usually quite painful, and the dorsum of the hand usually swells rapidly. Inpatient hospital care is the proper choice.

## The thumb

Dislocation can occur at either joint of the thumb. It is easy to reduce the distal joint, but it is frequently extremely difficult to reduce the proximal joint. Both joints have very strong supporting structures, and avulsion fractures can occur at a ligamentous attachment. Therefore, x-ray films must always be taken.

### The interphalangeal joint

TREATMENT. Dislocation of the interphalangeal joint is similar in every respect to dislocation of the fingers and can be reduced by traction in the line of the thumb and flexion at the joint after the bones have been adequately distracted. Immobilization by splinting is necessary for at least three weeks. After this time, active movements should be started, but the patient must be warned to expect very slow progress. The periarticular swelling will take several months to resolve. On rare occasions this dislocation cannot be reduced by closed means. Open operation shows that the usual reason is interposition of the palmar plate between the joint surfaces.

### The metacarpophalangeal joint

TREATMENT. Dislocation of the metacarpophalangeal joint frequently disturbs the anatomical arrangement around the joint to such a degree that locking will occur. The proximal phalanx is usually displaced dorsally and backward on the metacarpal head. Reduction should be attempted by increasing the hyperextension of the joint while pushing the metacarpal head dorsally and applying counterpressure to the dorsum of the base of the proximal phalanx. The thumb should then be moved into flexion and adduction. If reduction is not obtained after a good trial of this maneuver, further attempts should not be made. The dislocation is irreducible by closed

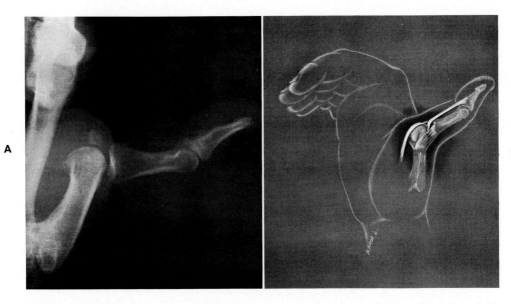

A          B

**Fig. 12-6.** *Dislocation of the metacarpophalangeal joint of the thumb.* **A,** The dislocation of this patient's thumb could not be reduced by closed manipulation. **B,** At operation it was found that the head of the metacarpal had pushed through a vertical slit on the palmar aspect of the joint capsule. Longitudinal traction tightened the grip of the buttonhole slit against the neck of the metacarpal.

methods, and relatively extensive surgery under ideal conditions is necessary to release it. The presence of an irreducible dislocation can be suspected if there is a dimple in the skin over the palmar aspect of the thenar eminence.

Locking of the joint is caused by the head of the metacarpal pushing forward through a vertical slit on the palmar aspect of the capsule (Fig. 12-6). This buttonhole in the capsule is made taut by longitudinal traction, and methods of reduction in which traction is employed usually fail because of this tightening. Occasionally the flexor pollicis longus tendon or the sesamoids around the joint may be interposed between the joint surfaces.

Surgical exploration cannot be done in the outpatient clinic. When the joint is explored under the proper conditions, it will still be found difficult to reduce. It is usually necessary to increase the length of the vertical slit slightly before reduction is possible. Sometimes not enough relaxation is obtained until a transverse cut is made in the capsule near its attachment to bone. After the joint has been reduced, there is no need to repair the hole in the capsule. The thumb should be immobilized in semiflexion for three weeks.

## The fingers

The majority of these injuries result from participation in sports, and they frequently recur if subjected to conditions similar to those producing the original injury. Bone injuries are rare, but it is wise to take x-ray films of all dislocations of the fingers as a precautionary measure. Strain films should always be taken because dis-

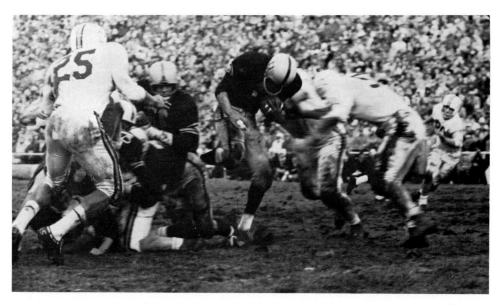

**Fig. 12-7.** *Simple dislocation of the interphalangeal joints.* This player suffered dislocations of the proximal interphalangeal joints of his left small finger and right ring finger one week prior to this game. The dislocations were reduced and reduction was maintained by using the adjacent fingers as splints to which the injured fingers were strapped. He continued to play football, made a full functional recovery in both fingers, and still played professional football fifteen years later.

location of these joints is almost always accompanied by total rupture of at least one ligament.

### Closed dislocation

TREATMENT. Metacarpophalangeal joint dislocation nearly always involves either the index or the small finger. Simple dislocations can be easily reduced and should be splinted for about three weeks. After a few days it can be taped to the adjacent finger and gentle movement encouraged. Irreducible dislocations can occur by the same mechanism as in the thumb and must be treated by open reduction under proper operative conditions.

The proximal interphalangeal joint usually dislocates dorsally and should be readily reducible by traction and flexion after distraction has been produced. After reduction the finger should be immobilized for three weeks in about 30 degrees of flexion. Frequently adequate immobilization can be supplied by buddy taping to an adjacent finger (Fig. 12-7).

Palmar or anterior dislocations of this joint occur and are frequently undiagnosed at the time because the joint is easily reduced. The problem with this injury is the avulsion of the central extensor slip from the base of the middle phalanx, which occurs at the time of injury. If this is not recognized, a boutonniere deformity will subsequently develop. Because of this risk open repair of the extensor insertion and

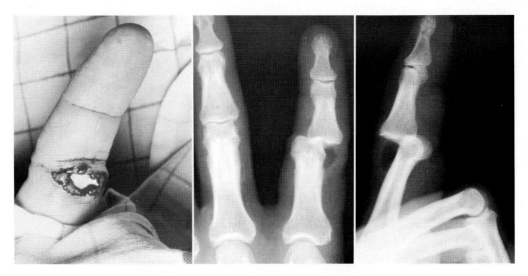

**Fig. 12-8.** *Open dislocation.* A violent hyperextension injury to this proximal interphalangeal joint tore open the flexion crease of the joint exposing the flexor tendon.

any torn collateral ligaments is the most satisfactory treatment. Splinting in extension for 4 to 6 weeks can be tried, but permanent stiffness may develop and the tendon may not properly reattach to the middle phalanx.

When exercising begins after immobilization of any of these joints, it must be active in type. Any attempt to increase the range by passive stretching will only tear the healing tissues with a resultant stiffness that is often worse than before manipulation was started.

### Open dislocation

Some dislocations are so violent that even the skin overlying the joint is torn. Because the dislocation is usually caused by a hyperextension injury, the palmar skin is torn and the flexor tendons are frequently exposed (Fig. 12-8). It is reasonable to expect massive periarticular scarring from these devastating injuries, and the joint may never regain its full range of motion. The principles of care are those of a simple dislocation combined with a meticulous wound toilet and careful surgical technique to ensure that the joint does not become infected.

### Recurrent dislocations

TREATMENT. Occasionally great difficulty is encountered in maintaining full reduction of a dislocated finger. The displacement will tend to recur to a varying degree. In such cases repeated attempts at reduction are useless, since the head of the proximal bone has buttonholed through the capsule of the joint. The capsular interposition between the two bone surfaces completely prevents proper reduction.

Open operation under full sterile conditions is necessary to allow reduction to be completed. It is wise to repair the hole in the capsule with one or two catgut sutures. After the reduction has been accomplished, the usual three weeks of immobilization will be necessary.

## OPEN INJURIES OF JOINTS

When a joint of the thumb or a finger is involved in a wound that is sufficiently extensive to expose the articular surfaces, the prognosis for the joint is bad. Many types of injuries can affect the joint, but the same principles of care apply to all injuries. The most important feature of treatment is to convert the open joint into a closed cavity. If possible, the joint should be covered by local skin flaps; if this is impossible, free skin grafts will have to be used. It must be remembered that the finger will be immobilized in the position of function, and consequently the skin cover must be planned with this position in mind.

After it is certain that adequate skin coverage is available, the other features of the wound can be treated. Any loose bone or cartilage must be removed from the joint cavity. If the collateral ligaments have been damaged, they should be repaired, using the minimum amount of suture. When a considerable amount of the articular surface has been destroyed, arthrodesis of the joint is inevitable. The problem is to decide when this should be done. The fundamental principle of first supplying adequate skin cover still applies. If such cover can be provided and the wound can be properly cleaned out, it is reasonable to remove the remaining portions of articular cartilage and thereby hasten the fusion of the joint. If the joint is transfixed with a Kirschner wire, the optimum position can be assured and the minimum amount of external splinting will be needed.

Open injuries are becoming increasingly more common with the increasing use of power tools. Friction burns, saw wounds, and abrasive wheel injuries can cause damage to such an extent that stiffness of the joint will result.

If there is the slightest doubt concerning the surgical cleanliness of the wound, no new bone areas should be exposed, and surgery should be restricted to obtaining primary skin cover.

## INTRA-ARTICULAR FRACTURES

Dislocations of the digital joints are quite frequently accompanied by very small chip fractures from around the joint margin. The presence of such small bone fragments is indicative of the extent of the original injury to the joint (Fig. 12-4, *A*). These fragments do not influence the treatment and make little difference to the ultimate prognosis. A slight separation of these fragments is acceptable to a good functional recovery, but recovery is always slow after these dislocations.

An intra-articular fracture that is not displaced is rare and should not be overtreated (Fig. 12-9). Early guarded movement is the best treatment and buddy taping is the best way to provide both protection and movement. Immobilization will almost inevitably lead to permanent joint stiffness.

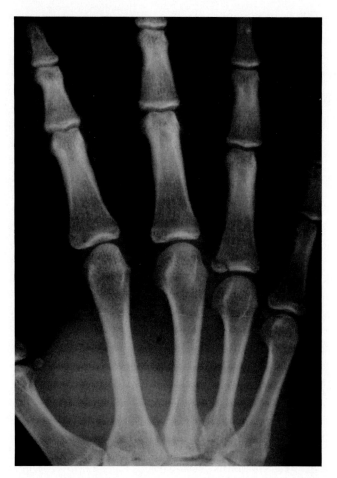

**Fig. 12-9.** *Intra-articular fracture.* Intra-articular fractures of the finger metacarpophalangeal joints do not always displace. This ring finger proximal phalanx fracture was treated by buddy taping. If the fragment had rotated away from the shaft, open reduction would have been necessary.

When the bone injury around the joint is extensive, or if a fragment is widely displaced and tilted out of position, the prognosis is poor (Fig. 12-10). Closed reduction is unlikely to produce an acceptable position, and certainly it will not produce an accurate anatomical reduction. If clinical examination shows that the fracture is associated with complete lateral instability of the joint, it is probable that the collateral ligament has been avulsed from its attachment.

I believe that better results are obtained in these injuries if the patient is admitted to the hospital and a very careful open reduction is done. Various techniques such as direct suture, Kirschner wire fixation, or use of a pull-out wire have been advised; a suitable choice can only be made by an experienced surgeon. The beginner should not inflict lack of judgment on these injuries.

Many of these injuries do not produce single large fragments of bone, and their

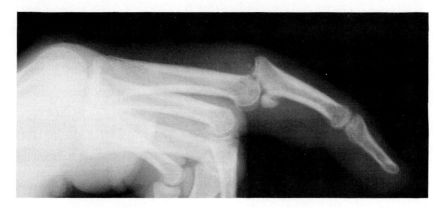

**Fig. 12-10.** *Intra-articular fracture.* Dislocations with large displaced fragments do not usually do well with closed reduction. Open reduction with careful matching of the fragments to produce a congruous articular surface is necessary.

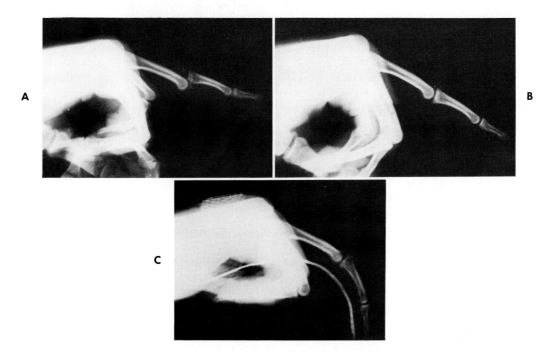

**Fig. 12-11.** *Fracture dislocation of proximal interphalangeal joint.* **A,** This dislocation produced both dorsal and palmar chip fractures. **B,** Reduction by traction was satisfactory. **C,** Splinting on a mildly curved splint did not maintain this reduction.

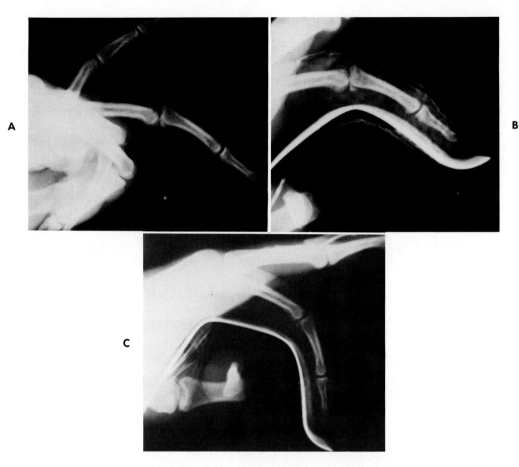

**Fig. 12-12.** *Fracture dislocation of proximal interphalangeal joint.* **A,** This dislocation produced both dorsal and palmar chip fractures. **B,** Immobilization on a curved splint did not maintain reduction. **C,** A further 10 degrees of flexion of the splint provided the proper balanced position.

treatment is very difficult. Great care must be taken in the follow-up care of these injuries if it is elected to treat them by closed reduction and immobilization. Reduction may be easy, but its maintenance is difficult (Fig. 12-11). It is essential to balance the extensor and flexor forces passing over the joint, and a considerable degree of flexion may be necessary in the splint (Fig. 12-12).

Some fractures such as the displaced condylar fracture virtually demand internal fixation, while others such as badly comminuted fractures should never be opened.

There is a very definite limit to what can be accomplished in the treatment of severely comminuted joints, and it is much better to attempt to produce a stable finger in the functional semiflexed position than to strive for complete anatomical reduction. The patient must be warned of the almost inevitable onset of degenerative arthritis and should be coached into a mood of thankful acceptance of whatever range of movement may result.

# 13 · FRACTURES

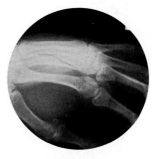

**Fracture**

**H**and fractures are the most common of all fractures and they most certainly are not minor injuries. However, in most cases they can be properly treated on an outpatient basis. Improper treatment can cripple a hand; these injuries demand a high degree of expertise and repeated visits to check whether the original reduction has been maintained.

## GENERAL REMARKS

A full and detailed diagnosis of the site and extent of bony injury is essential for proper treatment. X-ray films of the hand are an essential part of the physical examination; they are not a special examination. A posteroanterior x-ray view and a lateral view of overlapping fingers are totally inadequate. Three or four views clearly showing the injured digits are necessary; the posteroanterior and true lateral views should be supplemented with one or more oblique views to fully profile the injury.

Special views are also necessary when certain carpal fractures such as the scaphoid or hook of the hamate are suspected. If a joint surface is involved, the joint space can be seen in the posteroanterior film only if the distal bone of the joint is placed flat on the film.

The long bones of the hand constitute a series of lever arms joined together by joints and positioned in space by the action of the extensor and flexor muscles. When a long bone is fractured, a new "joint" is introduced into the system, and, since no further muscle control has been added, the system will buckle or collapse. The direction in which the angulation points is predictable in relation to the site of the fracture.

The angulation produced between the fractured bone ends has to be precisely reduced if function is to be restored. Usually this can be accomplished by closed means and external splinting. This splinting is directed to restoring the balance between the flexor and extensor muscles acting over the fracture. In some cases it may be necessary to include the wrist joint in the immobilization in order to balance these forces.

If a fractured finger is supported in the correct position, the immobilization will be so effective that all pain will rapidly disappear, and consequently adjacent fingers can be used. There is no justification in bandaging the whole hand for a fracture of a single digit.

Immobilization of a finger in full extension rapidly destroys the function of the hand.* In a finger immobilized in this manner, the fractures will tend to displace toward the palm, producing a malunion. In addition, the fingers adjacent to the immobilized digit will be severely restricted in their flexion movements because of the cross ties connecting the long extensor tendons. When several fingers are fractured the banjo splint is still occasionally used to "immobilize" the fingers. This barbaric apparatus suspends the fingers in extension and readily allows gross displacement of the fractured ends (Fig. 13-1).

Some fractures are inherently unstable and if the reduction cannot be maintained by closed means, then internal fixation is indicated. The use of pins or wires as internal splints to accurately maintain reduction in both stable and unstable fractures has become increasingly common. Inevitably this has led to an abuse of the use of this method, and it should be strongly stressed that a large number of hand fractures can be quite satisfactorily treated by closed methods.

Kirschner wires are the most commonly used means to provide internal stability for a fracture, but in recent years the use of very small plates and screws has been advocated. Perhaps there is an occasional justification for the use of a plate in a metacarpal shaft fracture, but I do not believe there is any indication for the use of plates for phalangeal fractures. It is unreasonable to expect the gliding mechanisms within a finger to function in the presence of relatively large metallic foreign bodies.

---

*Tongue depressors are for depressing tongues, not for splinting fingers.

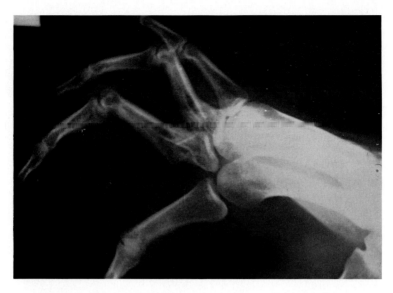

**Fig. 13-1.** *Phalangeal fractures and the banjo splint.* When a banjo splint is used to "suspend" fractures of the fingers, gross deformities will develop. Malunions such as these will cripple the hand. (From Flatt, Adrian E.: Alaska Med. **2:**34, 1960.)

There is general agreement that the common indications for internal fixation are when there is soft tissue interposition between the fractured ends, when the fracture is inherently unstable, when there is displacement close to or involving a joint, and in open fractures.

Several different methods can be used to impale the fracture. A Kirschner wire is more commonly used, but some favor Keith needles (Fig. 13-2). It is usually easier to use a power drill to supply the energy to penetrate the cortex. A short length of Kirschner wire held in a hypodermic needle mount is also commonly used.* The syringe carrying this wire can be readily controlled and the wire accurately introduced with one hand while the other holds the fracture reduced.

Usually one wire will be sufficient to maintain reduction of the fracture; sometimes a second may be needed to ensure mobilization. I have no hesitation in crossing the wires in such circumstances. Properly placed wires will hold the fracture securely; this method has been condemned as tending to hold the fracture apart. These wires are passive and will hold the bones in the position in which the operator held them. A properly maintained reduction during introduction of the wires will yield a good final reduction.

Deformity of a minor degree in the long bones of the arm or forearm usually has little effect on function, but within the hand relatively minor degrees of deformity may produce a significant disturbance of function. Fractures of the metacarpal shafts are not so potentially disabling as those of the middle phalanges, and fractures of

---

*Riordan Fixation Pin, manufactured by Zimmer, Warsaw, Ind.

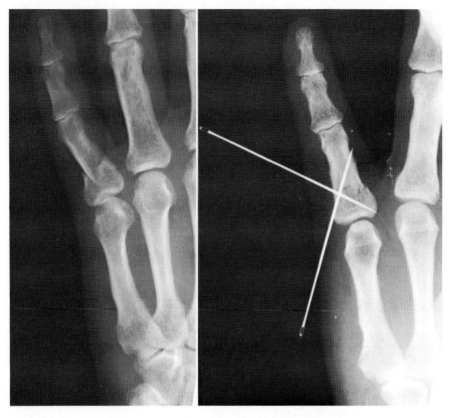

**Fig. 13-2.** *Pinning a phalangeal fracture.* Keith needles can be used to maintain the reduction of phalangeal fractures. Their method of employment is exactly the same as if a Kirschner wire had been used.

the middle phalanges are not so disabling as those of the proximal phalanges. The loss of function arises when the fracture is allowed to unite with angulation and when the tendons are damaged and adhere to the fracture site.

Angular deformities can sometimes be accommodated, but rotational deformities of even as small an amount as 10 degrees will significantly interfere with function. This rotation can occur in either the phalanges or the metacarpals (Fig. 13-3). It is a crippling deformity and must be carefully watched for during reduction. If the injured finger is taped to its neighbor, rotation can only be controlled if both fingers are flexed. This type of multiple immobilization has the additional advantage of controlling any tendency there may be for angular deviation to occur.

Many small chip fractures around joints represent the aftermath of a dislocation and severe soft tissue injury to the joint. The joint and not the bony fragment requires treatment; these injuries are discussed in the preceding chapter.

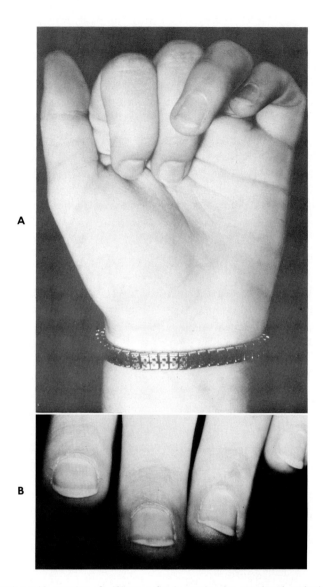

**Fig. 13-3.** *Malunion with rotation.* **A,** When a fist is made, the rotational malunion of the proximal phalangeal fractures of the ring and small fingers is clearly demonstrated. **B,** The plane of the ring and small fingernails is tilted, a sign of rotation after healing but also a useful guide during reduction and immobilization of these fractures. (From Furnas, D. W., Flatt, A. E., and McMurtry, R. Y.: The hand. In Liechty, R. D., and Soper, R. T., editors: Synopsis of surgery, ed. 3, St. Louis, 1976, The C. V. Mosby Co.)

## OPEN FRACTURES

Open fractures are common in the hand because all the bones are virtually subcutaneous. The principles of care are the same as in any other region of the body. Débridement and suture must be carried out, but in the hand, and especially the fingers, skin is so important that the minimum of skin edge should be excised during débridement. A fine monofilament wire or nylon suture should be used to close the wounds.

The major principles in the care of open fractures of the hand are to stabilize the skeleton, to treat the soft tissue injuries, and to close the skin wounds by whatever means possible, even if a skin graft is needed. The arbitrary time limit of six hours should be ignored, and, provided that the débridement has been thorough, the skin wounds can always be closed with little risk of subsequent infection. A sense of proportion is necessary in treating these wounds. It may be possible to suture the skin wounds of a finger in which there is a fracture combined with severe damage to the tendon and neurovascular structures. The best result possible in such a case is a stiff, insensitive skin cylinder containing a healed fracture. Amputation may be a better treatment.

An equally useless finger can be produced by prolonged immobilization of these injuries. It is vitally important that active exercises should be started as soon as the fracture callus is strong enough. Passive movements are dangerous; the extra sudden stress of such "therapy" may fracture the young callus. Active movements will supply motion graded to the patient's individual level of discomfort.

Problems will arise in the immobilization of multiple injuries. An individual finger can usually be successfully treated on a padded metal splint. If traction is considered necessary, the skin wounds may make it impossible to use adhesive tape traction. In such cases internal fixation of the fracture with a thin Kirschner wire should be used. When several fingers have open fractures, internal immobilization is the method of choice. By using this internal splint the fractures can be stabilized and the hand properly positioned in a large compression bandage (Fig. 3-10, p. 54).

## HEALING TIME

Union of transverse fractures of the phalanges is slow, and frequently five to six weeks of immobilization are needed before good callus is formed. Transverse fractures of the metacarpals also heal slowly in comparison with the oblique fractures, but normally only three to four weeks of immobilization are necessary before healing is well advanced. The actual time that fractures will need rigid protection depends upon the clinical and radiological assessment after three or four weeks of immobilization. It is the clinical assessment that is important. Open fractures take longer than closed fractures to gain the same degree of "stickiness." A closed fracture can be sufficiently "sticky" after three weeks of immobilization to discard the immobilization safely. The x-ray films at this time will hardly show the presence of callus and should be used more to assess position than as a guide to the strength of union of the fracture site.

## ACTIVE EXERCISE

Patients frequently misinterpret orders concerning the use of the fractured finger and will keep the whole limb at rest in a sling. It is important that the hand, arm, and shoulder be regularly exercised throughout the period of immobilization. A full course of exercises should be taught the patient before he leaves the office after his primary treatment. The exercises should be done at least twice a day.

It is said that mobility of the hand is of vital importance in the care of hand fractures. This is true. But this does not mean that the only and immediate treatment of all hand fractures is early movement. Fingers will recover a satisfactory and largely normal range of movement even after severe fractures if they are allowed a reasonable time to recover from the original trauma before the added irritation produced by movement. Early manipulation or passive stretching will definitely hinder progress. Early manipulations will rupture the granulation tissue of the healing area, with resultant hemorrhage and further scarring. Passive stretching of a joint will produce new adhesions around the area of the joint, and the ultimate fibrosis will limit the range of the joint even further.

Disuse of the hand can cause complications as serious as overenthusiastic mobilization. Often it will be necessary to encourage—or even actually bully—the patient into using the affected part after the cast or other form of immobilization has been removed. Lack of use can rapidly produce stiffness, pain, and atrophy. Unfortunately, the rate of recovery from these conditions is not proportional to the speed of their onset, and, once they have developed, it may take months of treatment to restore function to the hand.

## ANESTHESIA

Every year many thousands of fractures are reduced after local anesthetic has been injected into the fracture site. Such injections convert a closed fracture into an open fracture even after conscientious cleansing of the skin at the injection site. Infection at the fracture site is not common after this technique, but, when it does occur, it is a tragedy—a tragedy that could have been avoided if a little more time had been taken to administer the anesthetic by the appropriate regional block technique.

## CARPAL FRACTURES

Any of the carpal bones can be fractured, and the diagnosis and care of these injuries is difficult. Avulsion flake fractures are not uncommon and usually need no active treatment (Fig. 12-1, p. 208). Two carpal bones suffer fractures that can be hard to diagnose and are described in this section. The many other fractures that can occur are described in larger more specialized books and are not dealt with here.

### Scaphoid fracture

The carpal bone most commonly fractured is the scaphoid, yet its diagnosis and treatment is often difficult. The fracture usually occurs after hyperextension of the

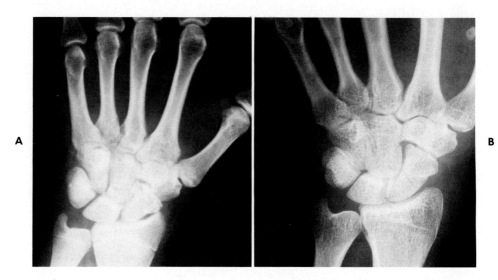

**Fig. 13-4.** *Scaphoid fracture.* **A,** Comminuted fractures of the scaphoid can be readily diagnosed. Note also the fracture of the head of the capitate. **B,** Single fracture lines in the waist of the bone may be hard to see.

wrist caused by falling on the outstretched hand. A fracture must always be suspected after such an injury, particularly if there is tenderness in the anatomical snuffbox. This tenderness can be deceptive because in the uninjured hand firm pressure into the base of the snuffbox is certainly uncomfortable. This tenderness is probably caused by direct pressure on the sensory branches of the radial nerve passing over the area.

X-ray films are essential in the diagnosis, and several "scaphoid" oblique views are necessary. Despite good-quality films, some scaphoid fractures are hard to see on the initial films (Fig. 13-4). However, if there is clinical evidence of a fracture, this lack of radiographic evidence must be ignored. If there is the least suspicion that there may be a fractured scaphoid, a plaster cast must be put on the forearm and hand, including the proximal phalanx of the thumb. The cast should be removed two to three weeks later and more x-ray films taken. If the new films do not show a fracture and if no discomfort is present on movement of the wrist, it is permissible to make a diagnosis of sprained wrist. Under such circumstances no time has been lost in treatment, since a sprained wrist would have had to have been immobilized in a similar position for the same length of time. On the other hand, if a fracture line is visible in the second set of films, then the correct treatment has been given from the start and the fracture has been given every chance to unite quickly (Fig. 13-5). The penalty the patient pays for delayed diagnosis and treatment of a fractured scaphoid is the significant risk of nonunion, aseptic necrosis, and the potential for degenerative arthritic changes in the hand.

Even with the best care, delayed or nonunion of this fracture occurs in a sig-

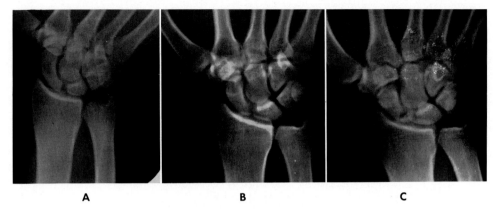

|     |     |     |
| :-: | :-: | :-: |
| **A** | **B** | **C** |

**Fig. 13-5.** *"Sprained wrist."* This athlete was told that he had a "sprained wrist" but was treated in a scaphoid fracture cast for two weeks. **A** and **B,** X-ray films of the carpus taken at the time of injury and when the cast was removed, respectively. Despite the obvious appearance of a fracture line in the scaphoid in **B** and despite the persistence of symptoms, the patient was allowed to continue playing football. The fracture line became even more obvious in the films taken two months later, **C;** at this time pain prevented his further participation in football.

nificant number of patients. This is because the pattern of the blood supply of the bone varies and the arterial supply mainly enters the tubercle and waist from the dorsum. Fractures of the proximal pole can therefore produce an avascular proximal fragment (Fig. 13-5).

The care of these fractures is difficult and because so many are associated with other carpal soft tissue injuries, it is sensible for the inexperienced to refer these problems to an experienced orthopedic surgeon.

## Hamate fracture

It is only in recent years that fracture of the hook of the hamate has been recognized as a cause of persistent discomfort in the ulnar side of the hand. Classically it occurs in club-swinging sportsmen and is usually reported in tennis, golf, and baseball players. The fracture is probably produced by a direct blow of the handle rather than by the ligaments and muscles attached to the hook. Firm pressure over the hook causes discomfort, but if the fracture is near the base, tenderness is usually more marked over the dorsoulnar aspect of the wrist.

If the fracture is suspected, an x-ray view of the carpal tunnel will demonstrate the fracture line. Conservative treatment is useless; the patient should be referred for excision of the fragment—a treatment that is curative.

## FRACTURES IN CHILDREN

The mechanism of production of fractures and their resulting deformity shows no real difference between child and adult although children more often sustain open crushing injuries. In fractures of the long bones the thick tough periosteum often remains intact and therefore aids both reduction and immobilization. These fractures frequently remain more stable within their tough periosteal sleeve than do their adult equivalents. Because of this, external plaster immobilization is usually satisfactory and open reduction or Kirschner wire fixation is rarely indicated.

Immobilization is always a problem in children, and it is wise to choose more extensive methods than might seem necessary for the fracture. A long-arm cast is frequently used (Fig. 3-13, p. 57). Children show little tendency to stiffen joints during immobilization, and the whole hand can be enclosed if it is necessary to frustrate attempts to explore and examine the injured area.

Epiphyseal injuries are common and occur more often in younger teenage children. These injuries are usually caused by indirect violence and are usefully classified into the five types described by Salter and Harris.

Type I—separation of the epiphysis from the metaphysis through the plate in a shearing manner

Type II—separation of the epiphysis, a small angle or metaphysis being broken off with it

Type III—an intra-articular fracture of part of the epiphysis without interference with the epiphyseal plate

Type IV—a vertical, displaced fracture passing from the articular surface through epiphysis, plate, and metaphysis

Type V—a compression fracture of the cartilaginous plate with no evident injury of epiphysis or metaphysis

Careful reading of the x-ray films will often show that the fracture line actually passes through the metaphysis adjacent to the growth plate. This is a fine academic distinction but of no practical value, since their care is the same as true epiphyseal injuries.

By far the commonest true epiphyseal injury is the Type II, in which a small triangular fragment of the metaphysis remains attached to the epiphysis on the side to which the finger is angulated. These fractures usually occur at the base of the proximal phalanx of the small and ring fingers and the thumb (Fig. 13-6).

Some of these injuries may be so slight as not to require reduction, but most do. I usually reduce the angulation, without anesthesia, by flexing the metacarpophalangeal joint to a right angle and then quickly but firmly pushing sideways and aligning the proximal phalanx with its neighbor. The finger should be "immobilized" by strapping it to an adjacent finger for ten to fourteen days, during which time the hand can be used freely (Fig. 13-6).

If the reduction is accurate, the prognosis is good in this type, as it is in Types I and III. Types IV and V directly affect the epiphyseal plate and may therefore cause growth disturbances (Fig. 13-7). The parents should be warned that there is this potential for arrest of part or all of the growth plate with resultant angulation or shortening of the bone.

In children the bone may avulse from the proximal epiphysis rather than frac-

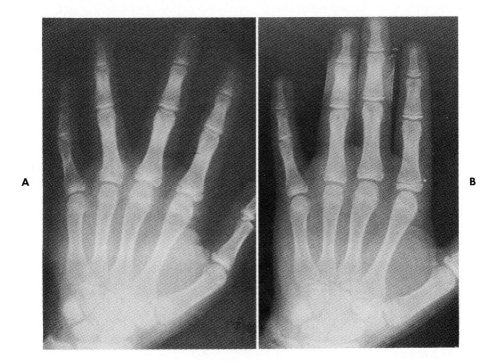

**Fig. 13-6.** *Epiphyseal injury.* **A,** The base of the ring finger proximal phalanx shows the typical tri-angular fragment that always appears on the side to which the finger is deviated in Type II injuries. **B,** Normal appearance after reduction; the reduction is protected by buddy taping the injured finger to its neighbor.

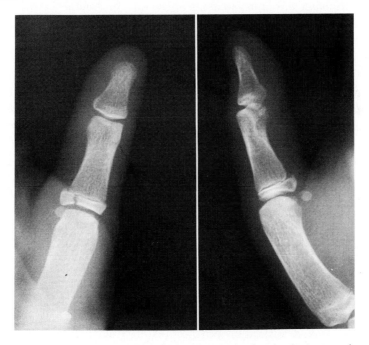

**Fig. 13-7.** *Epiphyseal injury.* A Type IV injury in the thumb of a teenage boy.

ture through the more distal portion. This avulsion of the epiphysis may occur in any of the phalanges but occurs more commonly in the distal phalanx. This is a dramatic looking injury because the broken surface frequently protrudes up through the nailbed. They are easily reduced and can be held reduced by suturing the nailbed.

If there has been complete separation at the level of the epiphysis, the prognosis for ultimate growth is good. The line of separation is not through the actual growth area of the epiphysis but through the metaphysis, and the injury is therefore treated like any other fracture by traction, reduction, and three weeks of immobilization.

## THE FINGERS
## The metacarpals

The radial two metacarpals are firmly fixed at their base to the carpal bones, while the more ulnar ring and small finger metacarpals have considerable mobility because of their movable carpometacarpal joints (Fig. 1-1, p. 4). Because of this mobility it is permissible to accept greater angular deformity in the ring and small metacarpals than can be tolerated in the index and long metacarpals (Fig. 13-3).

Another basic consideration in the treatment of fractured metacarpals is their relationship to each other. The metacarpals of the index and small fingers are the border bones, and their fractures are more difficult to treat than are those of the long and ring metacarpals, which are splinted by normal bones on either side of them. Although any portion of the bone can be fractured, the three commonest sites are the neck, midshaft, and base; each area has characteristic problems that need to be considered in the care of the fracture.

### Heads of the metacarpals

If a single large fragment has been separated from the head, it will need to be pinned in place if it is unstable. This is technically difficult to do and demands considerable experience in pinning techniques. If the fragment is not displaced, a simple plaster slab protection for about three weeks will be sufficient (Fig. 13-8).

More often the head suffers a depressed or a comminuted fracture from direct violence. There may be many small fragments that cannot be controlled either by manipulation or by pinning. The prognosis in these injuries is poor. Splint protection against pain for a few days is needed, and then active motion should be encouraged in the hopes that some form of congruous articular surface will form in relation to the proximal phalangeal base.

### Necks of the metacarpals

A fracture of the neck of a metacarpal is a serious injury. The head of the metacarpal usually tilts toward the palm, thereby producing a dorsal angulation of the fracture. Marked angulation can produce such an imbalance of the extrinsic and intrinsic muscles of the finger that function is severely limited if the fracture is allowed to unite in the unreduced position (Fig. 13-9).

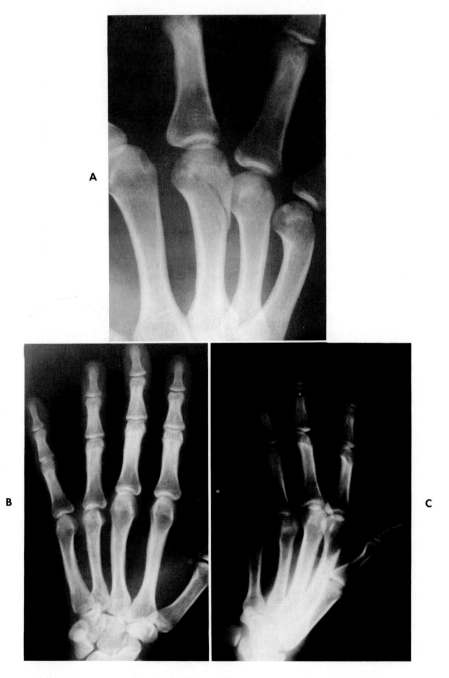

**Fig. 13-8.** *Metacarpal head fractures.* **A,** Fractures of the metacarpal head without displacement do well with minimum protection. **B,** Depressed or comminuted fractures of the head have a poor prognosis. **C,** They are often seen more clearly in an oblique view.

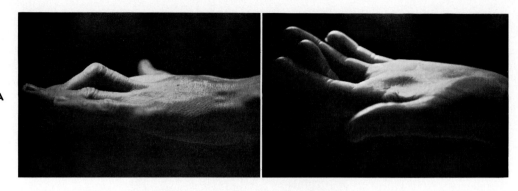

**Fig. 13-9.** *Metacarpal neck fracture.* **A,** Fractures of the metacarpal neck produce a dorsal angulation at the fracture site. **B,** The metacarpal head of the long finger is tilted into the palm and the tendon imbalance is so severe that function of the finger is grossly disturbed.

The extent of the displacement of the capital fragment will vary, but reduction is not difficult unless the head has been completely sheared off its shaft. These fractures are reduced by using the collateral ligaments of the metacarpophalangeal joint as a means of obtaining a grip on the short distal fragment. If the metacarpophalangeal joint is flexed to a right angle, the collateral ligaments of the joint will then be tightened (Fig. 1-5, p. 8). Manipulation of the proximal phalanx of the finger with the joint in this position will immediately transmit the movement to the small fragment consisting of the metacarpal head and neck.

CLOSED REDUCTION. The manipulation therefore should consist of flexing the affected finger to a right angle at the metacarpophalangeal and proximal interphalangeal joints. Pressure should then be applied backward in the line of the proximal phalanx, with counterpressure being applied on the dorsum of the hand. By this means the metacarpal head is pushed back, and the angulation is reduced.

OPEN REDUCTION. There are virtually no indications for actual open reduction, but percutaneous pinning with Kirschner wires is necessary when the metacarpal head is totally displaced from its shaft. Pinning may also be necessary when the reduction is unstable, usually because of comminution. Commonly the fracture can be held with one oblique pin, but occasionally it may be wiser to use two transverse pins passed across into the adjacent metacarpal. The two problems in the case of these particular fractures are to decide how much dorsal angulation can be accepted after reduction and to maintain the reduction. Minor degrees of angulation, particularly in the small finger, do not usually produce a significant amount of functional disturbance. Small degrees of angulation are acceptable in the small finger and even in the ring finger because their mobility at the carpometacarpal joints allows a slightly protruding head to move away from an object grasped in the hands. The index and long fingers have no comparable mobility, and if even a small angulation is allowed to persist, the protruding head will be a severe functional hindrance (Fig. 13-9).

It is hard to decide how much angulation is "acceptable." In the common boxer's fracture of the small finger metacarpal neck some physicians will accept up to 40 degrees of angulation; others have even accepted up to 70 degrees if there is no accompanying rotation at the fracture site. Clearly, the less angulation the better, but in no sense should one "treat the x-ray" and persevere until a perfect anatomical reduction is obtained. It is function that matters and in the ring and small fingers I accept up to about 35 degrees of angulation, particularly if I see the patient some days after injury when the fracture callus is already formed. Reduction in the index and long fingers has to be much better. Certainly, angulation greater than 10 degrees is unacceptable.

A useful test in deciding whether the angulation is acceptable is to get the patient to fully extend all the fingers. If the injured finger assumes a significant claw deformity (Fig. 13-9), then the angulation is not acceptable. Further reduction should be attempted, and it may be necessary to use percutaneous pinning for internal immobilization if repeated reductions have been necessary. Following reduction either by closed manipulation or by pinning, the finger must not be placed in the 90 degrees of acute flexion used in reduction.

The fracture should be protected by a gutter splint extending from the tip of the finger across the wrist to below the elbow. This can be either an ulnar or radial gutter splint incorporating two digits appropriately. When the index or long fingers are involved, a hole must be cut in the gutter splint to accommodate the thumb. Even if the fracture has been pinned, the gutter splint should be used to provide protection until the pins are removed in three or four weeks.

Follow-up care is vital because there is a great tendency for these fractures to displace unless they have been pinned. Another x-ray examination within the first week is essential. In most patients the splint can be removed for exercising at the end of the third week and abandoned at the end of the fourth week. The fracture is not fully healed at this time, but it is sufficiently "sticky" to allow gentle use of the hand. Only on very rare occasions will it be necessary to maintain immobilization beyond a month.

### Shafts of the metacarpals

The postural deformity following midshaft fractures is virtually the same as in fractures of the neck. Imbalance between the interosseus muscles and the long extensor tendons produces a dorsal angulation (Fig. 13-10).

Transverse fractures are caused by direct violence, but the more common oblique fractures result from a twisting or torsional force on the finger. In reduction of these fractures, rotational deformity must be carefully checked for if proper gripping power is to be restored.

#### *The inner fingers*

Fractures of the shaft of the long and ring fingers are so well splinted by their adjacent metacarpal shafts that very simple immobilization, consisting of a dorsal

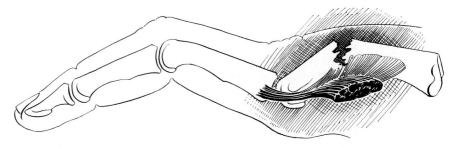

**Fig. 13-10.** *Midshaft fractures of the metacarpals.* The dorsal angulation is produced by the pull of the intrinsic muscles.

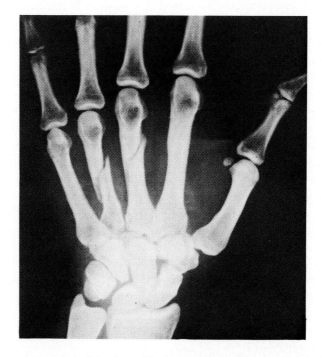

**Fig. 13-11.** *Inner metacarpal shaft fractures.* The long and ring finger metacarpals are splinted by the presence of intact metacarpals on either side. These spiral fractures will heal satisfactorily with only minimum protection.

plaster slab that leaves the fingers free, will be sufficient for their treatment. The plaster backslab should extend from the upper forearm to the level of the metacarpophalangeal joints.

Even if the fractures are spiral in type, with a minimum amount of shortening because of overriding, no other form of immobilization or treatment is necessary (Fig. 13-11). Angulation may occur occasionally in these fractures. It can be felt clinically and seen radiographically. It should be corrected by manipulation before the plaster slab is applied. The cast should be considered as a warning against excessive use rather than an essential part of treatment. It can be discarded after three weeks, but even during this time the patient can use the hand for light tasks. The phrase "light tasks" can be broadly interpreted. The fracture of the metacarpal shaft illustrated at the beginning of the chapter was incurred in major competitive football. The injury was no deterrent to the man concerned, and he continued to play football throughout the time the fracture was uniting. Union occurred at the normal time and with perfect position.

### The border fingers

Continuous traction is not a suitable treatment for these fractures; it does not necessarily maintain reduction, and it is liable to cause significant joint stiffness. These fractures frequently angulate and override because of the strong proximal muscle pull. Reduction is not difficult if the patient is seen soon after injury, but if treatment is delayed, hematoma formation may make it extremely difficult to manipulate the fractured ends. Good immobilization after a closed reduction can be provided by suitable application of a well-molded plaster cast.

Nonunion of transverse fractures, particularly of the index finger, is not uncommon, and maintenance of reduction with Kirschner wire fixation has become deservedly more popular. When properly done by an experienced surgeon in a good operating room, the reduction can be perfectly maintained and earlier hand motion permitted than if a plaster cast had been used (Fig. 13-12).

### Pinning metacarpal fractures

Transverse fractures of the metacarpal shafts of the border fingers, the index finger and small finger, are inherently unstable; an excellent means of immobilizing these fractures is transfixion with a Kirschner wire (Fig. 13-13). Open fractures can be successfully treated by this type of wiring, and even some comminuted fractures can be held adequately reduced by pinning with a Kirschner wire, although on some occasions more than one wire may be needed to maintain this reduction.

**OPERATIVE METHOD.** Kirschner wires, sizes 1 to 1.5 mm, should be used. The finger being treated must be flexed at the metacarpophalangeal joint to 90 degrees. The wire can then be introduced through the head in a proximal direction while the operator holds the fracture reduced between the thumb and fingers of one hand (Fig. 13-14). The wire should be so directed that it is passed in a slightly dorsal direction, coming out of the region of the base of the metacarpal and through the skin on the dorsum of the hand. A technical point of some importance is that before the wire is allowed to penetrate the skin on the dorsum of the hand, the skin should be pulled to one side so that ultimately the puncture wound of the skin will not lie directly over the cut end of the wire.

When the wire has penetrated through the dorsum of the skin, the chuck of the drill that is being used must be taken off the distal end of the wire and placed on the proximal portion. The wire must then be withdrawn through the dorsal puncture wound until its distal end has cleared the head of the metacarpal. This clear-

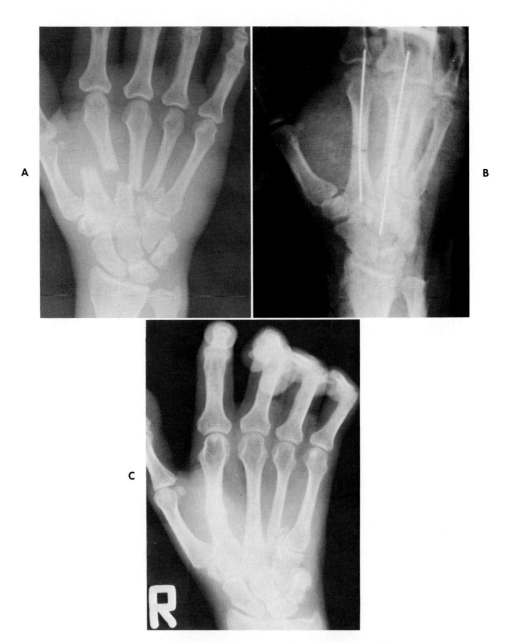

**Fig. 13-12.** *Border metacarpal fractures.* Fractures of the index and small finger metacarpals are inherently unstable. **A,** These fractures could not be held reduced by closed means. **B,** Kirschner wires in the index and long finger metacarpals provided good stabilization of the skeleton. **C,** The Kirschner wires were withdrawn after a month and healing was uneventful.

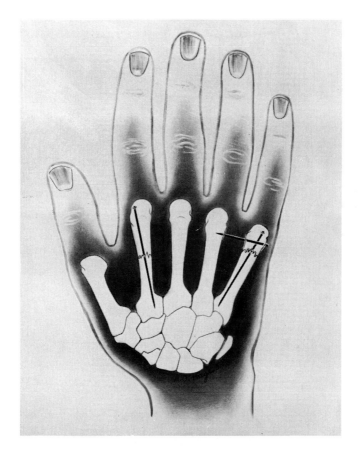

**Fig. 13-13.** *Pinning metacarpal fractures.* Kirschner wires can be used to immobilize fractures of the metacarpals. Midshaft fractures can be successfully treated with a single wire. Fractures of the metacarpal neck of the border fingers need an additional transverse wire through the head to prevent rotation.

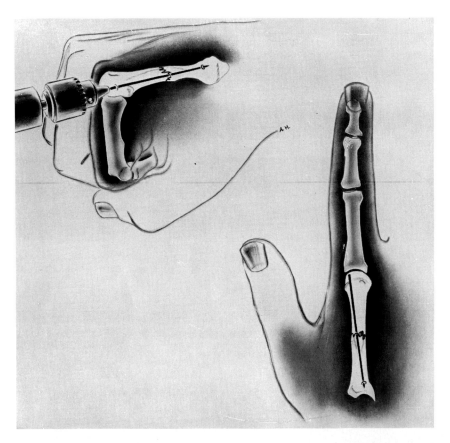

**Fig. 13-14.** *Placing a Kirschner wire in a metacarpal fracture.* The wire is introduced through the head of the metacarpal and passed upward and laterally so that the wire penetrates the dorsum of the bone near its base.

ance is shown by free passive range of movement in the metacarpophalangeal joint. When this movement has been demonstrated, the wire can then be cut off at its proximal end so that it lies beneath the skin. The length of wire left protruding from the bone is important. It must be sufficiently long for a pair of fine-nosed pliers to be able to grasp it but not so long that it causes pressure necrosis of the overlying skin. About 2 to 3 mm is usually a suitable length.

### Basal metacarpal fractures

These fractures, which are frequently missed, are often accompanied by dislocations or fracture-dislocations of the carpometacarpal joint of adjacent fingers. They usually occur in crushing or direct violence injuries that are accompanied by significant swelling in the area (Fig. 13-15). Both posteroanterior and lateral x-ray films are needed, but additional oblique films are often necessary to establish the full diagnosis. It is particularly important to determine whether or not a true fracture of one or more metacarpals is accompanied by dislocation of their own or nearby metacarpals.

The swelling in these injuries must be treated by elevation and a properly applied compression dressing reinforced by a palmar slab on which the fingers can be rested in a semiflexed position. The plane of the fingernails must be checked to ensure that no rotational deformity is being allowed to consolidate.

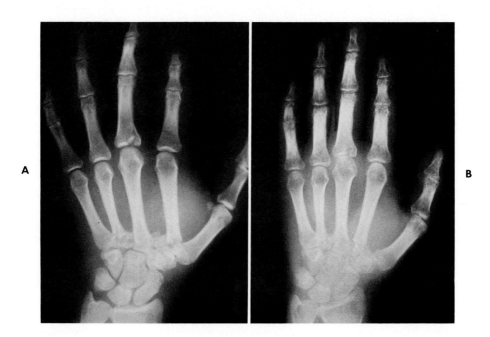

**Fig. 13-15.** *Basal metacarpal fractures.* **A,** In this crush injury the bases of the index and ring finger metacarpals were badly comminuted. **B,** Closed reduction and splinting produced an acceptable result. Note the basal fractures of the thumb metacarpal and the long finger proximal phalanx; both healed with minimal displacement.

When the fracture is unstable it should be pinned, usually by transfixing the shaft distal to the fracture to an adjacent metacarpal. Accompanying carpometacarpal dislocations should usually also be pinned so that motion of the fingers can be started without fear of displacement (Fig. 12-5, p. 214).

## The phalanges

The skin cylinder of a finger is so tightly packed with vital anatomical structures that fractures of the phalanges must necessarily involve the adjacent tissues. The flexor and extensor tendons are particularly likely to be damaged by sharp spikes of bone and to become adherent to the fracture site. The fractures are frequently open, and because the bones are relatively short, one of the three finger joints is often directly involved. Because of these factors, it is common for such injuries to result in some degree of permanent stiffness of the finger. The amount of stiffness is frequently inversely proportional to the amount of care given. These fractures are difficult to treat and require constant attention during the early days after injury.

Fractures of the phalanges require three to four weeks of immobilization before active movements can be started. The site of the fracture will have some bearing on the healing time. Fractures across the width of the phalanx pass through a large amount of cortical bone and little or no cancellous bone. Such fractures will therefore heal slowly. In contrast, fractures at the base of the phalanx heal rapidly because of the good blood supply in the area. Fractures of the head and neck heal relatively well—better than midshaft fractures but not so well as basal fractures.

There is no single correct way to treat each of the various phalangeal fractures. Those skilled in the care of these injuries achieve reasonable results using a variety of methods. Moreover, there is no disagreement about the principles to be used in reducing the fracture. It is the maintenance of reduction and aftercare that is contentious.

Most phalangeal fractures can be properly managed by closed reduction and external immobilization. Because the fracture creates an imbalance between extensor and flexor forces, stable reduction will only be obtained when the pull of these muscles is balanced. It can only be balanced by bringing the distal fragment into line with the proximal fragment, which lies in a balanced position in relation to the muscles attached to it. Traction on the finger or splinting it in an extended position will only exaggerate and perpetuate the angular deformity (Fig. 13-16).

If, however, the distal portion of the fractured finger is brought around and splinted in the balanced position, the fracture will remain reduced and rapidly heal (Fig. 13-17).

Immobilization is best obtained by including the wrist so as to remove the influence of those muscles arising in the forearm. A palmar slab starting below the elbow should incorporate a padded aluminum strip on which the finger can be placed. Accurate alignment of the padded strip in relation to the finger and the forearm is essential. The Burnham digital splint (Fig. 3-15, p. 58) is particularly useful for

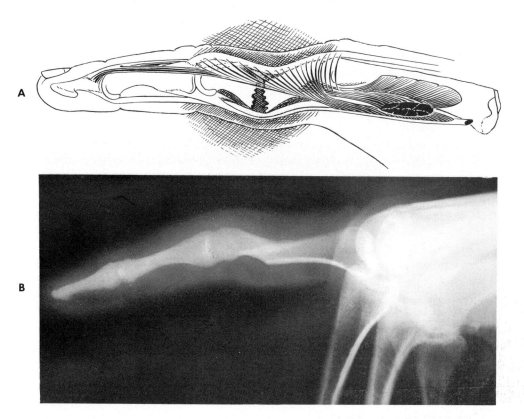

**Fig. 13-16.** *Fractures of the proximal phalanx.* **A,** Midshaft fractures of the proximal phalanx angulate to the palm. The angulation is produced and maintained both by the bony attachment of the intrinsics to the base of the phalanx and by the extensor elements passing onto the dorsum of the finger. **B,** Union in this deformed position will occur if proper reduction is not maintained.

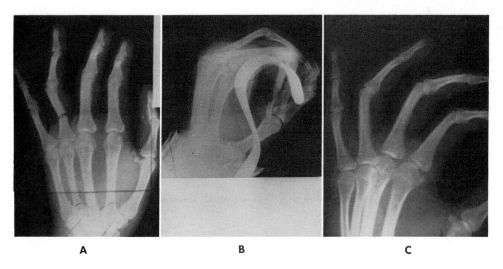

**Fig. 13-17.** *Proximal phalanx fracture.* **A,** Typical palmar angulation of the fracture. **B,** X-ray film taken with the fracture held reduced on a splint in the functional position. **C,** Film taken six months later shows the perfect result that can be expected from this treatment. (From Flatt, Adrian E.: Alaska Med. **2:**34-40, 1960.)

these fractures. Plaster of paris gutter splints can be used on either the ulnar or radial border of the hand. In each case two out of the four fingers are left free for use.

Immobilization of closed phalangeal fractures is usually needed for about three weeks; by this time the fracture will be "sticky," although the x-ray films may show little evidence of callus. Open fractures usually need another week of immobilization. Patients must not be abandoned during these weeks; redisplacement readily occurs, and periodic checks and x-ray examination are needed if there is judged to be the slightest risk of reangulation. Following the period of immobilization, protected active exercises are needed for at least another three weeks. Usually the best protection is buddy taping to an adjacent finger.

Because of the high incidence of proximal interphalangeal joint stiffness following these fractures, proponents of internal fixation with Kirschner wires suggest their use is particularly valuable in phalangeal fractures. In open fracture it is the method of choice if it will thereby allow better treatment of the surrounding soft tissue damage. Some fractures are inherently unstable and do benefit from internal immobilization; the majority can be properly treated by manipulation and splinting.

### Pinning phalangeal fractures

If it is necessary to maintain reduction by pinning, the site and type of fracture must influence where the pin is introduced. Proximal phalangeal fractures can usually be immobilized satisfactorily by one oblique Kirschner wire passed through the phalanx. In most circumstances the Kirschner wire is conveniently introduced through the head of the phalanx and passed from the distal to the proximal portion of the bone. The wire should be introduced by holding the finger flexed to 90 degrees at the proximal interphalangeal joint, and, after puncturing the skin, the wire should be directed to the more palmar part of the head and to one side of the midline (Fig. 13-18). It should then be passed obliquely across the shaft, aiming at the opposite corner of the base of the phalanx. It should come out of the dorsum of the phalanx near its base. It must not penetrate the articular surface of the metacarpophalangeal joint. When the point of the wire raises a lump in the skin, the skin should be rolled to one side on the point of the wire before it is punctured. By this means the skin puncture wound will not be directly over the end of the wire after it has been cut short.

The wire must be pulled in a proximal direction by reapplying the drill chuck to the pointed end. It must be withdrawn until there is free movement of the proximal interphalangeal joint. It should then be cut, leaving sufficient length for it to be grasped by a pair of pliers but not so long that it will cause pressure necrosis of the skin. Passing it obliquely in this manner will usually provide sufficient immobilization of the finger to allow early movement under supervision. It is usually advisable, however, to supplement this internal fixation with some form of splint on which the finger may rest in a position of function.

The wire should be left in place for at least three weeks, but the progress of the fracture must be tested by clinical and radiological means, and the wire can be removed when satisfactory "stickiness" of the fracture is obtained.

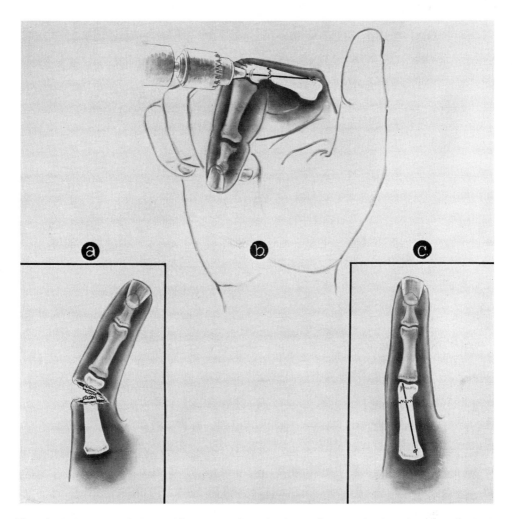

**Fig. 13-18.** *Pinning a phalangeal fracture.* **a,** Open fractures of the proximal phalanx are effectively treated by pinning. **b,** The finger is held in 90 degrees of flexion at the proximal interphalangeal joint to allow the wire to be introduced into the metacarpal head. **c,** The wire is placed obliquely in the bone and is allowed to come out on the dorsum of the proximal portion of the bone.

Middle phalangeal fractures can be treated in a similar manner, although the operation is technically more difficult to carry out because the middle phalanx is a somewhat smaller bone than the proximal phalanx.

Occasionally, fractures of the distal phalanx are treated by pinning. The indications are extremely rare and of somewhat doubtful validity.

### Proximal phalanx

Transverse fractures of the proximal phalanx at the midshaft level are relatively common. Occasionally the ends are impacted and the fracture is stable. However, this stability may conceal a rotational deformity of the shaft, and this must be care-

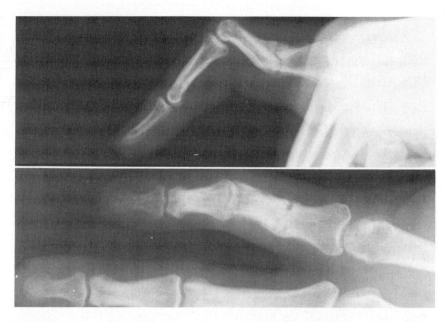

**Fig. 13-19.** *Transverse proximal phalanx fracture.* This transverse fracture was allowed to heal with the typical palmar angulation. It subsequently needed corrective osteotomy, but the flexion contracture of the proximal interphalangeal joint could not be corrected.

fully checked before the position is accepted and immobilization applied. More often, the fracture displaces with a palmar angulation (Fig. 13-19). This angulation is produced and maintained by the pull of the intrinsic muscles passing from the front of the metacarpal to the dorsum of the distal part of the proximal phalanx. It is vital that a good reduction be obtained in fractures of this type. If the angulation is allowed to persist, serious disability will be caused by the disturbance of the extensor mechanism of the finger and by restricted movements of the flexor tendons caused by their bow-stringing around the forward angulation.

TREATMENT. Reduction of transverse fractures of the phalanx is not difficult, but maintenance of the position can be troublesome. Traction on the flexed finger will reduce the angulation. The line of pull for the reduction is of great importance. It must be remembered that the fingers do not flex in a line parallel with the border of the palm or in the line of the forearm axis. Attempts to force them into this unnatural position will result in malunion and disturbances of grip. When a normal finger flexes into the palm, the nail points to the tubercle of the scaphoid. It is in this line that the traction and subsequent immobilization must be applied.

The fracture is usually stable when it is reduced into the functional position, and it can be held in this position on a Burnham digital splint (Fig. 13-17). It is useful to slide a Tubegauz cylinder over the finger, but not the splint, and to place the adhesive tape on top of this. If subsequent swelling of the finger makes the taping too tight, it is easy to release the construction by cutting between the Tubegauz and skin. More taping can subsequently be applied on top of the old.

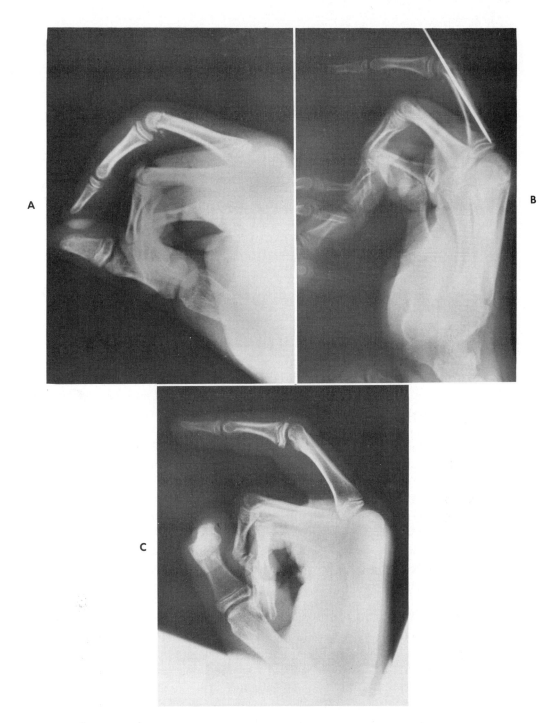

**Fig. 13-20.** *Transverse proximal phalanx neck fracture.* **A,** This fracture was easily reduced but proved to be unstable. **B,** The head was therefore pinned in place. **C,** Healing was uneventful and joint motion was maintained.

Occasionally the fracture is so unstable that the splinting and external taping cannot maintain an adequate reduction. Some would advocate constant traction by one of the many methods available, transfixing either a bone or the pulp of the finger. I believe that these unstable fractures require open reduction and internal fixation.

Three to four weeks of immobilization in the correct position will be sufficient to allow the fracture to become "sticky." After this time, active exercises can be commenced, but strong use should not be made of the hand for at least another four or five weeks.

Similar fractures near either end of the bone can often be satisfactorily reduced and maintained in a corrected position on a padded metal splint curved to the functional position. Sometimes instability demands internal immobilization (Fig. 13-20). Two or three weeks of immobilization are needed for these fractures to become sufficiently healed to allow active movements.

Oblique fractures of the phalangeal shaft are inherently unstable if the periosteal tube is completely torn. Occasionally the fragments do not displace, but usually the strong flexor and extensor mechanisms pull the distal fragment proximally, thereby leaving a sharp spine of bone near the side of the proximal interphalangeal joint (Fig. 13-21). If the fracture is allowed to heal in this position, the finger is considerably shortened, and an ugly troublesome lump protrudes distally (Fig. 13-22).

These fractures must be stabilized by pinning. This can be done by percutaneous pinning or open operation. In either case a skilled surgeon and an experienced assistant are needed to obtain a satisfactory reduction. Inevitably adhesions will develop between the extensor apparatus and the damaged periosteum; inept surgery must substantially increase the extent of these adhesions.

The pins can be left in place for three weeks and during this time protected movement of the finger is encouraged by taping it to an adjacent digit. After removal of the pins, buddy taping should be continued for another two to three weeks.

Comminuted fractures of the proximal phalanx are usually caused by crushing injuries. If the comminution is severe, the best treatment is traction on a curved splint. Even if the comminution is slight and undisplaced, the end result of the combined soft tissue and bony damage is usually a severe restriction of the range of motion (Fig. 13-23).

### Middle phalanx

Fractures of the middle phalanx are much less frequent than those of the proximal phalanx. The displacement of the two portions of bone are controlled by two important tendon insertions. The first is the dorsal insertion of the central extensor slip into the base of the phalanx, and the second is the long insertion of the flexor superficialis into almost the whole palmar aspect of the middle phalanx (Fig. 1-8, p. 13). These two insertions tend to counterbalance each other in the intact bone; in a fractured bone the stronger superficialis will tend to predominate. In fractures near the base of the bone the angulation will tend to be dorsal as the proximal pha-

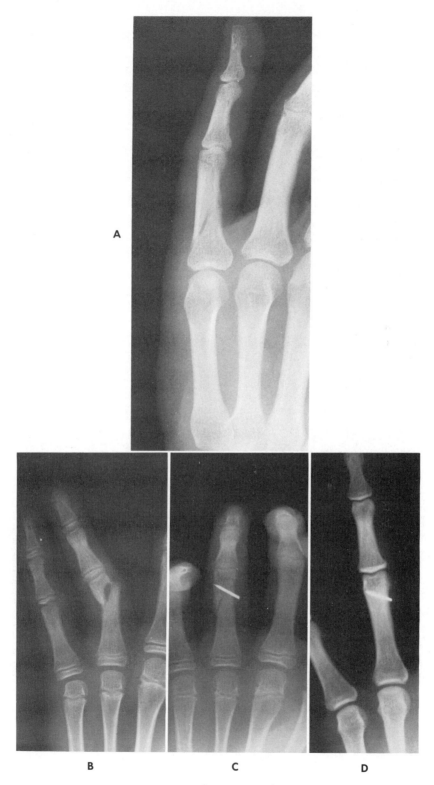

**Fig. 13-21.** *Oblique proximal phalanx fracture.* **A,** Oblique fracture of the shaft that did not displace because the periosteal tube remained intact. **B,** This oblique fracture displaced and reduction was maintained by pinning, **C. D** shows a ten-year follow-up with no adverse reaction to the presence of the pin.

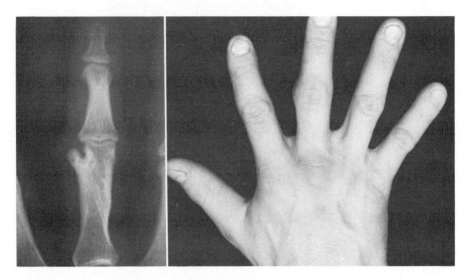

**Fig. 13-22.** *Displaced oblique proximal phalanx fracture.* This oblique fracture of the proximal phalanx shaft was allowed to heal with overriding. The troublesome hump had to be surgically removed.

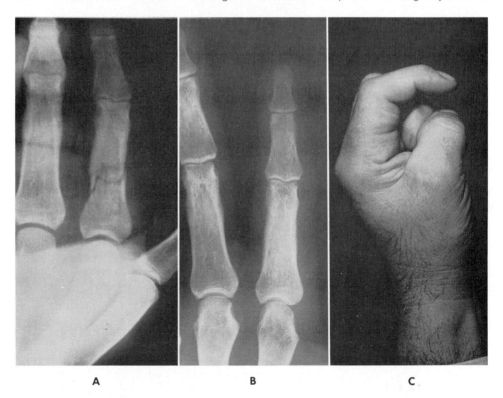

A       B       C

**Fig. 13-23.** *Comminuted phalangeal fracture.* This index finger was crushed in farm machinery, but the fracture was not compound. **A,** Multiple fracture lines in the proximal phalanx with little displacement of the fragments. **B** and **C,** Six months later: **B** shows perfect healing of the fracture, but **C** shows the far-from-perfect range of possible flexion.

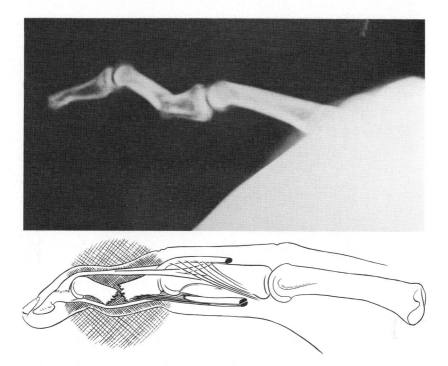

**Fig. 13-24.** *Fractures of the middle phalanx.* When the fracture occurs distal to the insertion of the flexor digitorum superficialis muscle, the attachment of the muscle will pull the proximal fragment toward the palm. The lever system will buckle, the distal fragment will angulate dorsally, and the distal interphalangeal joint will flex.

lanx is tilted upward. Along the shaft of the bone the fracture will angulate toward the palm (Fig. 13-24). Fractures in the middle two fourths of the bone can angulate in either direction but more commonly in a palmar direction. In neck fractures the main fragment will flex and the small distal head fragment will tilt upward.

These fractures can usually be treated quite satisfactorily by immobilization on a well-padded metal splint, but they need careful reduction. Traction combined with direct pressure over the fracture site will be sufficient to reduce the fracture. Reduction can be maintained on the splint with the metacarpophalangeal joint in about 60 to 70 degrees of flexion and the interphalangeal joints in sufficient flexion to maintain the reduction. Usually at least 20 degrees is necessary, and in some cases nearly double this amount may be needed to overcome the tendency to angulation. These fractures need to be immobilized for about three weeks before gentle active motion is started.

### Distal phalanx

Fractures of the distal phalanx usually result from crush injuries, and the treatment of the fractures is of secondary importance compared with the surrounding soft tissue damage (Fig. 13-25). Hematoma frequently builds up to a considerable

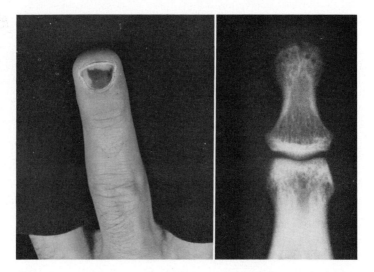

**Fig. 13-25.** *Fractured distal phalanx.* A colleague squashed his finger in a garage door and heard the fracture happen. His pain and subsequent inability to perform surgery was caused by the swollen painful pulp of the finger rather than the small comminuted fracture.

pressure within the pulp and beneath the nail. Apart from causing considerable distress to the patient, this pressure can be so great that it will cause necrosis by obliterating the blood supply to the bone. If the hematoma is wholly within the pulp, it will have to be drained through a small stab wound made on the side of the finger with a No. 11 blade, under local anesthesia. When the hematoma is largely subungual, the pressure can be released by trephining the nail or by making a drainage hole with the heated end of a paper clip. Many of these fractures are comminuted, and attempts can be made to mold the fragments into position after a few days. These attempts may possibly produce a slightly better looking x-ray film, but, since it is impossible to reposition the fragments accurately, there is little dramatic improvement in subsequent function to compensate the patient for the additional pain.

Transverse fractures of the body of the bone can usually be treated by a plaster cast. The distal fragment, to which the powerful flexor profundus tendon is attached, will be flexed in relation to the proximal fragment. It must be brought into line with the basal fragment and held immobilized for three or four weeks (Fig. 13-26).

Avulsion fractures of a small chip of bone on the dorsal surface of the distal phalanx, discussed on p. 199, represent a disruption of the extensor apparatus. Similar avulsion fractures on the palmar surface of the bone at the site of insertion of the flexor profundus tendon cannot be reduced by closed manipulation. Although it appears to be only a small chip of bone in the x-ray film taken in the lateral plane, this fracture is a serious injury. Clinical examination will show complete lack of voluntary flexion of the distal interphalangeal joint (Fig. 2-8, p. 36, and 11-2, p.

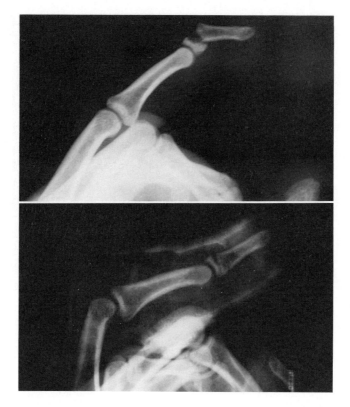

**Fig. 13-26.** *Fractured distal phalanx.* Transverse fractures of the main body of the phalanx can be treated by plaster immobilization if the distal fragment is reduced onto the proximal fragment.

189). It is essential for the function of the finger that the tendon be reattached to the bone. This restoration can be done satisfactorily only by open operation in hospital.

## THE THUMB

The function of the hand depends so greatly on the mobility of the thumb that fractures of this digit must be treated with great care. Malunion in the thumb can be considerably more serious than an equivalent deformity in one of the fingers.

Better immobilization of the thumb is obtained by a well-molded plaster cast than by most forms of splints to which the thumb can be strapped. The use of a cast implies that the palm of the hand and the wrist joint will be included in the immobilization. Such extensive immobilization is necessary to protect the thumb. There is no risk of permanent stiffness developing because the length of time that the fractures need such protection is usually only three to four weeks.

### The metacarpal

Most of the fractures involving this bone are incurred at or near the proximal end and for the purposes of treatment are divided into two groups, those involving the carpometacarpal joint and those in which the joint is not involved.

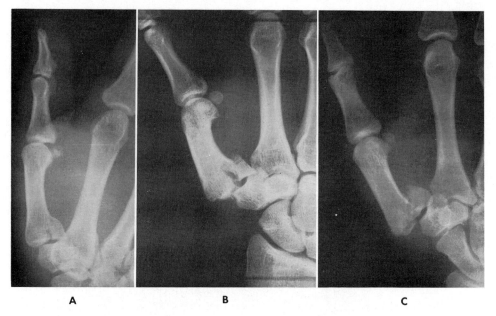

A                          B                          C

**Fig. 13-27.** *Bennett's fracture.* Three degrees of fracture are shown. **A,** Minimal displacement without separation of the two fragments. **B,** Separation of the two fragments with minimal distraction. **C,** Separation of the two fragments and proximal dislocation of the metacarpal shaft.

### Involvement of the carpometacarpal joint

Fractures involving the carpometacarpal joint, known as Bennett's fractures, are difficult to reduce, and it is even more difficult to maintain the reduction. Their treatment is difficult because the strong muscle power of the extrinsic flexors and extensors of the thumb tends to pull the thumb in a proximal direction, thereby increasing the displacement of the fracture as it rides over the saddle-shaped carpometacarpal joint (Fig. 13-27). These muscles are in fact dislocating the joint, and the injury should really be considered a fracture dislocation. As often happens in dislocations, a portion of bone is avulsed with the ligament. The size of the fragment and the degree of avulsion will vary, but the fracture line will always lie across the joint surface. If the fracture is allowed to heal with a gap between the fragments, it is inevitable that the integrity of the joint will be destroyed. If the proximal displacement of the metacarpal is not reduced, the articular end of the metacarpal must heal with an irregular surface.

There is considerable disagreement as to the "best" method of treatment for this injury. Advocates of closed methods of treatment are often prepared to accept the risk of joint incongruity. They reason that closed fractures are best treated by closed means and that over the years the incongruous surfaces will establish a working agreement without gross disability.

I can accept this reasoning in cases such as the one shown in Fig. 13-27, *A*, and possibly even those represented by Fig. 13-27, *B*, but clinical experience has convinced me that the best long-term results for cases as displaced as that shown in Fig. 13-27, *C*, can only be obtained by accurate reduction and internal fixation of the fragments.

TREATMENT. The selection of a suitable treatment should depend upon the degree of displacement at the fracture site (Fig. 13-28). In minor degrees of displacement, closed treatment may be satisfactory. This treatment is based upon the belief that it is possible to obtain traction from a cast applied to the forearm and hand and thereby pull the thumb distally, thus overcoming the proximal pull of the extrinsic flexor and extensor tendons. At the same time, pressure is applied at the proximal end of the metacarpal to reduce it toward the small fragment.

Operative treatment is indicated for grossly displaced fractures and for those fractures treated by closed means which x-ray examination shows have not been adequately reduced.

PLASTER CAST TREATMENT. The outpatient treatment of fractures involving the carpometacarpal joint can produce reasonable results if care is taken in the application of the plaster cast (Fig. 13-28, *B*). The cast must be applied so that it extends from the upper part of the forearm, across the wrist, and to the thumb. The plaster must be carefully molded around the base of the thumb, the palmar aspect of the head of the metacarpal, and the radial side of the thenar eminence. Skin traction tapes must be applied to the thumb on the proximal and distal phalanges and a wire hook incorporated in the cast. Elastic traction can then be used to produce a counterpull to overcome the strong extrinsic muscles of the thumb. When the proximal pull has been neutralized, the metacarpal shaft can often be replaced beside the small fragment by bringing the thumb over into opposition and a little adduction.

Skin traction is difficult to apply and even more difficult to maintain in an efficient state during weeks of traction. More efficient traction can be applied via a Kirschner wire that transfixes the metacarpal shaft in its distal part. It is usually recommended that bone traction on the thumb be applied through the shaft of the proximal phalanx. If this traction is used, the force must pass through the vitally important metacarpophalangeal joint, and there is serious risk that the joint may be damaged by prolonged traction. The traction apparatus will need constant supervision, and, if skin traction has been used, the circulation of the thumb and the state of its skin must be constantly checked.

The fracture must be immobilized initially for about one month. After this time the cast can be removed and x-ray films taken. Usually the fracture is sufficiently sticky to allow the traction apparatus to be left off, but it is necessary to reapply the plaster cast for about an additional three weeks to ensure good union.

OPERATIVE TREATMENT. This operation is difficult to perform. It cannot be done in the outpatient clinic and should be undertaken only by those experienced in this type of surgery. The key to success is to hold the thumb, or have it held, in opposition and a little adduction. Pressure on the base of the metacarpal toward the index metacarpal will approximate the main shaft to the fragment and it can often be felt to "click" into place. Percutaneous pinning can be tried and the result

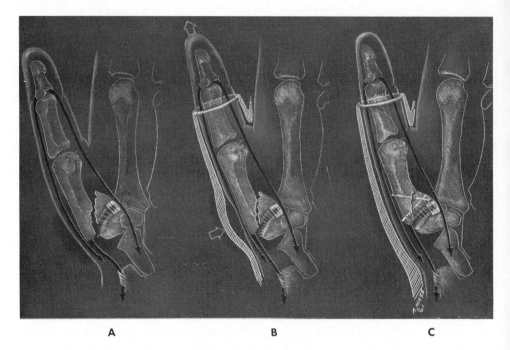

A                                B                                C

**Fig. 13-28.** *Treatment of Bennett's fracture.* **A,** The basic problem in the treatment of this injury is shown. A large bone fragment has avulsed from the main shaft, and the extrinsic tendons are pulling the metacarpal shaft proximally. **B,** Closed methods of treatment establish a distal pull on the thumb and apply pressure over the site of fracture. **C,** Operative repair holds the fracture reduced by internal fixation and protects the reduction with a plaster cast.

must immediately be checked by x-ray examination. If the reduction is not adequate, open reduction should be done.

In open reduction the fracture is approached through a small curved incision over the palmar aspect of the base of the thenar eminence. The joint space can be opened after the thenar muscles have been retracted medially. After the fracture has been reduced, it should be immobilized by some form of internal fixation. Stainless steel wire or Kirschner wires can be used (Fig. 13-28, *C*).

The reduction must be protected by a plaster spica that includes the metacarpophalangeal joint and holds the thumb in opposition. This should be worn for about six weeks. Active movement of the joint can then begin, but the pins should not be removed for at least another two weeks.

Rolando's fracture also involves the carpometacarpal joint, but in this injury there is comminution of the base of the metacarpal. The original injury was described as a T- or Y-shaped fracture line, but current practice uses the eponym to describe all intra-articular comminuted fractures. Congruous reduction cannot be obtained in these fractures either by closed or open methods. The thumb should be protected in a bulky dressing until acute discomfort has worn off and active movement encouraged. Eventually, some form of a new joint surface will develop,

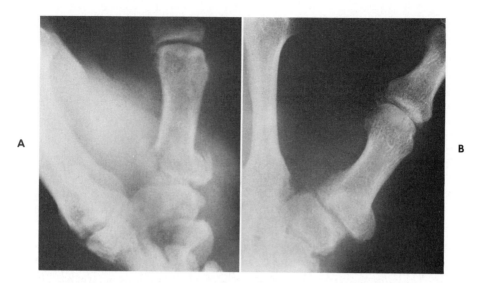

**Fig. 13-29.** *Rolando's fracture.* **A,** These comminuted fractures cannot be successfully treated by operative methods. **B,** Early protection and later use will eventually produce a new joint surface.

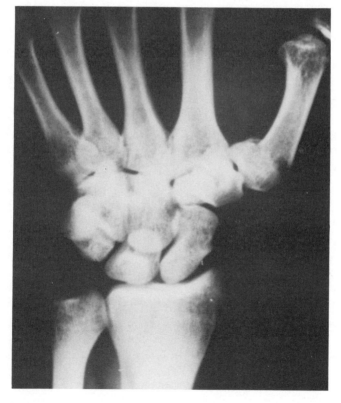

**Fig. 13-30.** *Thumb metacarpal fracture.* Fractures of the shaft but not involving the carpometacarpal joint usually angulate dorsally. Angulations up to about 30 degrees do not interfere with function.

but the patient must be warned to expect limited movement and residual discomfort (Fig. 13-29).

### Noninvolvement of the carpometacarpal joint

If the fracture line does not pass through the saddle joint, the treatment is essentially the same whatever part of the metacarpal shaft is involved. These fractures are more common than the intra-articular type. Because of the mobility of the undamaged carpometacarpal joint, angulation of 20 to 30 degrees can be accepted (Fig. 13-30).

TREATMENT. When necessary, the fracture is reduced by longitudinal traction and held in a position of reduction in a plaster cast that includes the forearm and hand. The cast should be applied with the thumb in the abducted position and the metacarpophalangeal joint slightly flexed. The plaster cylinder should be molded around the thumb and should include the metacarpophalangeal joint and the proximal phalanx, but the interphalangeal joint can be left free. The fracture is usually sufficiently consolidated after one month to allow the cast to be removed. Active exercises should be started, but active use of the thumb should be forbidden for an additional three weeks unless the patient's occupation is extremely light.

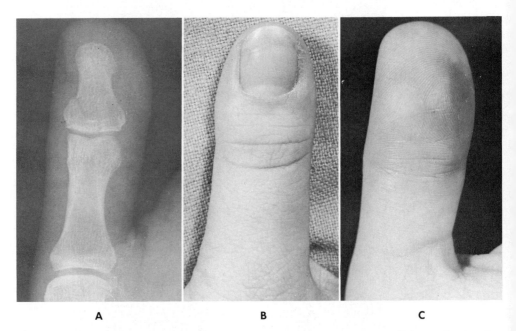

|        A        |        B        |        C        |

**Fig. 13-31.** *Thumb-distal phalanx fracture.* Direct violence to the tip that is sufficient to fracture the distal phalanx will cause considerable damage to the pulp. **A,** The fracture may be relatively minor but, **B** and **C,** the subungual and pulp hematoma will cause considerable pain.

# The phalanges
## Proximal phalanx

Fractures of the shaft of the proximal phalanx angulate in a fashion similar to those of the proximal phalanx of the fingers because of the pull by the thenar intrinsic muscles. This angulation can be reduced by longitudinal traction, and great care must be taken to ensure that the correction is maintained while the plaster cast is applied. It is best to put these fractures in a position of flexion with at least 45 degrees of flexion at the metacarpophalangeal joint and a slightly greater amount at the interphalangeal joint. Three weeks of immobilization are usually sufficient for these injuries.

## Distal phalanx

Fractures of the distal phalanx are produced by direct violence to the tip of the thumb. The fracture is usually comminuted, and no attempt need be made to reduce the fragments into a more normal shape. The soft tissue damage to the dorsum and pulp of the thumb is of much greater importance than the fracture (Fig. 13-31). If the soft tissue damage is properly treated, the bone will unite in a reasonable shape and will be further molded by subsequent use.

The long-term result of these injuries to the thumb is not always satisfactory. Persistent discomfort in the distal pulp is not due to the presence of small ununited chips of bone but is the aftermath of the original crushing injury, which has resulted in permanent scarring and contracture within the pulp.

# 14 · BURNS

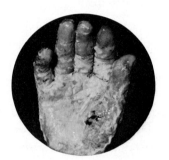

**Burn**

The hand is one of the most commonly burned areas of the body. Because of its vital functional importance, there is no room for doubt about its treatment.

The outpatient treatment of burns should be limited to small localized areas. Burns localized to a portion of a finger or well-demarcated localized burns on the palm or dorsum can be treated in the outpatient department provided that the patient will promise to return as frequently as necessary for aftercare.

Extensive burns, if they show only partial skin loss, should receive initial treatment in a hospital even if it is possible at a later date to continue treatment as an outpatient. If there is the slightest doubt about the advisability of treating the patient as an outpatient, no risks should be taken, and the patient should be admitted to a hospital.

The occupation of the patient will often have a significant effect on the type of burn and the degree of severity of the wound. Many industrial burns occur around the wrist since the hands are often protected by gloves, but most domestic burns occur on the unprotected palm or fingers.

Burns are caused by thermal, chemical, or electrical injuries. Dry heat from a variety of sources is the most common cause of burning and probably one of the most damaging. Moist heat, such as steam, will produce scalding. Chemical agents can produce serious injury, but one of the most destructive burn sources is electricity. Whatever agent produces the burn, the basic pathological changes are the same.

## PATHOLOGY

Burns can produce changes varying from mild erythema to frank cooking. In any tissue that is not actually charred, the basic reactions are the same. There is marked dilatation of the smaller blood vessels and increased capillary permeability. This increased permeability leads to extravasation of tissue fluid, which builds up rapidly in the first few hours after the burn, reaching its maximum in twenty-four to thirty-six hours. Thrombosis of many nearby smaller vessels will also occur and leads to the death of tissues surrounding the actual burn site. The burned area will rapidly undergo necrosis but will not usually begin to separate from the nearby viable tissue until about a week after burning. Total separation may take up to three weeks.

If the burn is extensive, the outpouring of tissue fluid will have a profound effect, both upon the patient's hemodynamics and electrolyte balance. The care of patients with extensive burns can only be undertaken in a properly equipped hospital, and discussion of such treatment is beyond the scope of this book.

## CLASSIFICATION

In former years elaborate classifications based upon a microscopic analysis of the depth of penetration of a burn were in use. Such classifications have no practical value (Fig. 14-1). The only information of use to the clinician is whether there has been partial or total loss of all epithelial elements.

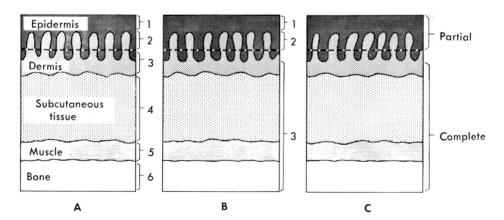

**Fig. 14-1.** *Degrees of burns.* The only information of practical use to the physician is whether or not there has been complete destruction of all epithelial elements. The most useful classification is shown in **C. A** and **B** represent earlier classifications that are still occasionally used.

## Partial skin loss

In partial skin loss there are still unharmed epithelial elements deep in the der-mis. These areas include the ducts of the glands in the dermis and hair follicles as well as the deepest parts of the epithelial papillae. After a latent period of three to five days the epithelial cells spread laterally across the granulating area and finally coalesce to provide a new epithelial cover.

## Total skin loss

In total skin loss all of the deep epithelial elements have been destroyed and re-epithelization is possible only by ingrowth from the periphery of the burned area.

•  •  •

A classification still in common use divides a burn into three degrees. The first and second degrees are used as subdivisions of the partial skin loss and are differ-entiated by the fact that blistering does not occur in first-degree burns, whereas it is common in second-degree burns. Third-degree burns are the same as total skin loss, since all epithelial elements have been destroyed. There is little purpose in this additional subdivision of the partial skin loss, since the essentials of treatment are exactly the same in both degrees.

## RECOGNITION OF THE DEPTH OF BURNING

The problem of deciding which portions of a burn show complete loss and which portions are only partially burned is extremely difficult, and no clinical tests have yet been devised that will establish without doubt the degree of burning. A careful history of the cause of the burn, the intensity of heat, and the duration of exposure will often be as valuable as the clinical examination.

The type of burn often helps in determining the extent of tissue damage. Dry heat usually produces mixed partial and complete loss; friction burns from wringers and rollers are also mixed in their degree of loss. Scalding usually produces only partial skin loss, as do flash burns and electrical spark burns.

Charred areas obviously represent total epithelial loss, but where the area shades out at the periphery the dividing line between partial and complete loss is difficult to define. Pressure on this area will show whether or not circulatory blanch-ing and filling occur, and the state of the nerves can be tested by pinprick. If there is neither circulatory return nor sensation in the skin, it must be assumed to be totally burned. It is sometimes helpful to palpate the burned area while wearing a sterile glove. Where there has been total skin loss, the area will feel indurated, and in areas of partial skin loss the surface will feel soft.

## PRINCIPLES OF TREATMENT

Burns produce both local and systemic effects. The patient's general condition must be treated just as actively as the locally burned area. A burn is an open wound that is virtually sterile immediately after burning. Treatment must be aimed at preserving this sterility and converting the open wound to a closed wound as soon as possible. Unless the burn shows total loss, there will be viable islands of tissue scattered over the raw surface that will provide the new skin to surface the burn if they are given the opportunity. These areas of partial skin loss can be easily converted into areas of total loss by the wrong treatment. The essentials of treatment are as follows:

1. First-aid treatment MUST protect the area from surface infection and must relieve pain.
2. Treatment should NOT consist of scrubbing or hard cleansing of the burned surface.
3. Solutions that will harm the viable cells by precipitation of protein (tannic acid) must NOT be used.
4. Infection MUST be prevented by application of sterile dressings, and swelling must be prevented by elevation and adding compression to the sterile dressings.

### First aid: cold-water immersion

Immediate immersion of a burned hand in ice-cold water as a first-aid measure has been advocated since 1799. In that year Sir James Earle, Surgeon Extraordinary to the King of England, reviewed current methods of treatment for burns and dismissed all except local cooling with water, which he felt gave good clinical results. This advice is still valid. Cold is an excellent antidote for pain, and total immersion of the burned area will effectively prevent airborne contamination of the raw surface. It is said that the cold inhibits capillary permeability, thereby decreasing edema and tissue destruction. Clinical experience, including members of my own family, has convinced me of the value of this treatment and I believe it to be an excellent first-aid measure.

The hand should be held under cold running water from the faucet while a large bowl of ice water is prepared. Ice cubes must be kept in the bowl throughout the time the hand is immersed. The length of time that the hand is cooled depends entirely upon the severity of the symptoms and should be left to the patient's judgment. Even children can judge the time necessary to relieve pain; premature removal will result in the return of pain, and the child will insist on further cooling of the hand. My own experience agrees with the views of several authors that the subsequent course of burns receiving this treatment is considerably more benign than that of comparable burns that did not receive early cooling. The amount of pain and tissue damage is remarkably reduced in hands that have been immersed in ice water.

### TYPES OF TREATMENT

One of two methods are usually employed: an occlusive dressing or exposure under controlled conditions. Whichever is used, strict attention to aseptic techniques is vital, since secondary infection by gram-negative organisms is a constant threat.

## Occlusive dressing technique

The commonly accepted method of treatment is to cover the burn with an occlusive dressing that is changed as necessary. Probably the most satisfactory topical dressing at the time is silver sulfadiazine (Silvadene).* Others use mafenide acetate (Sulfamylon cream).† Most small burns will heal under such a regimen providing local débridement is carried out regularly. In recent years there has been more frequent use of the exposure method.

## Exposure method

Although the exposure method is more applicable to burns of the trunk and proximal portions of an extremity, it can also be used in the treatment of local burns on the hand.

The rationale of this treatment is that the body is perfectly able to cover the burned area with its own sterile dressing in the form of a scab if the proper conditions are available. This early formation of a scab protects the wound against invasion by pathogenic organisms, provides a framework for the new epithelial cells, and provides a waterproof covering against the loss of proteins and salts in the exudate. If the burned areas are exposed to the air, the surface will cool to a temperature below that of the body, and the circulating air will dry the surface. These factors, together with exposure to light, combine to produce an environment unsuitable for bacterial multiplication. Antiseptics, which might damage the surviving epithelial cells, are not necessary. The area should be put at rest by splinting, and swelling should be controlled by elevation.

Humidity has little influence on this method of treatment, and it can be successfully used in regions with high temperatures and high humidities. In treating burns of the hand, the exposure method has only limited value, and it must definitely not be used in areas where there has been circumferential burning, because of the risk of a constricting tourniquet effect that may be produced by the contracting scab.

## DOMESTIC BURNS

TREATMENT. Most burns that occur in the home are of varying depth and have to be treated as mixed burns. Changing diapers and washing dishes are not appropriate tasks for a burned hand. If the patient cannot forego such duties, the risk of secondary infection is high, and occlusive dressings protected by a large rubber glove offer a better chance for successful treatment than the exposure method.

Children frequently grasp or touch extremely hot objects, such as electric irons or electric heating units. The severity of these burns will depend upon the duration of exposure, and usually contact with the hot surface is only momentary. In these cases the burns will probably represent only partial-thickness loss and can be treated either by the exposure method or by the closed dressing technique. Deeply burned

---

*Marion Laboratories, Inc., Kansas City, Mo.
†Winthrop Laboratories, New York, N.Y.

localized areas are best treated by prompt excision and replacement of the area with a split-skin graft.

A burn resulting from a book of matches flaring up in the hand is a combination flame and contact burn. In the main area of the burn there is usually only partial-thickness loss, but throughout this area there will be scattered sites of full-thickness loss. These areas are usually too small to justify excision and grafting. The burn should be treated by the exposure method if domestic duties will allow.

Burns caused by the spilling of hot liquids, such as water or cooking oils, are often extensive in area but usually cause only partial skin loss. Because of the relatively large area involved a significant degree of shock may be produced and should always be anticipated. Careful treatment is needed to prevent the occurrence of secondary infection, and these burns are not usually suitable for treatment by the exposure method.

## THERMAL BURNS CAUSING PARTIAL SKIN LOSS

TREATMENT. In thermal burns in which there is partial skin loss the necessary elements for new skin cover are present and must be protected to allow multiplication and spread. Whether the closed dressing technique or the exposure method of treatment is used, the preliminary treatment of the burn is exactly the same. Burns are painful, and suitable doses of analgesics must be given before any treatment is started. The burned area must be cleansed with rigid sterile surgical technique. Masks must be worn by all persons present during the dressing, including the patient. Sterile gloves must be worn and sterile solutions used for irrigation.

Frequently, domestic first-aid treatment consists of smothering the burned area in butter, cooking oil, or some thick proprietary salve. This greasy seal, which serves only to retain any dirt or contamination on the surface of the wound, must first be removed by gentle scraping or possibly even the use of ether to get to the level of the burned surface.

The burned area must be washed with a plentiful supply of sterile normal saline solution, and all foreign material and loose pieces of epithelium must be removed. Blisters should be opened and trimmed away around their periphery. Harsh scrubbing with brushes or sponges is not necessary and can be positively harmful, since it may destroy epithelial cells that would otherwise help in the process of re-epithelization. After the area has been thoroughly cleansed, it should be gently mopped dry with sterile sponges. The choice of dressings or exposure as the treatment will be influenced by many factors, principal among which are the age and intelligence of the patient, his occupation, and the ease with which he can return for subsequent care. The exposure method is suitable for the intelligent office worker, and closed dressings are better for the unruly child. The busy housewife, who frequently sustains this type of burn, has so many and varied occupations that neither method is really suited to her, but, on the whole, the closed dressing method is better; the dressings should be protected by a rubber glove when necessary.

CLOSED DRESSING TECHNIQUE. After the burn has been cleansed, the surface should be protected by a layer of topical antibacterial cream (silver sulfadiazine). In cooperative patients further dressings may not be necessary, but in general it is best to use several layers of fluffed-up gauze to act as a compression-absorbent dressing, which is held in place by a Kling bandage.

Careful and frequent follow-up is necessary when this method of treatment is used. If the initial dressing has been properly applied, it is unlikely that any clinically significant infection will occur from organisms beneath the dressings. Infection can readily be introduced from the outside if the bandages are allowed to get wet. They can become soaked from without, or they can become soaked from within by the exudate draining from the burned surface. In either case the wet dressings establish a direct connection between the burn and the outside and can thus act as a wick, allowing outside contaminants to grow inward to the burned surface. Because of this risk the patient must be warned against getting the dressings wet and must be told to report immediately if exudate appears to be soaking through. In any case the first dressing should be changed in one to two days so that any discharge that has accumulated in the dressings does not act as a culture medium. Dressings should not be changed very frequently, and the time interval between dressings will be dictated by the condition of the burned surface at the time of the first dressing. If the surface is moist and there is much exudate, another dressing will be necessary in at least forty-eight hours; but if there is little exudate, dressing times can be prolonged. Complete healing of an uncomplicated partial-thickness burn usually occurs between the second and third week.

Throughout treatment, active movements of the hand should be encouraged, but it is probably best to discourage actual use of the hand for occupational tasks, particularly if there is a risk of wetting the dressings.

Unfortunately, it is not always possible to be accurate in the diagnosis of the depth of a burn, and granulating areas, representing full-thickness loss, may be present. If these are small areas about the size of the end of a pencil, they can be safely left to epithelize from the periphery. The raw surface should be protected by dabs of antibacterial cream. As much as possible of the healed area should be exposed.

If the granulating areas are more than 2 cm in diameter, they will heal more quickly and more satisfactorily if they are covered with a split-thickness skin graft. The graft should be slightly larger than the area to be grafted. Since it is usually not technically possible to hold the graft in place with sutures, it should be smoothed out (raw surface upward) on a piece of petrolatum gauze. The gauze will then act as a splint and will prevent the graft from becoming curled up. When dressing the area after grafting, it is wise to avoid putting petrolatum gauze over fully healed areas. If the gauze is put on these areas, there is a risk of maceration of the new skin during the additional ten to fourteen days that the grafted areas will need to be protected. When grafts have to be used, the hand will need to be immobilized on a splint until the grafts take. The dressing procedure after grafting is identical to that used on skin grafts anywhere else on the hand (p. 110).

EXPOSURE TECHNIQUE. If it is decided to treat the burns by exposure, the area must be mopped completely dry with sterile sponges after cleansing. It is not necessary to add any active clotting agents to the burned surface. Occasionally cornstarch is lightly powdered over the area to help coagulate the surface exudate. Because of the risk of sensitivity reactions and the possibility of producing resistant bacteria, powders containing antibiotics are not recommended.

The burned surface will dry in twenty-four to forty-eight hours. While drying is proceeding, the patient's temperature may be slightly raised and there may be a slight reddening around the periphery of the burn, but these inflammatory signs will disappear as soon as the scab has formed. After the scab is complete, the patient must be warned to keep the hand dry at all times. During the second week after burning the crust will separate and reveal a completely healed surface. This separation often occurs in piecemeal fashion, and care should be taken to avoid damaging the new epithelium by too hastily tearing off the whole scab. It is wiser to use scissors to trim the edges of the scab as it separates. While the scab is in place, there must be limitation of function of the hand. Experience shows that this relatively short period of time does not produce any permanent limitation of function.

## THERMAL BURNS CAUSING FULL-THICKNESS SKIN LOSS

TREATMENT. A full-thickness burn represents an area of complete skin loss and therefore needs to be replaced just as much as an area of traumatic loss. Well-defined, obviously deep burns are not common, and it is often impossible to decide the depth and extent of the burned area during the first examination. However, if small clearly defined areas are present, the treatment of choice is immediate excision and replacement of the burned area with a thick split-skin graft cut from the flexor aspect of the forearm of the affected extremity. A sufficiently large graft should be cut to overlap the area of excision around its circumference. The graft should be sewed into place and the ends of the sutures left long to allow the compression dressing to be tied into place. The hand should be immobilized until the graft has taken, and the next dressing should be done on the fourth postoperative day. Details of the aftercare are the same as for grafts applied for traumatic defects and can be found on p. 109.

Even though the area of total loss has been excised, it is probable that there will still be a zone of inflammatory reaction around the excised area. The reaction produces edema, and even after the graft has taken, there may be a considerable length of time before the inflammatory reaction subsides and allows the grafted area to become supple. During this time, use of the hand is important, and it should be used to the point of discomfort for ordinary domestic and occupational tasks. Such use will frequently produce a better result more quickly than infrequent systematized occupational therapy or physical therapy.

## THERMAL BURNS CAUSING MIXED LOSS

The great majority of burns vary in depth over different portions of their surface and thereby are more difficult to manage than burns of a single thickness. Burning by flame is the most common cause of this varying depth of tissue loss, and these burns are usually too extensive to justify outpatient care.

TREATMENT. The overriding principle of care is to cover areas of complete skin loss with grafts at the earliest possible moment. This skin cover is particularly important in burns of the fingers where there is normally very little tissue covering the joints. If granulations are allowed to persist in these areas, a considerable degree of fibrosis will occur. Even if skin grafts are applied at a later date, the damage will have been done, and the joints will be fibrosed.

Initially the area will have to be treated as a partial-thickness loss and should be cleansed and dressed exactly as recommended for the closed dressing treatment of their burns. The dressings should be changed at intervals of about forty-eight hours under the strictest aseptic technique. Such frequent dressings are necessary so that removal or excision of dead tissue can be carried out as soon as possible. By this means, the areas of skin loss can be defined and prepared for grafting as soon as possible. The period of dressings will last about ten to sixteen days, and throughout this time there is a heavy responsibility on the physician not to introduce infection during the change of dressings. An additional responsibility is to maintain the hand in the position of function throughout treatment by means of appropriate splinting.

Because of the inevitable fibrosis in granulating areas, it is essential to apply skin grafts at the earliest possible moment, and the hand should certainly be covered with skin within three weeks from the time of burning. Split-skin grafts should be used, and wherever possible it is best to use sheet grafts, since small patch grafts leave intermediate areas of raw granulations that cannot be covered with skin until the grafts have consolidated and begun to proliferate from their edges. Pinch grafts are not suitable for use in the repair of burns of the hand.

## CHEMICAL BURNS

The agent producing a chemical burn will continue to act until it is so dilute that it can no longer cause any damage. It is only in this prolonged contact that chemical burns differ from thermal burns. There is usually great difficulty in determining the depth of the burn because so many variable factors affect the chemical action. Burns by acids coagulate the surface tissues and the result looks horrible, but in fact the chemical does not penetrate as deeply as an alkali, which will continue to extend and deepen the burn until it is sufficiently diluted or neutralized. Concentrated strong acids and alkalies will burn through the full thickness of the skin of the forearm or dorsum of the hand in 10 to 20 seconds. The thicker, palmar skin withstands the action for about 60 seconds. The rate of destruction will also be influenced by the actual concentration of the chemical, the amount of sweat on the hand, and the amount of protective dirt that may be present.

TREATMENT. Treatment will depend both on the chemical and its physical state. If the patient is seen soon after injury and the burning chemical is still present, as much as possible of it must be removed before any attempt is made at chemical neutralization. Running water is by far the best first-aid treatment for burns, but dry powders should be brushed off before the washing is commenced. Considerable quantities of water must be used, and in most cases this will be sufficient to remove the offending chemical. It would seem logical to use the appropriate neutralizing agent against the burning chemical, but in many cases ill-advised use of too concentrated a neutralizing agent has produced further chemical injury. Alkalies can be neutralized by citrus fruit juices, vinegar, or dilute acetic acid. Carbolic acid should never be used. In concentrated form it rapidly produces irreversible changes in the tissue protein. Its use in diluted form in wet compresses is equally dangerous since it will, at first, anesthetize the surface on which it is placed and later will produce gangrene from local arteriolar spasm. Acids may be neutralized by chalk, lime water, or sodium carbonate. Hydrofluoric acid is neutralized by the infiltration of the affected tissues by injection of 10% calcium gluconate until pain is completely removed.

### Phosphorus burns

TREATMENT. Unlike the liquid burning agents, solid phosphorus must be neutralized to prevent its continued action, since phosphorus will burn until it is totally deprived of oxygen. As a first-aid measure, the burning area can be submerged in a bucket of water while arrangements are made to obtain the appropriate neutralizing agent. Oily dressings must NOT be used as a first-aid compress, since phosphorus will dissolve in oil and the burning area will be enlarged. An aqueous solution of copper sulfate of any strength between 1% and 5% will react with the phosphorus, producing an inert coating of black copper sulfide. Since phosphorus glows in the dark, it is sometimes helpful to observe the area in a darkened room. Any glowing areas will show that further neutralization is necessary. The damage in a phosphorus burn is produced by the direct action of the heat of combustion and is not the result of chemical reaction. The aftercare is therefore exactly the same as for thermal burns of mixed depth. But the greatest care must be taken to ensure that all particles of phosphorus have been removed before the petrolatum gauze is put in place.

### ELECTRICAL BURNS

Electrical burns differ fundamentally from thermal burns because there is considerable depth to the tissue damage. The heat of an electrical burn is generated by the resistance of the tissues to the passage of the current. Although the entry burn may seem to be relatively small in extent, the burn may even involve muscles and bone, because the current will pass into the deeper tissues by means of the blood vessels, which are excellent conducting paths. Vascular damage can thus occur over a relatively widespread area and will lead to subsequent thrombosis and sloughing of the deeper tissues. Additional sloughing may occur because of the dehydration of tissues caused by the passage of the current.

TREATMENT. Treatment of electrical burns is difficult and should not be undertaken in the outpatient department. Although the entry burn will be well defined and quite clearly an area of total skin loss, it is unwise to treat this by excision and immediate grafting. The patient must be warned that more damage will become apparent later and that proper treatment cannot be planned until the full extent of skin loss is known.

## RADIATION BURNS

Localized, intense dosage of ionizing radiation can occasionally occur accidentally in persons handling isotopes or working in atomic stations. The safety precautions in handling these substances are so well organized that it is extremely unlikely that any physician not directly connected with the public health aspects of such hazards will be called upon to treat such a burn.

The signs to be expected are early edema and erythema followed by blistering, which frequently coalesces into large areas.

**TREATMENT.** Initial treatment is exactly the same as for partial-thickness skin loss. Subsequently, some areas that have received the major part of the radiation may slough. As in an electrical burn, it is difficult to predict the extent of such burns, and it is wise to wait for the slough to separate rather than to excise it at an early stage.

The ultimate prognosis in such burns is poor because the sclerosing effect of the radiation on the blood vessels will lead to subsequent atrophy and fibrosis.

# 15 · INFECTIONS

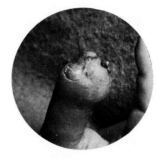

Infection

$S$urgical judgment is of paramount importance in treating an infected hand; judgment can only be acquired by experience, yet it is usually a junior house officer who is expected to care for these problems. The seriousness of the infection is frequently underestimated, and I believe that admission to hospital is the correct decision if there is any degree of doubt.

It is not sufficient to establish the anatomical site of the infection. The diagnosis must be further refined by identifying the responsible organism and establishing its antibiotic sensitivities. Appropriate surgery cannot be postponed for the results of these tests, but only when they have been completed can intelligent use be made of the multitude of anti-infective agents now available.

The hand is designed to withstand the insults of hard manual labor by being provided with a tough skin backed by fatty subcutaneous tissues that are subdivided into many small compartments by fibrous septa. Tendons and fascial tissues, of which there are many in the hand, have a very poor blood supply and a consequent low resistance to infection. These facts, combined with the patient's natural reluctance to stop work for an apparently minor injury, lead to rapid establishment of infection. Because of the tough nature of the skin and subcutaneous tissues of the hand, infection tends to spread widely along tissue planes in the depths of the hand rather than to point to the surface.

Many infections of the hand are caused by staphylococci, but other organisms can also cause infections. Among these organisms is the *Erysipelothrix rhusiopathiae*, which causes an infection that is a frequent source of misdiagnosis and overtreatment. If the patient works in a hospital or has recently been discharged from one, the strain of staphylococcus is likely to be resistant to penicillin, streptomycin, tetracycline, and sometimes erythromycin.

An unsuspected carrier is often the primary source of staphylococcal infections. If a patient's history shows that someone in his family is suffering from a pus-forming condition, such as an abscess, boil, carbuncle, sty, sinusitis, osteomyelitis, or impetigo, it is probable that this infection is the source of the staphylococcus. Even if the relative has recovered from the infection, he can still carry the organism in his anterior nares. When there is a history of such a contact, it is a wise precaution to take nasal swabs from all members of the family. Those found to be carrying the coagulase-positive staphylococcus should use bacitracin or neomycin nasal spray or apply ointment in the nose twice daily for ten days. Several days after this treatment is complete, a repeat nasal swab must be taken to ensure eradication of the organisms. Retreatment may be necessary. Unless such precautions are taken, there is a considerable risk of repeated reinfections of the hand, which may lead to permanent disability.

The ideal treatment for hand infections is prophylactic. No injury is so trivial that it can be ignored. Splinter and puncture wounds are particularly likely to lead to deep infection and should be watched carefully. Routine use of prophylactic chemotherapy is not justified. Cellulitis and lymphangitis must be treated by chemotherapy and rest.

The fundamentals of treatment are rest, elevation, and antibiotics. Surgery is only of value when pus has localized. Most early infections will respond within forty-eight hours to proper rest and adequate antibiotic blood levels. If, in this time there is not a considerable increase in comfort, then it is probable that pus is present. Pus should be considered present if the patient has already lost a night's sleep and complains of persistent throbbing pain. The risk of spread along tissue planes is great if one waits for "fluctuation" to appear or for the pus to "point." The former is a thoroughly unreliable sign in the hand, and the latter can only occur after considerable necrosis of deep tissues.

As soon as a presumptive diagnosis of pus has been made, incision and drainage of the area must be done. An adequate preoperative antibiotic level is essential so that any healthy tissues exposed during the exploration will be protected against infection. The majority of patients with hand infections can be safely operated upon under local anesthesia, the anesthetic being injected around nerve trunks well proximal to the site of infection. A short inhalation anesthetic is equally effective. A tourniquet should be used if bleeding so obscures the field that adequate surgery cannot be carried out.

# PARONYCHIA

Paronychia is an infection around the nail. It can be either acute or chronic and is usually caused by staphylococci. The infection is frequently introduced as a result of rough manicuring or picking at a hangnail. Pus collects in the space between the cuticle and the nail matrix and does not originally arise in the soft tissues around the nail. Occasionally an acute infection will track beneath the side of the nail and establish a subungual abscess.

## Acute paronychia

In the early stages of the infection there is pain, redness, and swelling of the subcuticular tissues at the side of the nail (Fig. 15-1). Lymphangitis and lymphadenitis are not commonly found. Usually acute paronychia will require surgical drainage. However, it is important to wait for localization of the infection. Incisions into areas in which the infection has not localized will only spread the organism into hitherto uninfected parts.

TREATMENT. Occasionally the infection can be aborted by the use of systemic antibiotics, but if such therapy does not succeed, treatment by hot-water soaks and rest will help to localize the infection into a bead of pus. The pus usually evacuates itself easily, but, if it does not, it should be released by a small incision. If the skin

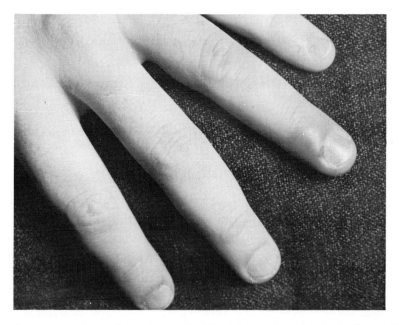

**Fig. 15-1.** *Acute paronychia.* In the early stages of this infection the subcuticular tissues at the side of the nail are red and swollen.

is first softened by soaking in hot water, the incision can be made without anesthesia. A sharp-pointed scalpel should be passed beneath the cuticle with the blade lying flat on the nail at the site of the pus collection. Occasionally, if the infection has become quite extensive, it may be necessary to incise and even to excise the nail at its side.

DRESSINGS. Small dry dressings are usually quite sufficient to cover the area of drainage. They can be held in place either by tape or bandage. They should be changed frequently until drainage ceases. If soaked dressings are left in place, the surrounding skin macerates, and the infection may become prolonged.

AFTERCARE. Healing usually occurs within one week, but it may be necessary to continue dressings into the second postoperative week. In most occupations the patient can safely return to work immediately after surgery.

## Subungual abscess

If acute paronychia is not treated early enough, the bead of pus may spread under the nail rather than drain to the surface (Fig. 15-2). The pus collects as a sub-

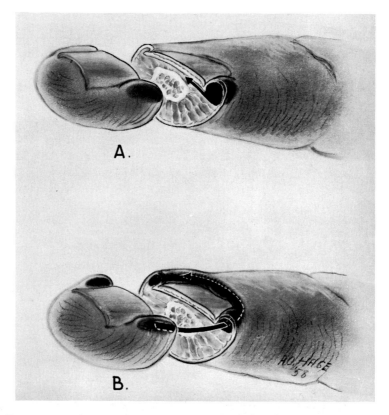

**Fig. 15-2.** *The progress of an acute paronychia.* **A,** The bead of pus may spread under the nail to produce a subungual abscess. **B,** The pus may spread all the way around the nail in the subcuticular tissues.

ungual abscess, which is usually easy to diagnose. If there is any doubt about the presence of a subungual abscess, transillumination of the finger will cause the pus to show up as an opaque area beneath the nail. If the infection has traveled toward the base of the nail, the skin overlying the nail root will be edematous and a bluish-red color. As the abscess increases in size, it will float the nail off the nail bed. The infection cannot be cured until the nail has been removed.

**TREATMENT.** Systemic antibiotics should be given. Regional or local anesthetic block should be used. Usually it will be found that the distal half of the nail is attached to the nail bed, thereby preventing drainage of the pus. An incision should be made transversely across the nail at the level of the lunula or just distal to the infection and the proximal part of the nail avulsed from its root (Fig. 15-3). The distal part of the nail should be left in place since it is the best available dressing for the unaffected part of the finger.

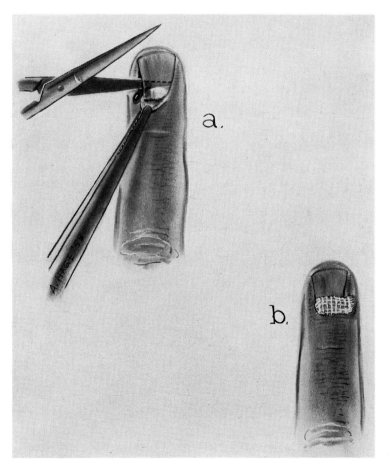

**Fig. 15-3.** *Treatment of subungual abscess.* **a,** An incision should be made transversely across the nail at the level of the lunula and the proximal part of the nail avulsed from its bed. **b,** The raw nail bed should be covered with a petrolatum gauze dressing.

DRESSINGS. The proximal part of the nail bed should be dressed with petrolatum gauze and a small pressure dressing. This dressing will have to be changed daily during the first few days until the nail bed dries over. A certain amount of pressure is needed during the healing period to keep the granulations sufficiently flat for the new nail to grow over without distortion.

## Chronic paronychia

Chronic paronychia, a low-grade persistent infection, is relatively common. It is often found in adults whose hands repeatedly get wet and in children who suck their thumbs. It may be due to small portions of dead and unremoved fingernail acting as a foreign body. It is usually caused by a low-grade staphylococcal infection and occasionally by a fungal infection. Most commonly the primary infection is a staphylococcus with a secondary colonization by *Candida albicans* in the moist skin folds. The cuticle is usually swollen, red, and macerated (Fig. 15-4). An intermittent seropurulent exudate will discharge from between the cuticle and the nail. The nail itself will be thickened, roughened, and distorted.

TREATMENT. The best treatment of chronic paronychia is a combination of systemic antibiotics and removal of the proximal part of the nail. The nail should be cut across at the level of the lunula and the proximal portion grasped in hemostats and avulsed. The infected granulation tissue beneath the cuticle should be scraped out before the dressing is applied.

DRESSINGS. The raw portion of the nail should be covered with petrolatum gauze and a small dry sponge dressing. The dressings are satisfactorily held in place by

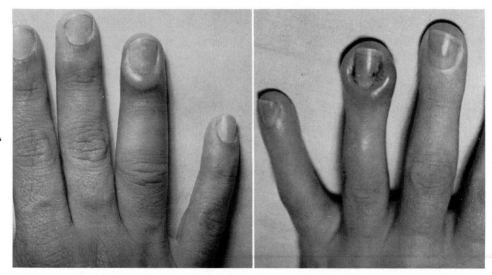

A

B

**Fig. 15-4.** *Chronic paronychia.* **A** and **B,** Two degrees of chronic paronychia. In the worse case, **B,** the cuticle is swollen, red, and macerated, and a discharge is coming from between the nail and the cuticle.

some Tubegauz bandage. The dressings will have to be changed daily, and it is advisable to maintain sufficient pressure to keep the nail bed surface flat until it dries. If it is allowed to heal with an irregular surface, the new nail will become distorted as it grows over the nail bed surface. If the infection persists despite this treatment, fungal infection should be suspected.

## FELON

A felon is an infection of the pulp space of the terminal phalanx of a digit. This pulp space is divided into a collection of virtually closed tissue spaces by the numerous fibrous septa passing from the skin to the periosteum of the terminal phalanx. This closed pulp space lies distal to the level of the epiphysis of the phalanx. Raised pressure in the space may close the blood vessels running to the distal four fifths of the phalanx and produce a bone necrosis. The blood supply to the actual epiphysis will remain unharmed, and viable bone will be available for regeneration should the distal portions be destroyed by osteomyelitis (Fig. 15-6).

The clinical picture of a felon is characteristic. Infection is commonly introduced by a puncture wound of the terminal pulp. This is followed by rapidly rising tension, which produces acute and increasing throbbing pain. The pain is made worse if the venous pressure is increased by lowering the hand. Conversely, elevation helps to relieve the pain. Sleep is often impossible, and the usual domestic analgesics are ineffective. Lymphangitis and lymphadenitis are common.

### Acute cases

TREATMENT. Treatment is almost invariably surgical. In treating a very early felon, it is permissible to try a twenty-four hour course of a broad-spectrum antibiotic. If the symptoms do not subside rapidly, there should be no hesitation in incising the finger and thereby decompressing the pulp space. One cannot wait for the pus to localize, and frequently little frank pus is seen at operation; such early surgery will prevent the pressure from building up to such a degree that osteomyelitis becomes inevitable. The pulp space should be approached by a direct incision over the point of maximum tenderness (Fig. 15-5).

Both fish-mouth and hockey-stick incisions traverse normal uninfected tissues, frequently fail to maintain drainage of the abscess, may damage the digital nerve, and leave bad scars. The fish-mouth incision is particularly bad, since it is carried completely across the pulp, separating the palmar and dorsal portions of the finger tip. This incision can seriously compromise the blood supply to the bony distal phalanx.

Direct drainage of the abscess is done through a small incision centered over the point of maximum tenderness and tension. A metacarpal block using 2% lidocaine is usually sufficient, and a tourniquet should be available since a bloodless field is useful in defining the limits of the abscess cavity. A small elliptical incision not more than 5 mm in length is made over the apex of the abscess. When the skin has been excised, the sinus track leading to the center of the abscess will be found.

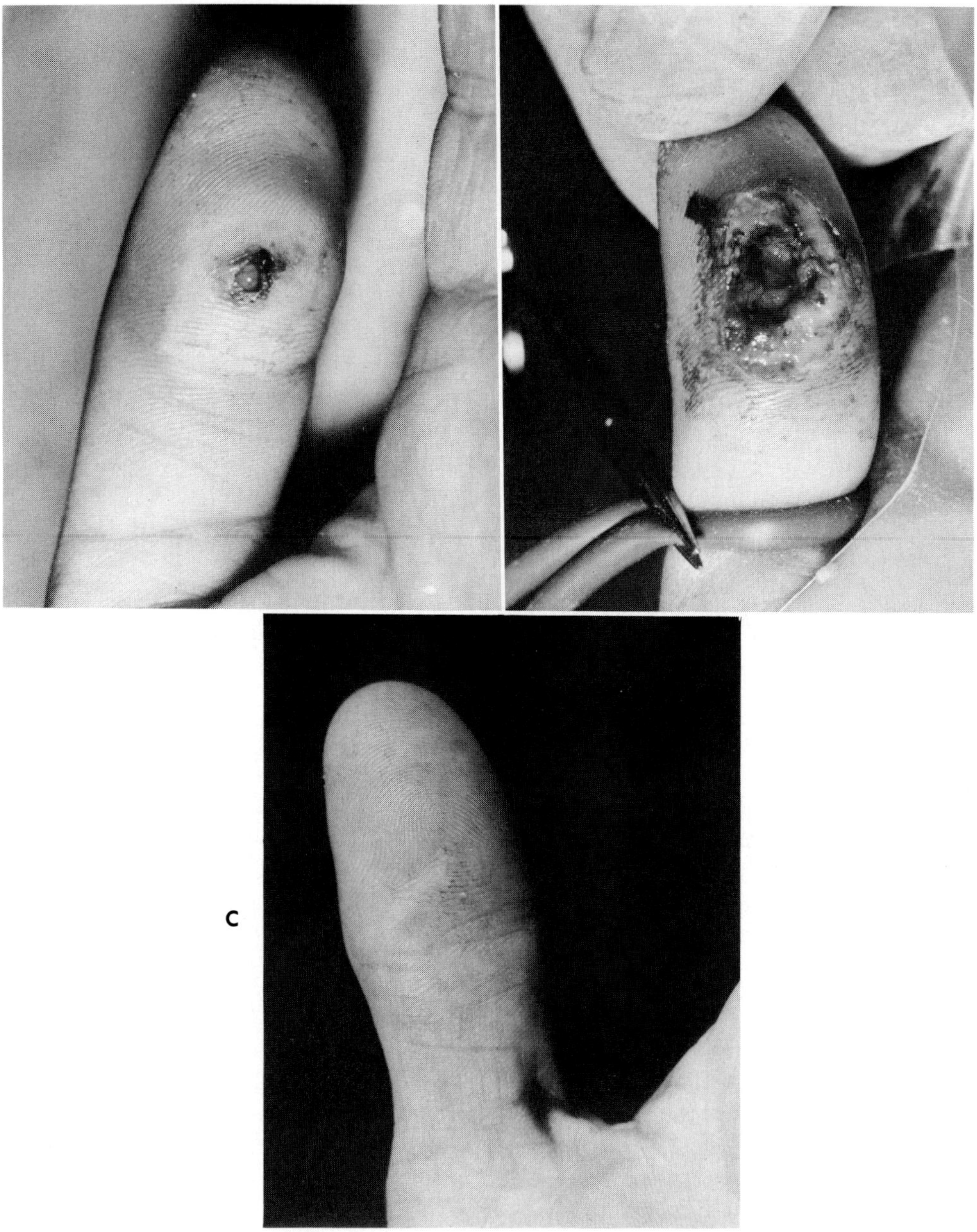

**Fig. 15-5.** *Felon.* **A,** This thumb felon had been present sufficiently long to "point" through the thick palmar skin. **B,** A conical excision or saucerization removed all the necrotic tissues and the wound was lightly packed. **C,** Six years later the thumb remains well healed and the scar is not tender. Note the improper use of a catheter as a tourniquet in **B.**

The slough must be completely excised. Since the area has been "saucerized" by excision of the skin ellipse, no drain is necessary (Fig. 15-5).

DRESSINGS. The wound should be covered with a layer of petrolatum gauze and several layers of cotton sponge. The dressings should be changed at two- or three-day intervals. The cavity will quickly fill in and usually heals within ten days. Scarring is minimal both within the pulp and on the skin surface.

## Late cases

TREATMENT. In treating late cases an x-ray film must be taken to show whether any sequestration of the terminal phalanx has taken place (Fig. 15-6). The finger must be opened through a direct incision and any obvious sequestra removed. Many areas of necrotic pulp will be found, and any such obviously dead areas must be removed before the finger is dressed. In children, bone that appears to be dead but that does not readily separate should be left in place, since children's bones show such remarkable recuperative powers.

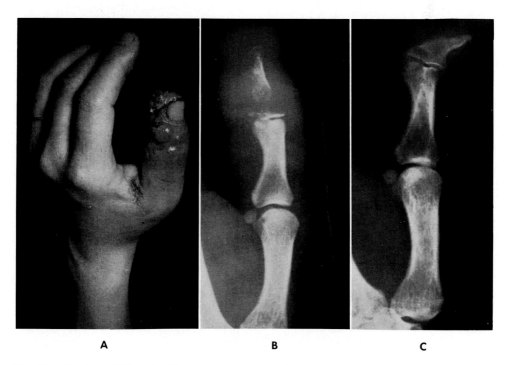

A                                    B                                    C

**Fig. 15-6.** *Neglected felon.* **A,** This patient pricked her thumb "quite a while" before she came for treatment. **B,** X-ray film showing the gross infection of the distal phalanx. **C,** Final state six months after sequestrectomy and excision of all dead tissue. Note how the proximal portion of the bone has completely regenerated, but destruction within the distal pulp space has resulted in a distorted bone.

## WEB SPACE INFECTIONS

The three triangular web spaces between the fingers can be infected by direct wounding or from an infected palmar callous at the base of the finger. The infection usually collects in the dorsal part of the web space, pointing through the thinner dorsal skin. If the pus is not released or the area does not drain, the infection will pass into the deeper tissues and may penetrate through a lumbrical canal into the palmar spaces. A well-developed web space infection shows a reddened, bulging area on the dorsal part of the web between two fingers that are held apart and cannot be adducted without pain, and the swelling will spread proximally from the infected web onto the dorsum of the hand (Fig. 15-7). This dorsal swelling is common and does not indicate a true palmar space infection.

TREATMENT. In the early stages of web space infections elevation, antibiotics, and analgesics help to relieve the pain. When the pus has localized, it must be drained. If the infection has entered through a callous that is obviously infected, it

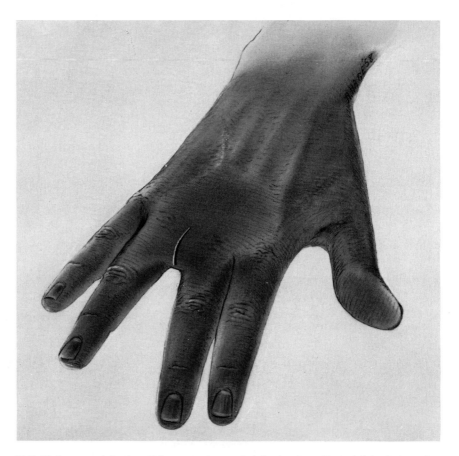

**Fig. 15-7.** *Web space infection.* When a web space infection is well established, there is a reddened, bulging area on the dorsal part of the web that forces two adjacent fingers apart. The swelling frequently spreads onto the dorsum of the hand.

should be excised. In other infections the incision should be placed vertically in the web space and does not normally need to be carried into the thicker palmar skin (Fig. 15-7). This incision has the virtue of direct access to the infection, avoids opening potentially normal palmar skin, but may heal more slowly than a palmar incision. If the pus does not ooze out when the skin has been adequately incised, the subcutaneous tissues should be separated by spreading with a pair of mosquito forceps. When the pus is reached, an adequate drainage hole must be made by the same method. Care must be taken not to plunge the tip of the forceps too deep or too proximal because of the risk of damage to the neurovascular bundles or the tendon sheaths. A rubber drain is not always necessary, but care should be taken to prevent the wound from sealing over too early.

DRESSINGS. Wet dressings over the incision in the web space covered by fluffed-up dry dressings will help set up a drainage gradient. They should be held in place by a light bandage, and the hand should be put at rest in a sling until drainage has stopped.

## SUBEPITHELIAL AND COLLAR BUTTON ABSCESSES

Superficial puncture wounds of the skin of the hand may introduce infection into the subepithelial tissues, where a small abscess will be formed. If these abscesses are not seen and treated early, they may penetrate into the underlying dermis and thus form a subdermal abscess. These abscesses resemble an hourglass or a collar button in shape, since the two abscess cavities are connected by a narrow waist (Fig. 15-8).

TREATMENT. A collar button abscess must always be suspected when there is a subepithelial abscess, particularly if the tissue reaction seems to be out of proportion to the size of the superficial abscess.

Anesthesia for patients with collar button abscesses is sometimes a problem. Since a local anesthetic cannot be injected directly into the abscess, it is difficult to anesthetize completely the deeper tissues without doing a multiple proximal nerve block. Often it is better to use a short inhalation anesthetic.

The skin over the subepithelial abscess must be cut away around the periphery

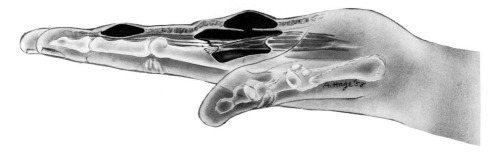

**Fig. 15-8.** *Subepithelial and collar button abscesses.* In this illustration a subepithelial abscess is shown over the palmar aspect of the middle phalanx. A similar infection has occurred over the proximal phalanx, but it has penetrated into the underlying dermis and has formed a collar button abscess.

and the superficial pus wiped away. The base of the abscess must be cleansed and searched for the small sinus that communicates with the subdermal abscess. If the opening cannot be easily determined, pressure around the periphery of the subepithelial abscess may cause a bead of pus to well up from the depths. Once the opening has been identified, the subdermal abscess must be drained by enlarging the opening with spreading mosquito forceps. After the pus has been drained out, it is often necessary to excise a small portion of the sinus opening to ensure that adequate drainage is possible during the healing process.

**DRESSINGS.** A rubber drain is not necessary if there has been sufficient excision of the circumference of the sinus. Petrolatum gauze or Telfa dressings should be placed next to the wound and changed daily until the exudate has ceased.

## TENOSYNOVITIS AND PALMAR SPACE INFECTIONS

Infection of the fingers and hand will spread along well-defined anatomical pathways, and such infections cannot be adequately treated if the applied anatomy is not clearly understood.

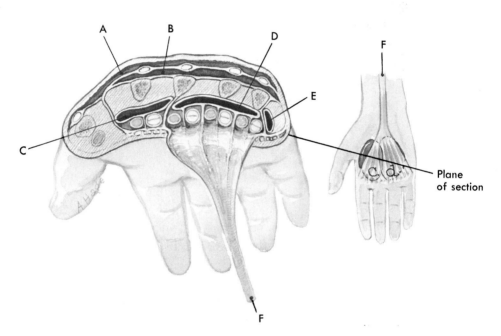

**Fig. 15-9.** *Hand fasciae and related spaces.* These potential spaces only become apparent after they have been distended with pus. The position and shape of the septa attached to the third and fifth metacarpals have been exaggerated to stress their relationships. **A,** Dorsal subcutaneous space; **B,** dorsal subaponeurotic space; **C,** thenar space; **D,** midpalmar space; **E,** hypothenar space; **F,** the palmaris longus tendon turned up to show the eight tunnels within which run the flexor tendons, the lumbricals, and the digital neurovascular bundles. (From Flatt, A. E.: Hand deformities. In Cantor, P. D., editor: Traumatic medicine and surgery for the attorney, vol. 2, © Butterworth, Inc., Washington, D.C., 1960. Reproduced with permission of Matthew Bender & Company, Inc.)

## Applied anatomy of hand infection

Several fascial planes in the hand are so arranged that they enclose potential spaces between their layers. In the normal hand these spaces are obliterated, but when infection occurs the pus distends the spaces and the fascial sheets determine the paths the pus shall take. There are two of these spaces on the dorsum (subcutaneous and subaponeurotic) and three (midpalmar, thenar, and hypothenar) on the palm of the hand.

These potential "spaces" are much better thought of as bursae developed to help the gliding movements of the tendons on the deeper tissues. These bursae are enclosed by extremely thin membranes, which are thicker in the hand of a manual laborer than in a delicately used hand. It must be remembered that the flexor tendons are enclosed in synovial sheaths. At the level of the metacarpophalangeal joints these sheaths do not have direct, open connections with either the lumbrical canals or the thenar and midpalmar bursae. However, the dividing membrane is so thin that it is easy for suppurative infections of the tendon sheaths to rupture into the adjacent bursa.

### Dorsal spaces

The extensor tendons are joined together in the transverse plane by several aponeuroses reinforced by a tough layer of fascia. Superficial to this layer is the subcutaneous space containing much of the lymph drainage of the borders of the palm, finger webs, and the fingers. The subaponeurotic space lies deep to the level of the extensor tendons between the tendons and the fascia covering the interosseous muscles and the metacarpal shafts (Fig. 15-9).

### Palmar spaces

The deep structures of the hand, such as flexor tendons, nerves, and arteries, lie on the floor of the hand, which is formed by the fascia overlying the metacarpal shafts and interossei. The roof is formed by the tough palmar fascia. Two septa pass from the borders of the triangle-shaped palmar fascia to the floor, dividing the palm into three spaces. The radial septum passes downward and in an ulnar direction, covering the transverse head of the adductor pollicis muscle and attaching to the midline of the shaft of the third metacarpal (Fig. 15-9). On the ulnar side of the palmar fascia the septum is attached to the fifth metacarpal shaft.

#### *The midpalmar space*

The midpalmar space lies between the radial and ulnar septa (Fig. 15-10). This potential space lies deep to the flexor tendons and lumbrical muscles of the long, ring, and small fingers. The flexor tendons, but not the lumbricales, are enclosed in the synovial sheath known as the ulnar bursa. The space can therefore extend distally along the lumbrical muscles toward the web spaces. Proximally it extends into the forearm under the flexor tendons and the flexor retinaculum.

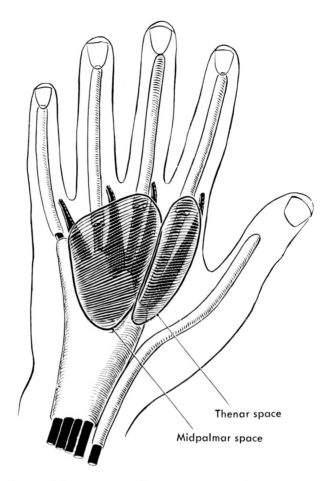

**Fig. 15-10.** *Midpalmar and thenar spaces.* Showing the close relationship of the midpalmar and thenar spaces. They are frequently connected within the carpal tunnel.

### The thenar space

The thenar space lies on the radial side of the septum, passing from the radial border of the palmar fascia. It contains the so-called radial bursa, which is the synovial sheath surrounding the flexor pollicis longus tendon. In addition, it contains the tendon and lumbrical muscle to the index finger, the thenar muscles, and the adductor pollicis muscle.

### The hypothenar space

The hypothenar space, which lies on the ulnar side of the membrane passing from the ulnar border of the palmar fascia, contains the hypothenar muscles.

## Dorsal space infections

The two dorsal spaces are not commonly infected, but there is normally a considerable degree of swelling on the dorsum of the hand when the palmar tissues are infected. This is because the lymphatic drainage of the hand largely flows to the dorsum and because the dorsal skin is not attached to the deeper structures as is the skin of the palm.

The skin itself may be subject to the usual infections such as boils and carbuncles. Occasionally, infections of the subaponeurotic layer may point dorsally as a collar button abscess and in such cases can be mistaken for a boil.

Infection of the subcutaneous space can occur following puncture wounds, and occasionally lymph-borne infections from the palmar area may settle in this space. The subaponeurotic space can also be infected by direct puncture wounds, but, in addition, it may become involved by direct extension from palmar infections as well as by lymph-borne infections.

CLINICAL PICTURE. A careful history is essential in the diagnosis of dorsal surface infections. At superficial examination the swollen red and convex surface of the dorsum will look the same whether it is caused by direct infection or by the presence of a palmar infection. The history may establish that appropriate wounding did occur to the dorsum. On the other hand, it may establish that there were signs of palmar infection prior to the development of the dorsal swelling. In "sympathetic" edema to palmar infections, the dorsal swelling may seem relatively nonpainful in spite of its clinical appearance. In true infection, the dorsum of the hand is painful and fluctuation of pus may be present.

TREATMENT. The best treatment in early stages of dorsal space infections is to attempt to prevent full development of the infection. The hand must be splinted in the position of function and put at rest in an elevated position; massive doses of a broad-spectrum antibiotic should be given.

When the infection is established and pus is present, there is no alternative to surgical drainage. Infections in both spaces must be drained by adequate dorsal incisions made parallel with the dorsal skin creases and at 90-degree angles to the long tendons. In subaponeurotic infections care should be taken to place the incision between the long extensor tendons.

DRESSINGS AND AFTERCARE. A thin rubber drain should be placed at the bottom of the infected area and left in place for the first few days. It should be withdrawn slightly each day to allow healing from the depths. Fluffed-up sponges should be used as a very mild compression dressing, and the hand should be bandaged in the position of function with a stretchable bandage. The dressings should be changed daily until the exudate dries up. Movements of the fingers should be encouraged as soon as the symptoms have subsided.

## Palmar space infections

Nowadays it is rare to see palmar space infections except in those totally devoid of medical care. When they do occur, it is usually caused by rupture of long-neglected tendon-sheath infections. The midpalmar space can be infected by direct wounding or by extension of infections of the long, ring, or small fingers or their web spaces. The thenar space is infected in a similar manner, except that the digits involved are the thumb and index finger. The hypothenar space is rarely infected.

The radial and ulnar bursae are adjacent in the carpal canal, and in the majority of cases a communication exists at this level between these two bursae. After an infection of one palmar space has involved its adjacent bursa, it can easily extend into the other space. It may pass proximally into the forearm and cause infection of the forearm fascial space known as Parona's space (Fig. 15-10).

### Midpalmar infections

Midpalmar infections occur in an area where the palmar skin is anchored to the deeper tissues by many fibrous septa. Tension, therefore, builds up rapidly and produces generalized malaise with raised pulse and temperature. There is a brawny swelling of the palm, which is extremely tender to the touch. The fingers and often the wrist are held in flexion. Attempts at passive extension of the fingers produce more pain. The dorsum of the hand is almost invariably swollen by "sympathetic" edema.

TREATMENT. A broad-spectrum antibiotic must be given before surgery. If subsequent tests of the organism show that it is more sensitive to a different agent, the treatment must be changed.

Midpalmar infections must be provided with early and adequate drainage through an incision placed parallel with and slightly proximal to the distal palmar crease (Fig. 15-11). Since the abscess is deeply situated, care must be taken not to damage the neurovascular structures lying in the depths of the wound. Once the palmar fascia has been opened, it is wiser to explore the depths by repeatedly passing a pair of mosquito forceps and opening the jaws as they are withdrawn. When the abscess has been opened, the pus should be cleaned out and any obviously dead pieces of fat or fascia excised.

DRESSINGS AND AFTERCARE. The incision must be kept open with a rubber tissue drain until all drainage has ceased. Voluminous dressings of fluffed-up sponges should protect and hold the hand in the position of function. The hand should rest in a sling until the wound is dry and begins to epithelize.

### Thenar space infections

Since there is no palmar fascia over the thenar space area, the skin can be raised up by the underlying infection until the whole thenar eminence is ballooned out. The position of maximum accommodation to the swelling is one with the thumb slightly flexed and in the abducted position. If tenosynovitis of the index finger or thumb was the original cause of the infection, the signs of this infection will also be present.

#### *Isolated thenar space infections*

TREATMENT. Isolated thenar space infection in the early stages can be treated by rest, elevation, and massive doses of chemotherapy. If pus is present, it must be drained. The incision is best placed in the web between the thumb and index finger (Fig. 15-11). It should be about 3 cm long and placed just to the dorsal side of the

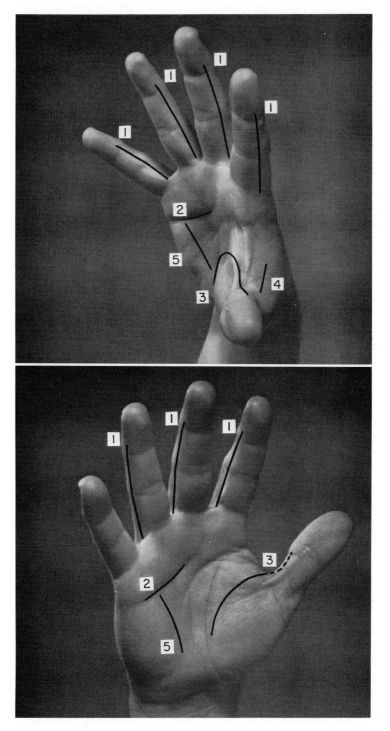

**Fig. 15-11.** *Incisions to be used in hand infections.* **1,** The neutral borders of the fingers for tenosynovitis. **2,** The distal palmar crease for the middle palmar space. **3,** The thenar crease and the neutral border of the thumb for tenosynovitis. **4,** The dorsum of the thumb web for the thenar space. **5,** The side of the hypothenar eminence for the ulnar bursa.

edge of the web. This incision opens the thinner dorsal skin, and the depths of the space can be easily reached by passing a hemostat proximally into the web space.

**DRESSINGS AND AFTERCARE.** Drainage should be maintained by a rubber drain until the discharge ceases, and the hand should be held in the position of function with bulky dressings or, when necessary, with a splint. Movements of the thumb should be encouraged throughout treatment.

### Infection secondary to tenosynovitis

**TREATMENT.** If the infection of the thenar space was caused by an extension of tenosynovitis of the thumb, the incision will have to be placed so that the two infections can be adequately drained. This incision should be made parallel with the flexor crease of the thenar eminence but a little to its radial side (Fig. 15-11). Great care must be taken not to bring the incision too far proximal and thus endanger the vital motor branch of the median nerve. This nerve runs horizontally across the hand about 2 cm distal to the distal wrist crease. The incision can be extended distally along the ulnar border of the thumb in a manner similar to the incisions along the neutral border of a finger.

The tendon sheath should be opened longitudinally by an incision placed near the bone and the pus drained out. If the tendon is dead, it must be excised at the time of the first incision. To leave it in place will only delay healing and necessitate further surgery to prepare the thumb for reconstructive surgery.

**DRESSINGS AND AFTERCARE.** A rubber drain should be placed in the infected area in the thenar space, but no drain is necessary along the tendon sheath incision. Damp dressings may be helpful for the first few days, but dry dressings should be used when the drainage has ceased and the drain is removed. Throughout the period of dressings, the hand should be kept in the functional position either by bandaging onto a splint or by bulky dressings.

Mobility must be maintained in the joints of the thumb by passive movements if the tendon has been excised. Active movements, using the tendon, should be started as soon as the local reaction has subsided sufficiently to allow movement without pain.

## Tenosynovitis

The synovial sheath of a digit can be infected primarily by a direct puncture wound or secondarily by extension of infection from felons, collar button abscesses, or palmar space infections. Secondary infection is the less common and is usually the less severe because the gradual involvement of the tendon sheath allows some degree of localization to develop.

**CLINICAL PICTURE OF PRIMARY TENOSYNOVITIS.** Despite the small area of infection, there is a marked generalized reaction, and the patient is ill. The temperature is usually elevated to 38.5° or 39.5° C because of toxic absorption. The tension in the finger is high, and the pain is acute. The finger is uniformly swollen on the palmar surface and is held in a semiflexed position. There is localized acute tenderness along the anatomical limits of the tendon sheath. The pain becomes excruciating if attempts are made to extend the finger passively.

Any finger that is acutely inflamed will be painful on passive extension. To establish that the pain is actually due to tenosynovitis the tendon must be moved within its sheath by holding the middle phalanx and passively extending the distal interphalangeal joint.

### Early cases

TREATMENT. Initial treatment is prophylactic to the extent that even small puncture wounds deserve careful cleansing and irrigation. Prophylactic antibiotic treatment is justified if there is the slightest suspicion that infection may develop.

Even in the early stages of tenosynovitis, if it is obvious that infection is probable, the finger should be put in a position of rest by splinting. The arm should be elevated in a sling and a broad-spectrum antibiotic given in generous doses. If the invading organism is sensitive to the antibiotic, the infection can often be controlled in the early stages. Unfortunately, few patients are seen sufficiently early to justify such treatment.

If rapid improvement does not occur, many surgeons now use direct irrigation and treatment of the tendon sheath with antibiotics through fine plastic catheters. This has shown good results in early cases. The diagnosis of primary tendon sheath infection must be properly established. There is little point in irrigating a tendon sheath that has been secondarily infected by a more superficial but untreated infection.

Through and through drainage is necessary in this technique, which therefore requires hospital admission. The principle of treatment is to make small transverse incisions over the proximal and distal ends of the infected sheath, introduce the catheter, wash out the sheath, and continuously bathe the tissues with the appropriate antibiotic solution. This method cannot "cure" an already necrotic tendon; considerable experience is needed in deciding to use this closed method rather than opening and inspecting the sheath and tendon by the more radical method described in the following paragraphs for established cases.

### Established cases

TREATMENT. Once pus forms it must be drained. The earlier it is drained, the greater is the chance that the tendons will survive. Early incision will also prevent the infection from spreading into the palm by rupture into a fascial space. The operation should be done under axillary block anesthesia or some short-acting general anesthetic because more meticulous surgery is required in these cases than in the other hand infections. General anesthesia allows a pneumatic type of tourniquet to be used to provide a bloodless field. A narrow rubber tube wrapped tightly around the base of the finger must never be used because of the risk of forcing a rupture of the infection into the palm of the hand.

The incision should be placed along the neutral border of the finger (Figs. 15-

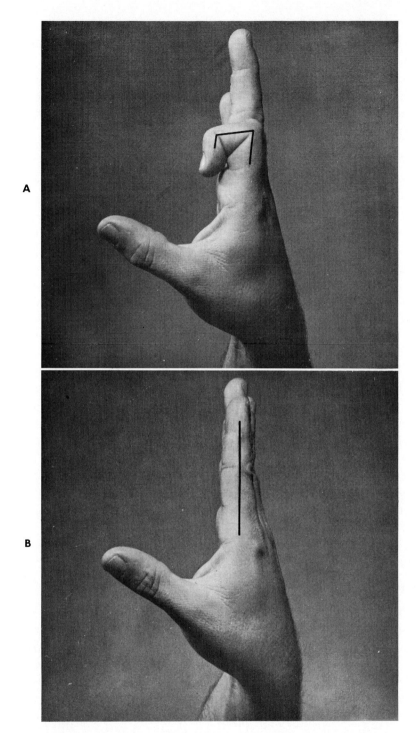

**Fig. 15-12.** *The neutral border of a finger.* **A,** This border is defined as a line joining the apices of the skin creases when both interphalangeal joints are flexed to 90 degrees. **B,** When the finger is extended, the line of the neutral border is shown.

11 and 15-12) and should extend at least between the proximal and distal finger joint creases. Any other approach to the tendon sheath will compromise future function of the finger. To use the "direct" approach illustrated in Fig. 15-13 is criminal and will inevitably lead to amputation. The neutral border incision will frequently need to be extended in a proximal and a distal direction to give adequate exposure. On the index and small fingers, it should be placed on the inner sides of the fingers so that scars are not left on the feeling borders of these fingers. When the skin is opened, the knife can be passed directly downward onto the bony phalanx. The neurovascular bundle is safely out of the way on the palmar aspect of the incision, and the only structure that needs to be watched for is the dorsal branch of the digital nerve, which crosses to the dorsum over the distal part of the proximal phalanx.

Once the tendon sheath has been exposed, it should be generously incised and the pus mopped out. The incisions should be placed to avoid the thickened portion of the tendon sheath, which acts as a pulley in the region of the middle of the phalanges. However, if proper drainage is not established by incision over the joint areas, the incision must be ruthlessly extended until the drainage is adequate. If

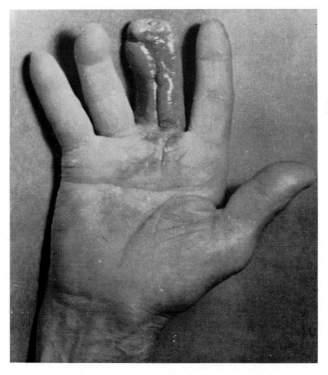

**Fig. 15-13.** *Tenosynovitis.* The infection in the tendon sheath of this finger was treated by a "direct" approach to the tendon. The patient was not satisfied and asked for different treatment. Amputation was the only possible treatment.

the tendon has been bathed in pus for any length of time, it will be avascular and necrotic. The gray fibrillated areas must be excised so that healing will proceed rapidly and with the minimum of fibrosis. Occasionally it will be necessary to transect the tendon in order to remove all of the necrotic tissue.

**DRESSINGS AND AFTERCARE.** The wound must be drained for a few days with a fine rubber tissue drain. It is often helpful to place nylon sutures at intervals of about 0.5 cm along the length of the wound and to leave the ends of the sutures long but not tie the knots. Damp dressings are often helpful during the first few days. As soon as the drainage appears to have almost ceased, the drain should be removed and dry dressings substituted for the damp ones. If no significant drainage occurs during the next forty-eight hours, the sutures should be loosely tied and dry dressings continued. This method of secondary suture will considerably shorten the healing time and decrease the amount of fibrosis.

Movement of the finger should be encouraged as soon as the pain and swelling have diminished enough to allow this. Active movements should be carried out by the patient if the tendon was not excised. If the tendon was excised, passive movements are necessary to provide the range of movement necessary to allow later reconstructive surgery.

### Very late cases

**TREATMENT.** Occasionally tenosynovitis has been present for so long that the bones or joints of the finger are also involved. In such instances it is permissible to consider amputation if only one finger is involved and the infection remains localized to that finger. The thumb is never amputated for this condition.

Wholesale amputations cannot be carried out, and if several fingers are involved, attempts must be made to save some or all of them. Surgery will have to be relatively ruthless, and adequate drainage for the infection must be provided. Multiple incisions along the neutral borders allow a good view of all the structures within a finger. Tissue that is obviously dead, whatever its nature, must be excised, and drains must lead down to the deeper tissues.

If infection is established elsewhere in the hand, it must be treated by the same principles and with equal vigor. Good surgical débridement and drainage combined with massive doses of chemotherapy will give the best result possible under the circumstances. To identify the most effective agent, cultures must be taken and tested for sensitivity to the full range of chemotherapeutic agents.

## LESS COMMON INFECTIONS

Infections in the hand have been reported as being caused by virtually every pathogenic organism known to man. Some of the less exotic are related to occupation and the working environment. Nurses and dentists are prone to herpes simplex infections, slaughterhouse workers to *Erysipelothrix rhusiopathiae*, and nurses, housewives, cleaners, and others whose hands are constantly in water are prone to *Candida albicans*. Other fungal infections by organisms such as *Sporothrix schenkii* and *Blastomyces* and *Coccidioides* species may be seen in gardeners and agricultural workers.

*Pseudomonas aeruginosa* may produce a dramatic blue-green discoloration frequently mistaken for gangrene. Atypical mycobacteria that used to be regarded as saprophytes are now being indicted in human infections. *Mycobacterium marinum* is the most common in this group. *Pasteurella multocida* lives in the mouths of dogs and cats and can cause an acute painful papular or vesicular inflammation following a bite. Gonorrhea is probably the most common cause of acute septic arthritis in the young adult, and it also causes acute tendon sheath infections. Drug addicts frequently use the dorsal veins of fingers and hand as a portal of entry; unfortunately, they have little regard for sterility, and severe infection frequently occurs at these sites.

## ERYSIPELOID INFECTION

Erysipeloid infection is deceptive, because it produces a reaction that resembles a very acute infection needing urgent treatment. In fact, if left untreated, it will heal spontaneously within a month to six weeks.

*Erysipelothrix rhusiopathiae* is the cause of swine erysipelas. It is also found as a commensal in the gut of pigs and other animals. The most common occupational groups involved are farmers, veterinarians, butchers, slaughterers, and handlers of fish. The infection occurs most commonly between May and September and is uncommon after the mean temperature falls below 65° F (18° C).

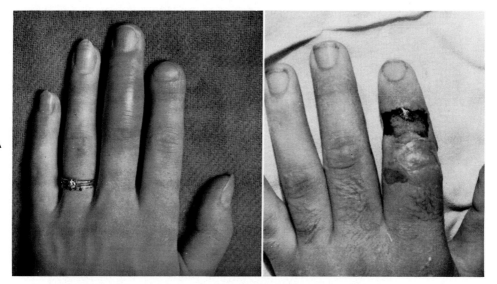

**Fig. 15-14.** *Erysipeloid infection.* **A,** Typical swollen discolored area in an early stage of the infection (in this case, infection occurred as a result of cleaning fish). **B,** Late stage of the infection (infection resulted from handling raw meat).

CLINICAL PICTURE. The infected finger swells, and a patch of purplish erythema spreads out from the site of entry of the organism (Fig. 15-14). The swelling may spread proximally onto the dorsum of the hand. Although a mild throbbing pain is often present, the symptoms and general reaction are not so great as one would expect with an acute infection.

TREATMENT. Surgery must be avoided at all costs. If these areas are incised, they will almost invariably become secondarily infected. The treatment of choice is rest, reassurance, and inactivity. Those who cannot resist prescribing some form of therapy should know that sulfonamides are of no value but that the organism is sensitive in vitro to penicillin and streptomycin. Clinical trials appear to show that penicillin shortens the clinical course of the disease.

## HERPETIC INFECTION

Infection of a finger by the virus of herpes simplex is a lesion that is becoming increasingly recognized and has been called an "aseptic felon." Nurses, doctors, and dentists are particularly exposed to this condition because of the nature of their work.

CLINICAL PICTURE. The primary infection is a relatively minor but often painful illness that can closely resemble the clinical picture of a pyogenic infection. However, lymphangitis, glandular enlargement, and constitutional symptoms do not usually occur. The simple herpetic lesion is a solitary clear vesicle on an inflamed base. The vesicle may be replaced by a small group of vesicles, and the area may become bullous and hemorrhagic. When the distal finger pulp or the paraungular folds are affected, the lesion can be as painful as a pyogenic felon (Fig. 15-15).

In the early stages the diagnosis can be made by the demonstration that the

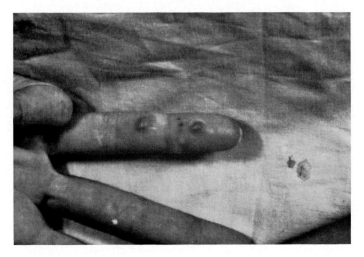

**Fig. 15-15.** *Herpetic infection.* Herpes simplex infection usually produces a single clear vesicle or a group of vesicles each on an inflamed base.

vesicles are bacteriologically sterile. In later stages, especially if the lesions are hemorrhagic or necrotic, the diagnosis is more difficult but can be helped by the absence of local or general signs associated with pyogenic infections.

TREATMENT. The infection usually takes ten to fourteen days to run its course. The affected areas must be kept dry and protected from secondary infection by painting with a solution such as spirits of camphor. There is no indication for surgical intervention unless secondary infection has produced a true pyogenic felon. As with other forms of primary herpes, recurrences are common. They should be treated in the same manner as the primary infection and can be expected to recover in seven to ten days.

# 16 · MISCELLANEOUS INJURIES AND WOUNDS

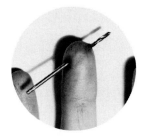

Discussed in this chapter are a variety of conditions that do not readily fit into the average classification of hand injuries. The majority are not frequently seen, but each has certain features in its care that need emphasis if adequate treatment is to be given.

## PRESSURE BLAST INJURIES

Tools delivering high-pressure blasts of air, grease, paint, or abrasive materials are occasionally misdirected so that they injure the hand. The pressures used are so great, being on the order of 600 to 7000 pounds per square inch, that the nozzle does not have to touch the skin. A fine spray can enter through apparently intact skin and fill up a large area of pulp in an incredibly short time.

Physicians seeing such an injury for the first time must beware; the small wound of entry bears no relation to the destruction that has occurred within the hand (Fig. 16-1). The instant ballooning of the tissues causes local ischemia, and the injury may be painless for many hours. Within twenty-four hours profound secondary

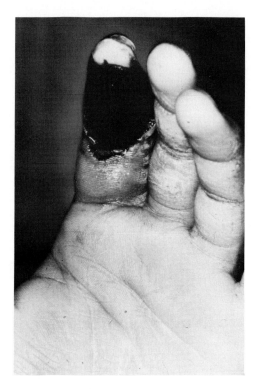

**Fig. 16-1.** *High-pressure injection injury.* This painter was referred to the hospital several days after his finger "slipped while cleaning the gun." Paint solvent entered the finger, and the area of loss is now demarcated. (From Sprague, B. L., and DeCesare, W. F.: J. Iowa Med. Soc. **65**(11):461-464, 1975.)

changes take place and throbbing becomes severe, forcing the patient to seek help. By this time damage may be irreversible, and therefore conservative treatment for the patient seen immediately after injury is not correct. Proper evaluation of the extent of damage and prompt surgical decompression and débridement of the expanded tissues can ultimately make the difference between good function and severe disability.

The key to diagnosis is an appreciation of the extent of the tissue planes within the hand. A penetration of the distal finger pulp can deposit foreign material in the palm because it travels along the tendon sheath; a palmar wound can force the injected substance through the carpal tunnel, into Parona's space, and even as far as the elbow. Small exploratory incisions over the point of entry are therefore valueless. Hot soaks are equally futile because they are liable to increase the metabolic demands of tissues that are already ischemic.

These injuries cannot properly be treated on an outpatient basis. The patient must be convinced of the seriousness of his injury, admitted to hospital, and offered thorough surgical exploration of the wound. The principal value of an operation is the opportunity to decompress the area, define the extent of damage, and remove any chemical irritant that may have been injected. This decompression will provide the best chance to save the circulation and prevent infection.

## Care after admission to hospital

An experienced surgeon to whom one of these injuries has been referred will be well aware of the principles outlined below. They are included because less experienced physicians may be forced by circumstances they cannot control to undertake these primary surgical care measures because if the hand is to be saved, the affected area has to be decompressed (Fig. 16-2).

GENERAL COMMENTS. Although a proper surgical toilet is the best defense against the development of infection, the risks are so great in many of these injuries that prophylactic antibiotics should be given. It is wise to take precautions against tetanus

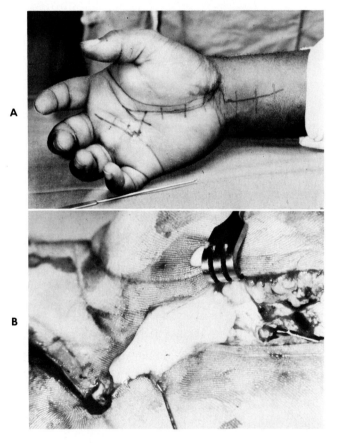

**Fig. 16-2.** *Paint gun injury.* **A,** The point of entry can be seen where the apex of the cross-hatched inkline crossed the distal palmar crease. The hand was opened the full length of the planned incision. **B,** When the incision was made, the paint extruded under great pressure. (From Sprague, B. L., and DeCesare, W. F.: J. Iowa Med. Soc. **65**(11):461-464, 1975.)

infection. The dressings should be changed every other day until it is obvious that the wound is healing cleanly. Superficial débridement with forceps and sponges may be necessary on several occasions because particles of foreign material work up to the surface.

ANESTHESIA. Anesthetic block should be established well proximal to the area of damage. An axillary block or even general anesthesia is a sensible choice.

DRESSINGS. Petrolatum gauze from which most of the grease has been removed should be packed lightly into the wound. The wound should be covered with several layers of dry sponges, which should be laid over rather than packed into the wound. Fluffed-up sponges should then be placed over the whole area and the dressings held in place by Tubegauz or a compression bandage.

It is extremely difficult to maintain apposition of the wound edges through layers of compression dressings. Despite this difficulty, circumferential adhesive-tape dressings should not be used because of the risk of constricting the blood supply to the area. For all except the smallest injury the hand should be placed in the optimum position, illustrated in Fig. 3-8, p. 52.

AFTERCARE. Most of these injuries demand such extensive exploration that it is wise to confine the patient to bed for a day or two and to keep the hand elevated at all times.

Patients should not be allowed to return to work too soon. These wounds tend to heal slowly, and if the tissues are subjected to further trauma during the healing phase, it is quite possible that further areas of necrosis will develop.

## Airblast injuries

The air pressure is frequently being used as a vehicle to carry some form of abrasive or other foreign body, and these particles will be found implanted throughout the damaged area. The limits of the damaged area can usually be defined clinically by palpation of the crepitus caused by the air within the tissues. The wound must be considered "untidy" because of the extensive damage to the subcutaneous tissues, even though the entry wound may be small and well defined.

After thorough cleansing of the skin of the area, the periphery of the entry wound should be excised. The incision will have to be extended sufficiently to give adequate exposure of the deeper tissues. Extensive cleansing and débridement must be carried out, and any pockets of gas under pressure must be incised. It is usually impossible to remove all the fine particles that have been tattooed into the tissues, and only the larger accumulations should be excised. There is usually so much edema of the tissues that it is impossible to close the wound primarily, but sutures may be placed across the wound so that secondary suturing can be carried out at a later date.

## Grease and paint gun injuries

The immediate damage is caused by the explosive force of the pressure spreading through the tissues. Later damage is caused by the chemical irritation provoked by the grease or paint or the solvents carrying them. Thus both the immediate pressure and the subsequent inflammatory reaction can cause vascular obstruction, which may be followed by thrombosis and eventual gangrene. If the injury is not seen until several days after the accident, sterile abscesses may have formed. These will be followed by sloughing of the skin and deeper tissues.

If the injury is neglected for several weeks, multiple small sinuses may appear, through which the foreign material and necrotic tissue will drain. Some particles may become encapsulated in fibrous tissue and never drain to the surface.

Once the correct history has been obtained, the diagnosis is easily made. A lateral x-ray film of an involved finger may show well-defined translucent areas of grease or radiopaque paint lying between the skin and bone. The wound is classified as "untidy" because of the extensive and irregular damage done to the deeper tissues. The skin incision should extend over the most involved area and along a skin crease. It should pass through the entry wound, which should be excised (Fig. 16-2).

Badly damaged tissues and all obvious foreign material must be removed. It will be too widely dispersed for total removal and lightly stained, but viable tissue should not be excised. If the tendon sheath has been entered, it must be incised and the material expressed. Removal of even small volumes will appreciably lower the interstitial pressure, allow the circulation to improve, and prevent the spread of thrombosis and gangrene.

After thorough débridement, the wound should be closed as much as possible. Catgut cannot be buried in the deep tissues, and the skin edges should not be sutured because of the risk of infection and swelling of the tissues. The closure will have to be produced by careful application of the dressings.

The ultimate scarring within the pulp of the finger injured by these substances can be extensive and can cause considerable disability. If the tendon sheath had been entered, there will almost certainly be a considerable restriction in range of movement.

## BITES

Bites from either animals or human beings are among the dirtiest wounds it is possible to receive. The mouth contains such a variety of dirty flora that its organisms are capable of producing an overwhelming infection in the area of the bite. The principles of treatment are not greatly different from those of wounds that appear to be of similar type but were not infected by organisms from a mouth.

### Animal bites

Wounds caused by animal teeth are usually rather deep and of the untidy variety. The first step in treatment is to locate the animal that caused the wound. Rabies can be carried by a variety of animals, including dogs, cats, squirrels, chipmunks, foxes, skunks, and bats.* If the animal can be caught, it must be isolated and ob-

*In the Midwest the cow is the second most common animal to be rabid; a fearsome thought, but in fact they do not attack humans. The most common? The skunk.

served for the development of rabies. Usually this implies restraining the animal in some form of cage under trained observation during the subsequent two weeks to see whether or not the infection will develop. If the animal is dead, the body must be obtained and the brain examined for the characteristic Negri bodies. If there is the slightest doubt that the animal is a contact or carrier of rabies, then it is wiser to immunize the person who has been bitten despite the fact that it can be an extremely uncomfortable and prolonged procedure.

Although great care must be taken to exclude the possibility of rabies, it should be remembered that *Pasteurella multocida* occurs in the mouth, nose, and throat of both dogs and cats. The cat carries a more virulent organism than the dog; both strains of the organism are sensitive to hydrogen peroxide and penicillin therapy.

In general, patients with animal bites go to a doctor's office very shortly after being bitten, and it is therefore possible to carry out adequate early treatment.

**OPERATIVE TREATMENT.** Every bite must be considered a badly bruised, potentially infected area, and adequate cleansing of the wound area, together with débridement of any possibly ragged pieces of skin, must be carried out. Because of the potential lack of viability in the surrounding tissues, it is wrong to use strong antiseptic solutions to wash out the bite area. There is no need to use proprietary solutions for the irrigation. A neutral soap solution is just as effective as the many more expensive products nowadays used for cleansing in the operating room.

The best surgical procedure for any animal bite is immediate and thorough cleansing of the skin surrounding the bite area followed by excision of any obviously nonviable tissue and cleansing and irrigation of the bitten area. It is not advisable to do a primary suturing of the wound because of the risk of encouraging an anaerobic infection. The area should be protected with an occlusive dressing of petrolatum gauze and dry sponges held in place by Tubegauz or stretchable bandage. Penicillin should be given in massive doses, since it is an extremely effective agent against the majority of organisms found in the mouth. It is best given as a heavy loading dose of rapidly absorbed solution, followed by a booster dose of the slow-release type.

## Human bites

A patient with a human bite tends to be somewhat shy of his trophy and may wait several days before presenting himself for treatment. Such delay is unfortunate and dangerous because of the many virulent aerobic and anaerobic bacteria that have been introduced into tendinous tissue of low blood supply through a bruised, ragged, and untidy wound (Fig. 16-3).

The vast majority of these wounds, though classified as bites, are in fact open wounds on the dorsum of the hand caused by striking an opponent in the mouth with a clenched fist. Although this wound is not technically a bite, the results of the wound are similar. The wound is incurred with the hand in the fist position. Thus, organisms can be inoculated deep into the tendon tissues and frequently penetrate into the metacarpophalangeal joint. There is about 15 mm excursion of the extensor tendons between their extremes of movement. It follows, therefore, that extension of the fingers will close the joint and move the damaged and contaminated portion of the extensor tendons to a more proximal site, where an anaerobic infection can develop. When the hand is in extension, the skin wound does not bear any relationship to the area of damage to the underlying tendons.

After the true history of the wound has been obtained, surgical care must be devoted to attempting to localize the infection that is inevitably present and to helping the patient overcome the virulence of the infection.

**OPERATIVE TECHNIQUE.** The hand must be restored to the position in which it was held when the injury was incurred. Thus, most patients will have to be treated with the hand held in a fist position. The most important immediate procedure is cleansing and débridement of the wound. A culture must be taken from the depths of the wound before this is started. The wound itself must be extended in a proximal direction to make quite certain that ascending infection of the tendon or the tendon sheath is not present.

The extension of the wound must be quite ruthless until it can be shown clearly that the tendon which can be seen in the floor of the wound is of normal appearance. If the tendon is completely cut across or is extremely ragged, no attempt should be made to repair it at this operation. The capsule of the joint must be carefully examined for a wound. If the capsule has been penetrated, the opening must be enlarged sufficiently to allow proper irrigation of the depths of the joint with sterile saline. A thorough débridement must be carried out, potentially dying and certainly

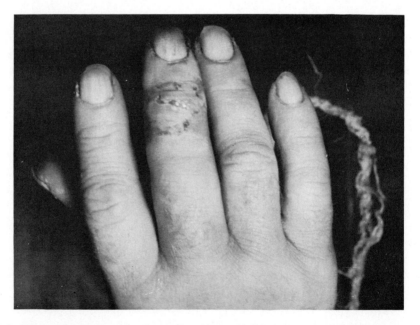

**Fig. 16-3.** *Human bite.* The patient reported to the hospital five days after his opponent in a brawl had bitten his finger. He found it necessary to gouge his opponent's eye in order to release the finger. Despite energetic treatment, the finger had to be amputated.

necrotic tissues must be removed, and the wound must be well irrigated. The skin edges must not be sutured together.

**DRESSINGS.** A light occlusive dressing must be placed on the hand and held in place with a stretchable bandage. The hand itself must be splinted in a modified fist position so that the original wounded areas are adjacent and so that the risks of an anaerobic infection developing are reduced.

**AFTERCARE.** The patient must be impressed with the seriousness of the injury, and the hand must be placed at rest in a sling. Massive doses of a broad-spectrum antibiotic must be given. The wound should be dressed every day, and if it does not appear to be improving rapidly, additional cultures must be taken so that the organisms can be identified and tested for sensitivity to antibiotics. Regular applications of moist heat interspersed with hydrogen peroxide irrigations will usually control any residual infection left in a wound that has had proper primary treatment. Secondary closure of the wound can be considered but is usually unnecessary because once the infection is controlled, the wound will granulate in and epithelize rapidly.

### Late cases

Unfortunately, the patient frequently presents with a wound that is already swollen and from which a profuse and foul discharge is oozing. Gangrene may have already appeared peripherally, and as it progresses it will tend to leave an adherent

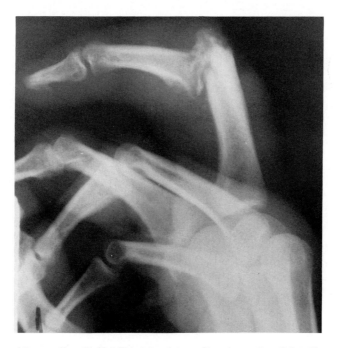

**Fig. 16-4.** *Human bite: septic arthritis.* This lateral x-ray film shows the dislocation and destruction of a proximal interphalangeal joint which had been bitten two months previously. The infection could not be eradicated and the finger was eventually amputated.

slough in the center of the wound. In addition, gangrene may also appear in areas that are seemingly remote from the original site of infection as a result of the infection moving along adjacent fascial planes and settling in these areas.

In such late cases flare-ups of infection may occur at irregular intervals many weeks or months after the original infection and even after all apparent infection has subsided. These flare-ups occur because there is a symbiosis between the anaerobic saphrophytic organisms and the pyogenic organisms. Treatment must be directed to a débridement of the original site of the wound from which the infection first spread. Other obviously infected areas must also be laid wide open and the whole area irrigated with hydrogen peroxide, and massive doses of broad-spectrum antibiotic must be given. Joints that have been penetrated are particularly prone to develop septic arthritis, which is virtually impossible to eradicate (Fig. 16-4).

In treating late cases of human bite, it is advisable to give a very guarded prognosis as to how long it will take to clear up the infection and as to the restoration of function. When the infection has finally subsided and the skin is healed, it will be found that the extensor tendon excursion is not greatly hindered provided there was not an actual break in continuity of the tendon at the time of the original injury.

## COLD INJURY

Frostbite is caused by severe cold that lasts for a sufficient length of time for ice to form within the affected area (Fig. 16-5). In many respects its pathology is not unlike a burn because it results from cellular injury over a relatively long period of time.

The best treatment is rapid rewarming to body temperature in water kept at 42° C. There is very little good evidence that local anesthetic blocks of the appropriate sympathetic supply have much influence on the recovery of the frozen area.

After the area is thawed, portions will be found to be gangrenous, and the difficult decision must be made as to how much should be excised. In general one should be cautious in excising tissues. The part should be kept dry and exposed to the air, and a waiting policy should be adopted. Much tissue that at first sight appears to be dead subsequently is found to be viable. The surface necrosis does not go through the depths of the finger, and if the superficial layers only are excised, an appreciable amount of recovery will occur during the week after thawing. In some cases amputation will inevitably be necessary, but it should not be done as a primary measure. When the areas of loss are finally defined, the appropriate treatment will be either amputation or skin grafting of the remaining granulating areas.

Digital epiphyses can be damaged by cold not severe enough to produce true frostbite. Children playing out in severe weather frequently come indoors with "fingers like ice." The interference with growth does not show until early teenage years, and nothing can be done to correct the situation at this stage (Fig. 16-5). The treatment is truly prophylactic and presupposes proper protective gloves that cannot readily be removed by the child.

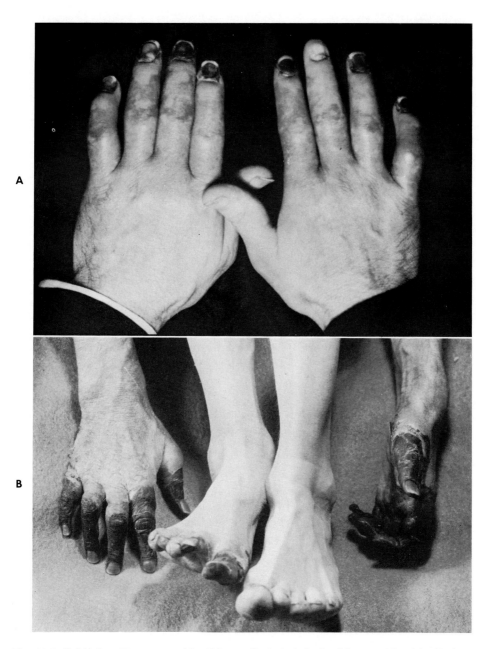

**Fig. 16-5.** *Cold injury.* Two cases of frostbite are illustrated. **A,** A mild case of frostbite. **B,** A severe case of frostbite. In **B** the darkened areas of skin can be seen to be separating, showing that the surface necrosis does not go into the depths of the tissues.

*Continued.*

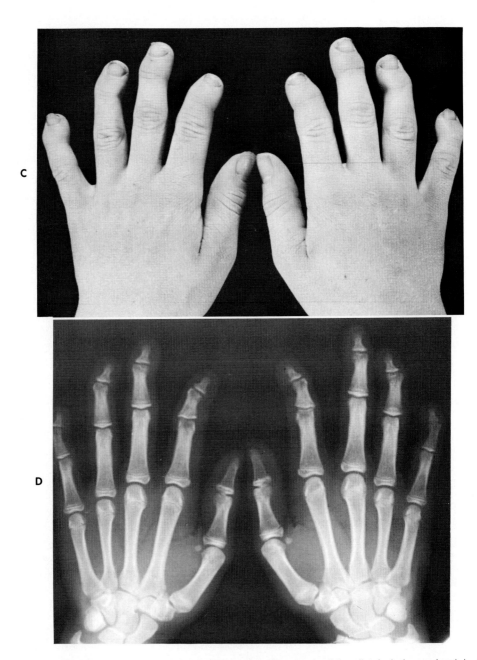

**Fig. 16-5, cont'd.** *Cold injury—children.* Damage to the growth of the distal phalangeal epiphyses can occur in children's hands without frank frostbite appearing. **C,** The obvious deformity in a teenager's hands. **D,** The x-ray film shows that all epiphyses are still open except those of the affected distal phalanges.

## FOREIGN BODIES

Foreign bodies in the hand are better out than in. However, foreign bodies in certain positions may be so innocuous that the surgery necessary for their removal would probably cause more trouble than the foreign body itself.

Of overriding importance in considering the treatment for foreign body in the hand is an accurate history of the circumstances under which it entered the hand. Every foreign body must be considered potentially infected, and if the foreign body entered through dirty skin or is known to have come from a dirty area, then the wound must be treated with great caution.

Even a small puncture wound is sufficient for the tetanus bacillus to gain an entrance, and, if there is the slightest doubt that such organisms might have entered the hand, full precautions must be taken. The dangers from infection of the hand are so great that, if in doubt, it is wise to try to lay open the track of the foreign body and possibly to excise it rather than to adopt a wait-and-see policy.

ANESTHESIA. If operation is to be attempted, this can usually be carried out quite satisfactorily under local anesthesia. A metacarpal block can be used for a digit, and a more proximal block should be used if the wound is in the palm or dorsum of the hand.

TREATMENT. The major problem will be the localization of the foreign body. If it is radiopaque, localization is made relatively easy by strapping a small metal ring over the entry wound and taking x-ray films in two planes. By this means the site of a foreign body can be localized from the surface. It is often helpful to directly impale the site by passing a needle down until it touches the foreign body. The needle then becomes an accurate guide for the scalpel, which enlarges the wound.

If the foreign body is not radiopaque, then xeroradiography may help in its localization. It has been reported that shining a high-intensity fiberoptic light source through the hand in a darkened room may silhouette the foreign body. When exploring this type of wound, an attempt should be made to define the track with a blunt needle or probe and to inject some methylene blue down the entry track. In this way, at least some indication of the direction the foreign body took can be obtained. It is useless to attempt to do this type of surgery unless there is a bloodless field.

### Radiopaque foreign bodies
#### Metal

As a result of hammering, small metallic splinters frequently enter the hand through very small entry wounds and are often extremely difficult to find on surgical exploration. If left in place, they usually become encapsulated by scar tissue and produce no symptoms. This waiting course is probably quite justified in such types of foreign bodies, particularly because the heat generated by the production of the splinter will usually make the foreign body itself virtually sterile. This wait-and-see advice is even more strongly justified if the foreign body lies deep within a hand, but size and sharpness must have some bearing on the decision (Fig. 16-6).

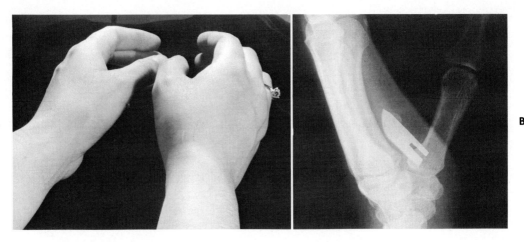

**Fig. 16-6.** *Metallic foreign body.* This physician, when a student in biology class, "cut" the base of her right thumb. Her instructor treated the wound with a Band-Aid. **A,** Five years later a swelling appeared beneath the small scar. **B,** X-ray revealed the cause of the foreign body reaction and the blade was removed.

### Glass

Fragments of glass that are radiopaque should probably be removed, unless they are extremely small. They have a great tendency to travel and can possibly do further damage to important structures deeper in the hand. If they are not removed, they are a frequent source of discomfort and actual pain in the hand, and usually patients will eventually demand their removal.

Despite the fact that the glass may have lead in it and therefore be radiopaque, it is extremely difficult to see in the tissues, and, unless the field is absolutely bloodless, it may be almost impossible to localize; surgical removal of such pieces of glass should not be undertaken lightly, and the patient should be warned that it may be a long and tedious procedure.

### Shotgun pellets

Gunshot wounds are a major problem and do extensive damage. They are not suitable for outpatient care. It must always be remembered that the wad of a shotgun shell may be made from low-grade animal materials that are a potential source of both tetanus and gas gangrene infection. Isolated pellets can be removed if they are easily localized, but there is little value in attempting to remove large numbers of pellets scattered at different levels in the tissues. The surgery necessary to carry out such a removal would do far more harm than would be caused by the actual pellets.

## Nonradiopaque foreign bodies

Organic foreign bodies such as wood splinters, thorns, and fish bones do not usually show on an x-ray film. All these foreign bodies should definitely be removed; they must be considered dirty, and the risk of infection is high if they are left in place.

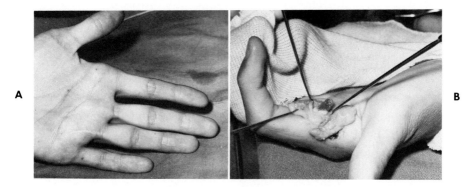

**Fig. 16-7.** *Wood in hand.* **A,** The swelling at the base of the index finger was uncomfortable, and its owner thought he had a "splinter." **B,** The intense tissue reaction around the broken-off shaft of an arrow embedded in the hand.

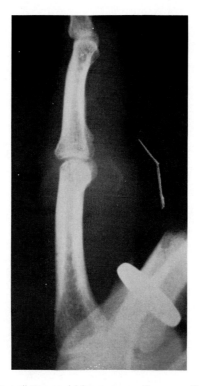

**Fig. 16-8.** *Wood splinter.* This splinter could be seen on the x-ray film because one surface was coated with lead paint. It was removed before the surrounding infection had penetrated the flexor tendon sheath.

Wood splinters should always be removed. The body reacts adversely to buried wood, and massive tissue reactions and abscesses are common if the foreign body is not removed (Fig. 16-7). Luckily these splinter wounds are usually so painful that patients come for their immediate removal.

Splinters beneath a fingernail must be properly exposed so that the end can be firmly grasped before attempting its withdrawal. To do this either cut a V-shaped notch in the end of the nail or shave it down with a razor blade until sufficient splinter is exposed for it to be grasped with rat-tail or multi-teeth forceps. If small portions are left behind, subsequent abscess formation is almost certain.

Splinters penetrating the soft tissues have a tendency to travel parallel with the skin surface so that their track is relatively superficial, and they can be excised after infiltration of a local anesthetic (Fig. 16-8). It is a temptation simply to withdraw the splinter with a pair of fine forceps, but as a general rule this is not advisable. It is much wiser to lay open the track down which the wood passed or in which it lies and to clean this out thoroughly rather than to risk leaving behind a nidus of infection at the distal point of a wood splinter. Deep splinter tracks should be excised under local anesthetic. It is unwise to irrigate these tracks because of the risk of forcing infection between tissue planes. It is particularly bad to irrigate the wound

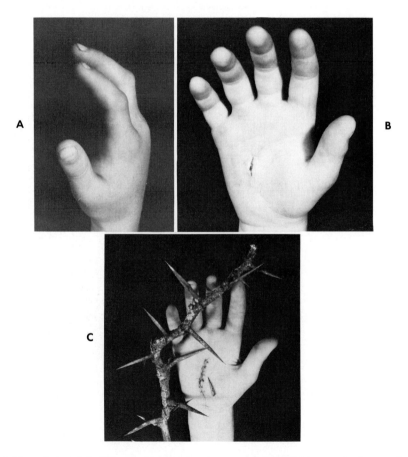

**Fig. 16-9.** *Thorn in hand.* **A,** This very swollen hand occurred within 24 hours of a thorn entering the palm. **B,** The entry wound had been enlarged when futile attempts were made to find the foreign body. **C,** The parent branch, the thorn, and the incision through which it was removed.

with some of the detergent solutions now available. These agents are quite capable of producing a severe chemical inflammation in surrounding tissues.

Many perennial shrubs possess long thorns that can break off within the hand (Fig. 16-9). These are always better removed. The narrow thorns of the blackthorn seem to provoke an excessive nonsuppurative chronic foreign body reaction (Fig. 16-10).

An infinite variety of foreign bodies can impale a finger, such as twist drills, large needles, and similar cylindrical objects. In general, these should be removed from their point of entry. It will be found that those which have penetrated the bone of the phalanx are often extremely well embedded, and some instrument such as a regular pair of pliers may be needed to loosen them from their bony bed. After their removal, their track should be flushed out with hydrogen peroxide and explored sufficiently to ensure that no foreign matter has been left behind. Fish hooks with a one-way barb which have caught a finger should be thoroughly cleansed in situ. The skin around their estimated point of exit should be anesthetized with 2% procaine. After this has taken effect, the hook should be passed onward until it comes out of the skin. As soon as the point of the hook can be grasped through its

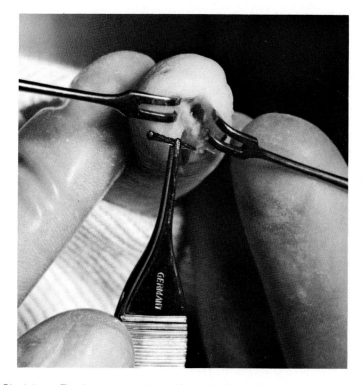

**Fig. 16-10.** *Blackthorn.* The long narrow thorn of the blackthorn bush can break off within a finger and cause a chronic foreign body reaction shown by the hole from within which this thorn was removed.

exit wound, the other end should be cut off flush and the hook pulled through.* If such a procedure is impossible, then the whole area must be extensively infiltrated with local anesthetic and an incision made down onto the hook. The wound can be safely closed with nylon sutures after any damaged tissues surrounding the tip of the hook have been excised and after the area has been thoroughly cleansed. The risk of subsequent erysipeloid infection must be recognized, and the patient must be warned to report back should any form of redness appear. The treatment of this infection is described on p. 295.

## PEN AND PENCIL WOUNDS
### Ball-point pen wounds

Ball-point pen wounds leave tattoo marks similar to those which used to be made by fountain pens. There is no need to perform surgical excision of the area since it will rapidly heal. The composition of the colored inks used in ball-point pens varies with the different manufacturers, but none of the inks would appear to be irritative to the tissues, with the possible exception of some of the purple inks. If crystal or methyl violet is present in the ink, this may cause an inflammatory reaction similar to that seen in skin puncture by indelible pencils.

### Indelible pencil wounds

The lead of indelible pencils contains the toxic aniline dye methyl violet or methyl blue. If the point of the lead has broken off in the tissues, it must be removed by surgical excision. Complete healing can be obtained only when all the pieces of pencil lead and the surrounding stained tissues have been excised. If this is not done, there will be very slow healing at the skin surface and a steadily increasing necrosis of the deeper tissues.

## THE RING AND THE SWOLLEN FINGER

Any circumferential constriction around a finger will cause distal edema and may make it impossible to slip off that which was put on so easily. A great variety of objects has been indicted, including string, elastic bands, pop-top can openers, and more formal jewelry. For lesser degrees of swelling a little soap may be sufficient lubricant to allow removal. When the finger is grossly swollen, all but the formal jewelry can be cut off. Although it is sensible to cut off such rings, patients frequently demand that everything be tried to save the ring, giving little thought to efforts being made to save the finger.

A useful method for removing rings from fingers that have a normal bone structure but are grossly swollen is one in which a small aneurysm needle and a reel of thick ligature silk (No. 1 or No. 2) are employed (Fig. 16-11). One end of the silk is passed under the ring with the help of the aneurysm needle, which should be lubricated before it is passed beneath the ring. After the end of the silk has been secured

---

*This is the way I do it; the literature is replete with other more ingenious methods.

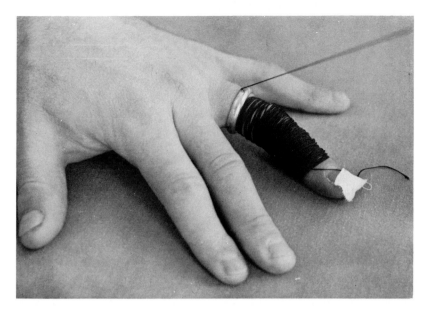

**Fig. 16-11.** *Removing a ring.* In this posed photograph the finger is not swollen and the ring, there-fore, appears relatively loose. In practice, one hand will be needed to push off the ring while the other unwinds the silk.

on the dorsum of the hand by adhesive tape, the reel of silk is slowly unwound as the finger is tightly wound from the ring to the tip of the finger (Fig. 16-11). The silk must be wound evenly on the finger, and the process may take several minutes. The additional tension caused by the binding of the finger can be very distressing to the patient. Warnings must be given about this discomfort, and a mild sedative may occasionally be indicated. When the finger has been wrapped as far as the distal interphalangeal joint, the silk should be cut and the end taped to the skin. The proximal end of the silk should be lifted up and held pointing in the distal direction. If the silk is now unwound from the finger and the ring is pushed gently distally, it will be found that the soft tissues are milked beneath the ring in a proximal direction and that the ring can be removed with ease. As a refinement, some physicians ad-vocate the subcutaneous injection of hyaluronidase into the swollen area near the finger. The solution should be dispersed by massage before the finger is bound with the silk. Usually this injection is not necessary, and it is absolutely contraindicated in fingers in which there is evidence of sepsis.

## Making a ring safe

Dr. William Frackelton and his colleagues have devised a simple inexpensive method of slotting a ring in three quadrant locations to protect the wearer. Should the ring catch on a projection, it will spread open and the finger will be saved. I know this to be true. I retain my own left small finger because my slotted ring opened when it caught on a projecting nail as I slipped off my garage roof.

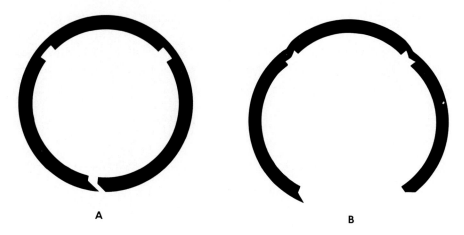

A                                                              B

**Fig. 16-12.** *Making a ring safe.* **A,** The ring should be cut through and the slots made at the sites indicated. **B,** If an accident occurs, the ring will open and the finger will not be degloved. (Courtesy Dr. William H. Frackelton, Hilton Head Island, S.C.)

This modification procedure does not spoil the ring, and it can be readily done by any jeweler using a fine metal saw (Fig. 16-12).

### Procedure

Step 1:  If the ring is overly tight, it should be first "sized" by the jeweler to the correct enlargement.

Step 2:  At 2:30 and 9:30 o'clock positions, two slots are cut partially through from the inside. At 6:00 o'clock position, a slot is cut from the inside, *at right angles*, one third through the thickness. The remaining two thirds are cut through obliquely. (If the ring is a thin band, this slot may be made diagonally and obliquely only).

## REPLANTATION OF AMPUTATED PART

There has been tremendous progress in the techniques of microvascular anastomosis and the replacement of amputated parts in the last decade. Surgery of this type is done by highly skilled surgeons in specialized centers. Their success depends on the proper selection of cases and the optimal care of victim and amputated part while they are being transported to the special center.

### Contraindications

Absolute contraindications to replantation are extensive crushing of the amputated part or significant additional wounds to the part or the amputation stump. Preexisting serious disease such as recent myocardial infarction or heart failure in the victim is also a contraindication, but a frequent and preventable problem is improper care of the amputated part during transportation.

In major amputations with a large muscle bulk a warm ischemia time of six or more hours should be considered a contraindication to replantation.

There are a number of relative contraindications to replantation, but the decision regarding these rests with the operating surgeon and not the referring physician. Such features as heavy soil contamination, warm ischemia time over four to six hours, distal damage to the amputated part, and lack of patient motivation must all be discussed with the surgeon before a decision is made to transport the patient, and part, to the special center.

## Transportation of patient and part

All common sense measures such as control of hemorrhage, evaluation of general status, support of vital functions, and provision of appropriate medications must be taken while rapid transportation is being arranged.

The amputated part must be gently cleaned, wrapped in a sterile dressing, and placed in a plastic bag that is sealed after the air has been evacuated. It should be placed in an ice chest, but ice should not be in direct contact with the part. It is improper to place the part in a nonphysiologic solution or a dry ice container, since cellular disruption will result.

# Recommended reading

What is originality? Undetected Plagiarism.

**W. R. Inge**

**P**lagiarism is a heinous sin, but in such a well-ploughed field as the treatment of hand injuries, repetition of previously published material is inevitable. If I have unconsciously appropriated some apt phrase, I trust the author will consider such theft a sufficient tribute.

I have drawn freely upon the writings of many surgeons, and from their work I have selected a few representative references as additional reading for those who have the time and inclination to expand their knowledge. Several books on the care of the injured hand are already available. They are all more comprehensive than this book and, therefore, make appropriate additional reading.

## GENERAL REFERENCE BOOKS

Bunnell, S.: Surgery of the hand, ed. 5, Philadelphia, 1970, J. B. Lippincott Co.

Kilgore, E. S., and Graham, W. P.: The hand: surgical and non-surgical management, Philadelphia, 1977, Lea & Febiger.

Lister, Graham: The hand: diagnosis and indications, London, 1977, Churchill Livingstone.

McGregor, Ian A.: Fundamental techniques of plastic surgery, ed. 5, Edinburgh, 1972, E. & S. Livingstone.

Moberg, Erik: Emergency surgery of the hand, Edinburgh, 1967, E. & S. Livingstone.

Rank, B. K., and Wakefield, A. R.: Surgery of repair as applied to hand injuries, ed. 3, Edinburgh, 1968, E. & S. Livingstone.

Robins, R. H. C.: Injuries and infections of the hand, London, 1961, Edward Arnold Ltd.

Rockwood, C. A., and Green, D. A.: Fractures, vol. 1, Philadelphia, 1975, J. B. Lippincott Co., Chapter 6.

## SPECIFIC REFERENCES
### Chapter 1. Functional anatomy

Barron, J. N.: The structure and function of the skin of the hand, The Hand 2:93-96, 1970.

Bell, Sir Charles: The hand; its mechanism and vital endowments as evincing design, London, 1852, John Murray.

Braithwaite, F., Channell, G. D. Moore, F. T., and

Whillis, J.: The applied anatomy of the lumbrical and interosseous muscles of hand, Guy. Hosp. Rep. 97:185-195, 1948.

Chase, A.: Surgical anatomy of the hand. In Converse, J. M., editor: Reconstructive plastic surgery, Philadelphia, 1977, W. B. Saunders Co., Chapter 69.

Fetrow, Kenneth O.: Practical and important variations in sensory nerve supply to the hand, The Hand 2:178-184, 1970.

Kaplan, Emanuel B.: Functional and surgical anatomy of the hand, ed. 2, Philadelphia, 1965, J. B. Lippincott Co.

Kuczynski, K.: The proximal interphalangeal joint anatomy and causes of stiffness in the fingers, J. Bone Joint Surg. 50-B:656-663, 1968.

Landsmeer, J. M. F.: Anatomical and functional investigations on the articulation of the human fingers, Acta Anat. (supp. 24) 25:1-69, 1955.

Littler, J. W.: Architectural principles of reconstructive hand surgery, Surg. Clin. North Am. 31:463-476, 1951.

Napier, J. R.: The prehensile movements of the human hand, J. Bone Joint Surg. 38-B:902-913, 1956.

Walsh, J. Francis: The anatomy and functions of the muscles of the hand and of the extensor tendons of the thumb, Philadelphia, 1897, Charles H. Walsh.

Wood-Jones, Frederic: The principles of anatomy as seen in the hand, ed. 2, London, 1946, Baillière, Tindall & Cox.

## Chapter 2. Examination of the injured hand

Bunnell, S.: Surgery of the hand, ed. 5, Philadelphia, 1970, J. B. Lippincott Co., Chapter 4.

James, J. I. P.: The assessment and management of the injured hand, Hand **2**:97-105, 1970.

Littler, J. W.: Examination of the hand. In Converse, J. M., editor: Reconstructive plastic surgery, Philadelphia, 1977, W. B. Saunders Co., Chapter 70.

## Chapter 3. Principles of care

Burnham, P. J.: Regional block at the wrist of the great nerves of the hand, J.A.M.A. **167**:847-850, 1958.

Burnham, P. J.: Simple regional nerve block for surgery of the hand and forearm, J.A.M.A. **169**:941-943, 1959.

Cullen, S. C.: Anesthesia in general practice, ed. 5, Chicago, 1957, Year Book Medical Publishers, Inc.

De Jong, R. H.: Axillary block of the brachial plexus, Anesthesiology **22**:215-225, 1961.

Eaton, R. G., and Butsch, D. P.: Antibiotic guidelines for hand infections, Surg. Gynecol. Obstet. **130**:119-122, 1970.

Haas, L. M., and Landeen, F. M.: Improved intravenous regional anesthesia for surgery of the hand, wrist, and forearm: the second wrap technique, J. Hand Surg. **3**:194-195, 1978.

James, J. I. P.: Common, simple errors in the management of hand injuries, Proc. R. Soc. Med. **63**:69-71, 1970.

Mason, M. L.: Rehabilitation of the hand, American Academy of Orthopaedic Surgeons Instructional Course Lectures, Ann Arbor, Mich., 1949, J. W. Edwards, vol. 6, pp. 95-106.

Parkes, A.: The management of injuries of the hand, Practitioner **186**:692-699, 1961.

Peacock, E. E., Jr.: Management of conditions of the hand requiring immobilization, Surg. Clin. North Am. **33**:1297-1309, 1953.

Smith, I. M., and Rabinovich, S.: A guide to commonly used antibiotics and related compounds, ed. 2, New York, 1970, Ayerst Laboratories.

Stone, N. H., Hursch, H., Humphrey, C. R., and Boswick, J. A.: Empirical selection of antibiotics for hand infections, J. Bone Joint Surg. **51-A**:899-903, 1969.

## Chapter 4. Surgical techniques

Boyes, J. H.: Operative technique in surgery of the hand. In Pease, Charles N., editor: American Academy of Orthopaedic Surgeons Instructional Course Lectures, Ann Arbor, Mich., 1952, J. W. Edwards, vol. 9, pp. 181-195.

Kilbourne, B. C., and Paul, E. G.: Do's and don'ts in the treatment of hand injuries, Surg. Clin. North Am. **38**:139-154, 1958.

McGregor, I. A.: Fundamental techniques of plastic surgery, ed. 5, Edinburgh, 1972, E. & S. Livingstone, Chapters 1 and 3.

## Chapter 6. Wounds of the skin

Barron, J. N.: The skin of the hand, Postgrad. Med. **23**:453-468, 1947.

Beasley, R. W.: Reconstruction of amputated fingertips, Plast. Reconstr. Surg. **44**:349-352, 1969.

Beasley, Robert W.: Local flaps for surgery of the hand. Orthop. Clin. North Am. **1**:219-225, 1970.

Bevin, A. G., and Chase, R. A.: The management of ring avulsion injuries and associated conditions in the hand, Plast. Reconstr. Surg. **32**:391-400, 1963.

Frackelton, W. H., and Doctor, J. P.: Plastic surgery of hand injuries, American Academy of Orthopaedic Surgeons Instructional Course Lectures, Ann Arbor, Mich., 1955, J. W. Edwards, vol. 12, pp. 131-159.

Harrison, S. H.: Reconstructive surgery of the hand with special reference to skin cover, Br. Med. J. **2**:746-750, 1956.

Horn, J. S.: The use of full thickness hand skin flaps in the reconstruction of injured fingers, Plast. Reconstr. Surg. **7**:463-481, 1951.

Lie, K. K., Magargle, R. K., and Posch, J. L.: Free full thickness skin grafts from the palm to cover defects of the fingers, J. Bone Joint Surg. **52-A**:559-561, 1970.

Porter, R. W.: Functional assessment of transplanted skin in volar defects of the digits, J. Bone Joint Surg. **50-A**:955-963, 1968.

Reid, D. A. C.: The immediate replacement of skin loss in digital injuries, Transactions of the International Society of Plastic Surgeons, First Congress, Baltimore, 1957, The Williams & Wilkins Co., pp. 430-434.

Robins, R. H.: The primary reconstruction of the injured hand, Ann. R. Coll. Surg. Engl. **14**:355-370, 1954.

Smith, J. R., and Bom, A. F.: An evaluation of fingertip reconstruction by cross-finger and palmar pedicle flap, Plast. Reconstr. Surg. **35**:409-418, 1965.

Snow, J. W.: The use of a volar flap for repair of fingertip amputations, Plast. Reconstr. Surg. **40**:163-168, 1967.

Sturman, J. J., and Duran, Robert J.: Late results of fingertip injuries, J. Bone Joint Surg. **45-A**:289-298, 1963.

## Chapter 7. Injuries to the nail

Burke, H. J., and Gonzalez, R. I.: Fingernail reconstruction, Plast. Reconstr. Surg. **30**:452-461, 1962.

Harty, M.: The dermal papillae in the fingertip, Plast. Reconstr. Surg. **45**:141-145, 1970.

Kleinert, H. E., et al.: The deformed fingernail, a frequent result of failure to repair nailbed injuries, J. Trauma **7:**177-190, 1967.

## Chapter 8.  Pulp loss

Cronin, T. D.: The cross-finger flap, Am. Surg. **17:** 419-425, 1951.

Curtis, R. M.: Cross-finger pedicle flap in hand surgery, Am. Surg. **145:**650-655, 1957.

Durdin, M., and Pangman, W. J.: The repair of surface defects of fingers by transdigital flaps, Plast. Reconstr. Surg. **5:**368-371, 1950.

Gatewood: Plastic repair of finger defects without hospitalization, J.A.M.A. **87:**1479, 1926.

Hoskins, H. Dean: The versatile cross finger pedicle flap, J. Bone Joint Surg. **42-A:**261-277, 1960.

Tempest, M. N.: Cross finger flaps in the treatment of injuries to the finger tip, Plast. Reconstr. Surg. **9:**205-222, 1952.

## Chapter 9.  Amputations

Atasoy, E., et al.: Reconstruction of the amputated finger-tip with a triangular volar flap, J. Bone Joint Surg. **52-A:**921-926, 1970.

Clifford, R. H.: Finger tip injuries, Surg. Clin. North Am. **33:**1311-1316, 1953.

Fisher, R. H.: The Kutler method of repair of finger tip amputations, J. Bone Joint Surg. **49-A:**317-321, 1967.

Freiberg, M. D., and Manktelow, R.: The Kutler repair for fingertip amputations, Plast. Reconstr. Surg. **50:**371-375, 1972.

Kutler, W.: A new method for finger tip amputation, J.A.M.A. **133:**29-30, 1947.

Metcalf, W., and Whalen, W.: The surgical, social and economic aspects of a unit hand injury, J. Bone Joint Surg. **39-A:**317-324, 1957.

Snow, J. W.: The use of a volar flap for repair of fingertip amputations, Plast. Reconstr. Surg. **40:**163-168, 1967.

Tempest, M. N.: The emergency treatment of digital injuries, Br. J. Plast. Surg. **7:**153-161, 1954.

## Chapter 10.  Crush injuries

Allen, H. S.: Crushing wounds of the hand, Am. J. Surg. **80:**780-783, 1950.

Josh, B. B., and Chaudhari, S. S.: Dorsal relaxation incision in burst fingers, The Hand **5:**135-139, 1973.

Mason, M., and Allen, H. S.: Crushing injuries of the hand, Instructional Course Lectures, American Academy of Orthopaedic Surgeons, Ann Arbor, 1952, J. W. Edwards, vol. 9, pp. 195-202.

Primiano, G. A., and Reep, T. C.: Disruption of the proximal carpal arch of the hand, J. Bone Joint Surg. **56-A:**328-332, 1974.

## Chapter 11.  Tendon injuries

Boyes, J. H.: Immediate and delayed repair of the cut digital flexor tendons, Ann. West. Med. Surg. **1:** 145-152, 1947.

Carroll, R. E., and Match, R. M.: Avulsion of the flexor profundus tendon insertion, J. Trauma **10:** 1109-1118, 1970.

Elliott, R. A.: Injuries to the extensor mechanism of the hand, Orthop. Clin. North Am. **1:**335-354, 1970.

Hauge, M. Foss: The results of tendon suture of the hand, Acta Orthop. Scand. **24:**258-270, 1955.

McFarlane, R. M.: Treatment of extensor tendon injuries of the hand, Can. J. Surg. **16:**1, 1973.

Nemethi, C. E.: Extensor tendons in the industrially injured hand, Industr. Med. **25:**113-119, 1956.

## Chapters 12 and 13.  Joint injuries and fractures

Barton, N.: Fractures of the phalanges of the hand, Hand **9:**1-10, 1977.

Burnham, P. J.: Physiological treatment for fractures of the metacarpals and phalanges, J.A.M.A. **169:** 663-666, 1959.

Campbell, C. S.: Gamekeeper's thumb, J. Bone Joint Surg. **37-B:**148-149, 1955.

Casscells, S. W., and Strange, T. B.: Intramedullary-wire fixation mallet finger, J. Bone Joint Surg. **51-A:** 1018-1019, 1969.

Dewar, F. P., and Harris, W. R.: Open reduction of Bennett's fracture, Can. J. Surg. **1:**33-36, 1957.

Gedda, K. O., and Moberg, E.: Open reduction and osteosynthesis of the so-called Bennett's fracture in the carpo-metacarpal joint of the thumb, Acta Orthop. Scand. **22:**249-257, 1953.

Green, D. P., and Anderson, J. R.: Closed reduction and percutaneous pin fixation of fractured phalanges, J. Bone Joint Surg. **55-A:**1651-1654, 1973.

Green, D. P., and O'Brien, E. T.: Fractures of the thumb metacarpal, South. Med. J. **65:**807-814, 1972.

Hunter, J. M., and Cowen, N. J.: Fifth metacarpal fractures in a compensation clinic population, J. Bone Joint Surg. **52-A:**1159-1165, 1970.

James, J. I. P.: Fractures of the proximal and middle phalanges of the finger, Acta Orthop. Scand. **32:** 401-412, 1962.

Lamphier, T. A.: Improper reduction of fractures of the proximal phalanges of fingers, Am. J. Surg. **94:** 926-930, 1957.

London, P. S.: Sprains and fractures involving the interphalangeal joints, Hand **3:**155-158, 1971.

McCue, F. C., et al.: Athletic injuries of the proximal interphalangeal joint requiring surgical treatment, J. Bone Joint Surg. **52-A:**937-956, 1970.

McElfresh, E., Dobyns, J. G., and O'Brien, E. T.: Management of fracture-dislocation of the proximal interphalangeal joints by extension-block splinting, J. Bone Joint Surg. **54-A:**1705-1711, 1972.

Moberg, E., and Stener, B.: Injuries to the ligaments of the thumb and fingers, Acta Chir. Scand. **106:**166-186, 1953.

Neviaser, R. J., Wilson, J. N., and Lievano, A.: Rupture of the ulnar collateral ligament of the thumb (gamekeeper's thumb): correction by dynamic repair, J. Bone Joint Surg. **53-A:**1357-1364, 1971.

Swanson, A. B.: Fractures involving the digits of the hand, Orthop. Clin. North Am. **1:**261-274, 1970.

## Chapter 14. Burns

Boswick, John A.: Management of the burned hand, Orthop. Clin. North Am. **1:**311-319, 1970.

Condon, K. C., and Kaplan, I. J.: A method of diagnosis and management of the burned hand, Br. J. Plast. Surg. **12:**129-149, 1959.

Editorial: Cold water for burns and scalds, Lancet **1:**578-579 and 695, 1968.

Larson, D. L., et al.: Contracture and scar formation in the burn patient, Clin. Plast. Surg. **1:**653-666, 1974.

McCormick, R. M.: Problems in the treatment of burnt hands, Clin. Plast. Surg. **3:**77-83, 1976.

ÓFeigsson, Ó. J.: Observations and experiments on the immediate cold water treatment for burns and scalds, Br. J. Plast. Surg. **12:**104-119, 1959.

Shulman, Alex E.: Ice water as primary treatment of burns, J.A.M.A. **173:**1916-1919, 1960.

## Chapter 15. Infections

Bolton, H., Fowler, P. J., and Jepson, R. P.: Natural history and treatment of pulp space infection and osteomyelitis of the terminal phalanx, J. Bone Joint Surg. **31-B:**499-504, 1949.

Carter, S. J., and Merscheimer, W. L.: Infections of the hand, Orthop. Clin. North Am. **1:**455-466, 1970.

Cortez, L. M., and Pankey, G. A.: *Mycobacterium marinum* infections of the hand: report of three cases and review of the literature, J. Bone Joint Surg. **55-A:**363-370, 1973.

LaRossa, D., and Hamilton, R.: Herpes simplex infections of the digits, Arch. Surg. **102:**600-601, 1971.

Linscheid, R. L., and Dobyns, J. H.: Common and uncommon infections of the hand, Orthop Clin. North Am. **6:**1063-1104, 1975.

Lowden, T. G.: Prevention and treatment of hand infections, Postgrad. Med. **40:**247-252, 1964.

Petrie, P. W. R., and Lamb, D. W.: Severe hand problems in drug addicts following self administered injections, Hand **5:**130-134, 1973.

Sneddon, J.: The care of hand infections, Baltimore, 1970, The Williams & Wilkins Co.

Stern, H., Elek, S. D., Millar, D. M., and Anderson, H. F.: Herpetic whitlow, Lancet **2:**871-874, 1959.

## Chapter 16. Miscellaneous injuries and wounds

Dickson, R. A.: High pressure injection injuries of the hand. A clinical, chemical and histological study, Hand **8:**189-193, 1976.

Farmer, C. B., and Mann, R. J.: Human bite infections of the hand, South. Med. J. **59:**515-518, 1966.

Gelberman, R. H., et al.: High pressure injection injuries of the hand, J. Bone Joint Surg. **57-A:**935-937, 1975.

Kelly, J. J.: Blackthorn inflammation, J. Bone Joint Surg. **48-B:**474-477, 1966

Lee, M. L. H., and Buhr, A. J.: Dog bites and local infection with *Pasteurella septica*, Br. Med. J. **1:**169-171, 1960.

Mann, R. J., et al.: Human bites of the hand: twenty years of experience, J. Hand Surg. **2:**97-104, 1977.

Mason, M. L., and Queen, F. B.: Grease gun injuries of the hand, Q. Bull. Northwestern University Med. School **15:**122-132, 1941.

Mills, W. J., Jr., and Whaley, R.: Frostbite experience with rapid rewarming and ultrasonic therapy, Part I, Alaska Med. **2:**1-4, 1960.

Mills, W. J., Jr. Whaley, R., and Fish, W.: Frostbite experience with rapid rewarming and ultrasonic therapy, Part II, Alaska Med. **2:**114-124, 1960; Part III, Alaska Med. **3:**28-36, 1961.

Palmieri, T. J.: High pressure injection injuries of the hand, Bull. Hosp. Joint Dis. **35:**18-35, 1974.

Smith, M. G. H.: Grease-gun injury, Br. Med. J. **2:**918-920, 1964.

Stark, H. H., Wilson, J. N., and Boyes, J. H.: Grease gun injuries of the hand, J. Bone Joint Surg. **43-A:**485-491, 1961.

Tanzer, R. C.: Grease gun injuries of the hand, Surg. Clin. North Am. **43:**1277-1283, 1963.

Tempest, M. N.: Grease gun injuries, University Leeds Med. J. **2:**125-129, 1953.

# INDEX

Boldface numbers indicate pages with illustrations.

**323**